Dermal Absorption and Decontamination

Aileen M. Feschuk • Rebecca M. Law
Howard I. Maibach

Editors

Dermal Absorption and Decontamination

A Comprehensive Guide

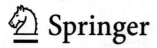
Springer

Editors
Aileen M. Feschuk
Faculty of Medicine
Memorial University of Newfoundland
St. John's, NL, Canada

Rebecca M. Law 🆔
School of Pharmacy
Memorial University of Newfoundland
St. John's, NL, Canada

Howard I. Maibach
Department of Dermatology
University of California San Francisco
San Francisco, CA, USA

ISBN 978-3-031-09224-4   ISBN 978-3-031-09222-0   (eBook)
https://doi.org/10.1007/978-3-031-09222-0

This Springer imprint is published by the registered company Springer Nature Switzerland AG
The registered company address is: Gewerbestrasse 11, 6330 Cham, Switzerland

Preface

Chemical warfare agents (CWAs) are chemical substances used to incapacitate, harm, or kill others in terrorist attacks, war, or other military settings [1]. CWAs have been used throughout history dating back to at least 600 BC and were utilized in World War I and World War II [1]. Since then, CWAs have been used in the Iran-Iraq wars, Japanese underground rail station attacks, and in individually targeted attacks like those on Kim Jong-nam, Sergei Skripal, and Alexei Navalny [2, 3]. Although a great deal of CWA research has been conducted by military bodies, much is unavailable in the public domain. However, one of our editors was privileged to have read a great deal of research in this area, conducted by the American Government, and found it highly remarkable. In addition to threats posed by CWAs, approximately 100,000 different chemicals are used in industrial settings daily in the United States [4].

The skin is the first line of defense against many CWAs and TICs; however direct contact with the skin may result in the penetration of these insults through the dermal layers and into the circulatory system [5]. The passage of a topically applied substance into the bloodstream is known as percutaneous absorption [6]. Percutaneous absorption can be the result of diffusion across skin layers, or the result of entry through the hair follicles or sweat ducts, known as the transepidermal and appendageal pathways, respectively [7]. Chemical dermal decontamination on the other hand is the removal and/or neutralization of chemical insults from skin [8]. The potential for exposure to CWAs or toxic industrial chemicals (TICs) highlights the importance of a comprehensive understanding of percutaneous penetration and decontamination. Despite this importance, these areas of dermatology are highly under-researched.

This book evaluates factors which influence percutaneous penetration of chemical substances, and the efficacy of water/soap and water decontamination protocols (which are often considered the gold standard of dermal decontamination) against a multitude of chemical contaminants, using a variety of study designs (e.g., animal and human models, and in vitro and in vivo protocols). These manuscripts also explore the efficacy of other dermal decontamination methods, again, using a wide array of study designs.

Although dermal penetration and decontamination is a topic that draws little publicity, Matta et al. [9] investigated the percutaneous absorption of multiple commercially available sunscreens and found that they exceeded thresholds set by the US Food and Drug Administration (FDA). These FDA thresholds had exempted sunscreen from undergoing some nonclinical toxicology assessments (e.g., systemic carcinogenicity and developmental and reproductive studies). These findings should be a wake-up call to the medical public about the clinical importance of dermal penetration and decontamination.

It is the authors' hope that this book may guide the development of a universally accepted decontamination protocol and may provide insights into areas of research such as topical application of consumer grade products (e.g., cosmetics, lotions, sunscreens), as well as medicaments, transdermal drug systems, and dermatotoxicology.

The editors welcome corrections or comments regarding this book.

St. John's, NL, Canada   Aileen M. Feschuk
St. John's, NL, Canada   Rebecca M. Law
San Francisco, CA, USA   Howard I. Maibach

References

1. Chauhan S, Chauhan S, D'Cruz R, Faruqi S, Singh KK, Varma S, Singh M, Karthik V. Chemical Warfare Agents. Environ Toxicol Pharmacol. 2008;26(2):113–22. https://doi.org/10.1016/j.etap.2008.03.003.
2. Greathouse B, Zahra F, Brady MF. Acetylcholinesterase inhibitors toxicity. In: StatPearls. Treasure Island, FL: StatPearls Publishing LLC.; 2021.
3. Okumura T, Takasu N, Ishimatsu S, Miyanoki S, Mitsuhashi A, Kumada K, Tanaka K, Hinohara S. Report on 640 victims of the Tokyo subway sarin attack. Ann Emerg Med. 1996;28(2):129–35. https://doi.org/10.1016/s0196-0644(96)70052-5.
4. Tomassoni AJ, French RNE, Walter FG. Toxic industrial chemicals and chemical weapons. Emerg Med Clin North Am. 2015;33(1):13–36. https://doi.org/10.1016/j.emc.2014.09.004.
5. Blickenstaff NR, Coman G, Blattner CM, Andersen R, Maibach HI. Biology of percutaneous penetration. Rev Environ Health. 2014;29(3):145. https://doi.org/10.1515/reveh-2014-0052.
6. Idson B. Percutaneous absorption. J Pharm Sci. 1975;64(6):901–24. https://doi.org/10.1002/jps.2600640604.
7. Sobańska AW, Robertson J, Brzezińska E. Application of RP-18 TLC retention data to the prediction of the transdermal absorption of drugs. Pharmaceuticals. 2021;14(2):147. https://doi.org/10.3390/ph14020147.
8. Clarkson ED, Gordon RK. Rapid decontamination of chemical warfare agents from skin. In: Handbook of toxicology of chemical warfare agents. London: Academic Press; 2020. p. 1233–47. https://doi.org/10.1016/b978-0-12-819090-6.00073-8.
9. Matta MK, Zusterzeel R, Pilli NR, Patel V, Volpe DA, Florian J, Oh L, Bashaw E, Zineh I, Sanabria C, Kemp S, Godfrey A, Adah S, Coelho S, Wang J, Furlong L-A, Ganley C, Michele T, Strauss DG. Effect of sunscreen application under maximal use conditions on plasma concentration of sunscreen active ingredients. JAMA. 2019;321(21):2082. https://doi.org/10.1001/jama.2019.5586.

Contents

Chapter 1
Skin Decontamination with Water: Evidence from In Vivo Human Studies

Nadia Kashetsky, Rebecca M. Law, and Howard I. Maibach

Introduction

Chemical dermal decontamination is the removal and/or neutralization of chemical contaminants from the skin [1]. Contamination occurs by occupational exposure to chemicals, such as pesticides; chemical warfare agents, such as vesicating agents used in World War I and the Iran-Iraq conflict and nerve agents used by the Syrian military in 2013; and by targeted chemical attacks, such as the assassination of Kim Jong-Nam and the assassination attempt targeting Sergei Skripal and his daughter with nerve agents [1, 2]. Contamination may result in acute injury such as burns or mortality, and long-term sequelae, such as delayed ocular, respiratory, and cutaneous effects from sulphur mustard [2]. With the constant possibility of occupational exposures, chemical warfare, and targeted attacks, increased attention has been given to determining effective and timely dermal decontamination strategies to decrease morbidity and mortality.

Many proposed decontamination solutions for different chemical agents exist. These include water solutions, sodium hypochlorite, powder decontamination material (M291 SDK), Sandia foam, Diphoterine®, Reactive Skin Decontamination Lotion® (RSDL), polyurethane sponge, and immobilized enzyme badges [1]. Models to evaluate efficacy of decontamination solutions have relied largely on animal models and in vitro experiments [1, 3]; however, these studies may not always reflect what occurs in human clinical circumstances [3]. Historically, it has been assumed that soap and water, the most commonly used decontamination

N. Kashetsky (✉)
Faculty of Medicine, Memorial University, St. John's, NL, Canada
e-mail: nkashetsky@mun.ca

R. M. Law
School of Pharmacy, Memorial University of Newfoundland, St. John's, NL, Canada

H. I. Maibach
Department of Dermatology, University of California San Francisco, San Francisco, CA, USA

© The Author(s), under exclusive license to Springer Nature
Switzerland AG 2022
A. M. Feschuk et al. (eds.), *Dermal Absorption and Decontamination*,
https://doi.org/10.1007/978-3-031-09222-0_1

1

solution, will remove a variety of dermal chemical contaminants; however, recently, it has been suggested that decontamination may be incomplete and washing may sometimes increase percutaneous penetration [4]. Brent [3] summarized limited clinical studies on human corrosive dermal exposures and concluded that aggressive water lavage is associated with the best clinical outcomes, with no comparable body of clinical evidence for other decontaminating solutions [3]. Of note, alkali metals (metallic lithium, sodium, or potassium) are exceptions to water-based decontamination solutions, as they form their corresponding base when hydrated [3].

There has yet to be a review of experimental studies reporting decontamination with water-only and soap and water-based solutions of dermal contaminants in in vivo human skin. This systematic review summarizes experimental studies reporting decontamination with water-based solutions of dermal chemical contaminants with in vivo human data.

Methods

The Preferred Reporting Items for Systematic Reviews and Meta-Analysis (PRISMA) guidelines were followed [5].

Search Strategy

A literature search utilized Embase, MEDLINE, PubMed, Web of Science, and Google Scholar databases on June 4, 2021, using the search terms ("cutaneous" or "skin" or "dermal" or "percutaneous" and "decontamination" or "decontaminant" or "skin decontamination"). No date, geographical, or language restrictions were used.

Eligibility

Articles were included if they reported (1) chemical contamination of the skin, (2) decontamination with water and/or soap and water, (3) experimental studies, (4) in vivo human subjects, and (5) had data in the English language.

Data Screening

Title and abstract screening were completed by two independent researchers (R.L. and H.M.) and conflicts resolved by discussion with a third (N.K.). Full-text review was completed independently by two researchers (N.K. and H.M.), and conflicts were resolved by discussion with a third (R.L.). References from relevant articles were manually checked to identify any additional studies.

Data Extraction and Analysis

Data extraction was completed by one researcher (N.K.) and verified by another (H.M.), and conflicts were resolved by discussion with a third researcher (R.L.). Data was extracted on study and participant characteristics, chemical contaminant information, decontamination information, and outcomes. Skin residence time was defined as time between contact with contaminant and decontamination. Due to data heterogeneity, meta-analysis was not conducted, and only descriptive analysis was performed.

Results

Study and Participant Characteristics

After title and abstract screening of 3017 studies and full-text review of 51 studies, ten met eligibility criteria and were included, representing 18 chemical contaminants and 199 participants (Fig. 1.1, Table 1.1) [6–15]. Several studies used multiple

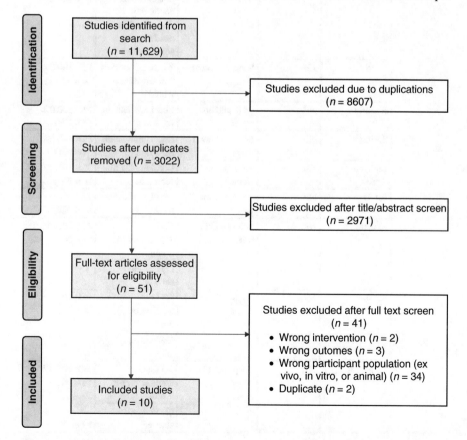

Fig. 1.1 Selection process for study inclusion

Table 1.1 Summary of chemical contaminants, number of participants, decontamination solution, and associated outcomes

Chemical contaminant		Number of participants	Decontamination solution	Method of decontamination	Corresponding outcome
Pesticide	Propoxur	36	Soap and cold water	Washing hands as workers normally would	PD: 100.0% ($n = 36/36$)
	Chlorothalonil	16	Soap and cold water	Washing hands as workers normally would	PD: 100.0% ($n = 16/16$)
	Mancozeb	36	Soap and cold water	Washing hands as workers normally would	PD: 100.0% ($n = 36/36$)
	Captan	15	10% isopropanol distilled water	Shaking hands in polyethylene bags containing 250 mL of the handwashing solution for 30 s	PD: 100.0% ($n = 15/15$)
	Chlorpyrifos	12	10% isopropanol distilled water	Shaking hands in polyethylene bags containing 250 mL of the handwashing solution for 30 s	PD: 100.0% ($n = 12/12$)
	Acephate	12	Soap and water	Washing hands as workers normally would	PD: 100.0% ($n = 12/12$)
	Azodrin	NR	Soap and hot water	Local application for 2 min	PD: 100.0% ($n = $ NR)
	Ethion	NR	Soap and hot water	Local application for 2 min	PD: 100.0% ($n = $ NR)
	Lindane	NR	Soap and hot water	Local application for 2 min	PD: 100.0% ($n = $ NR)
	2,4-D	NR	Soap and hot water	Local application for 2 min	PD: 100.0% ($n = $ NR)
	Malathion	NR	Soap and hot water	(1) Local application for 2 min (2) Full-body shower	PD: 100.0% ($n = $ NR)
	Baygon	NR	Soap and hot water	(1) Local application for 2 min (2) Full-body shower	PD: 100.0% ($n = $ NR)
	Parathion	NR	Soap and hot water	(1) Local application for 2 min (2) Full-body shower	PD: 100.0% ($n = $ NR)

Chemical contaminant		Number of participants	Decontamination solution	Method of decontamination	Corresponding outcome
Chemical simulants	Oil-based mock chemical/ biological agent: optical brightening powder suspended in baby oil	20	Warm water (temperature, 35 °C)	Shower with a hose (60–70 psi) for 30 s	CD: 100.0% ($n = 20/20$)
	1:1 mixture of methyl salicylate and vegetable oil	12	Water (temperature, 18.5 °C; volume, 5 L) and 0.5% detergent solution	Two washes of three stages: rinsing with water, wiping with a sponge and detergent solution, and rinsing, for 3 min	PD: 100.0% ($n = 12/12$)
Cleaning agent	Cream cleaning agent containing 10% fluorescent sodium salt	18	Warm water (temperature, 40 °C)	Application of water (1 L) for 20 s, followed by gentle tapping five times with gauze	PD: 100.0% ($n = 18/18$)
Cosmetic agent	Zinc oxide nanoparticles and capric/ caprylic triglycerides	3	Soap and water	Three washes (unspecified details)	PD: 100.0% ($n = 3/3$)
Therapeutic agent	1.62% testosterone gel	24	Soap and water	Washing for up to 10 min	PD: 100.0% ($n = 17/17$)

CD complete decontamination, PD partial decontamination, NR not reported

decontamination protocols leading to 351 total decontamination outcomes. Three studies included data from decontamination with water (10.8%, $n = 38/351$ decontamination outcomes), seven with soap and water (68.4%, $n = 240/351$ decontamination outcomes), and two with 10% isopropanol distilled water (20.8%, $n = 73/351$ decontamination outcomes) (Tables 1.2, 1.3, and 1.4).

Water-Only Chemical Decontamination

Overall, results of dermal decontamination using water showed complete decontamination (CD) outcomes in 52.6% ($n = 20/38$) and partial decontamination (PD) in 47.4% ($n = 18/38$) (Table 1.2). Contaminants included an oil-based mock

Table 1.2 Water-only decontamination: study and participant characteristics, chemical contaminant and decontamination information, and outcomes

Study characteristics		Participant characteristics	Chemical contaminant information			
Author (year)	Sample size	Age (years), sex (F/M), occupation	Chemical contaminant	Location of application	Method of contamination	Amount or dose of contaminant
Moffett et al. (2010) [12]	20	Age: NR Sex: NR Occupation: military personnel	Oil-based mock chemical/biological agent: optical brightening powder suspended in baby oil	Ventral forearm	Pesticide sprayer for 3 s	NR
Aoki et al. (2018) [6]	18	Age: 21–22 Sex: 0/18 Occupation: NR	Cream cleaning agent containing 10% fluorescent sodium salt	Lower leg (radius, 3.5 cm)	Researcher using two fingers for 30 s	0.6 g

Study characteristics		Decontamination information				Decontamination outcome	
Author (year)	Sample size	Skin residence time (min)	Washing solution	Method of washing	Analysis of decontamination	Results of decontamination	Corresponding decontamination outcome (CD, PD, none)
Moffett et al. (2010) [12]	20	5	Warm water (temperature, 35 °C)	Shower with a hose (60–70 psi) for 30 s	Absence of visible fluorescent particles from two out of three graders under UV light source	90% ($n = 18/20$) of participants achieved decontamination in 30 s and 100% ($n = 20/20$) in 90 s	CD: 100.0% ($n = 20/20$)
Aoki et al. (2018) [6]	18	NR	Warm water (temperature, 40 °C)	Application of water (1 L) for 20 s, followed by gentle tapping five times with gauze	Amount of fluorescence remaining on hair root and hair bulb	Cleaning agent residual indexes: 60.94 at hair root and 54.75 at hair bulb	PD: 100.0% ($n = 18/18$)

CD complete decontamination, *PD* partial decontamination, *F* female, *M* male, *NR* not reported

Table 1.3 Soap and water decontamination: study and participant characteristics, chemical contaminant and decontamination information, and outcomes

Study characteristics		Participant characteristics	Chemical contaminant information			
Author (year)	Sample size	Age (years), sex (F/M), occupation	Chemical contaminant	Location of application	Method of contamination	Amount of contaminant
Maibach and Feldmann (1975) [13]	6	Age: NR; Sex: male; Occupation: NR	Azodrin, ethion, malathion, parathion, lindane, Baygon, 2,4-D	Forearms, palm, or forehead	Micropipette	4, 40, or 400 $\mu g/cm^2$
Marquart et al. (2002) [11]	24	Age: NR; Sex: NR; Occupation: NR	Propoxur	Hands	Occupational harvesting tasks	Estimated with a model relating dislodgeable foliar residue to exposure levels using transfer factors
	36	Age: NR; Sex: NR; Occupation: agricultural workers	Chlorothalonil ($n = 16$ participants); Mancozeb ($n = 24$ participants)	Hands	Applied during harvesting tasks	Estimated with a model relating dislodgeable foliar residue to exposure levels using transfer factors
	24	Age: NR; Sex: NR; Occupation: NR	Mancozeb ($n = 12$ participants); Propoxur ($n = 12$ participants)	Hands and wrists	Applied to the hands and wrists using a pipette	Mancozeb in three doses (5, 15, and 30 mg; $n = 4$ participants each); propoxur in three doses (2.5, 5, and 7.5 mg; $n = 4$ participants each)
Curwin et al. (2003) [7]	12	Age: NR; Sex: 0/12; Occupation: tobacco harvesters	Acephate	Hands	Occupational exposure during tobacco harvesting	NR

(continued)

Table 1.3 (continued)

Study characteristics	Sample size	Participant characteristics	Chemical contaminant information			
Lin et al. (2012) [10]	3	Age: NR Sex: NR Occupation: NR	Zinc oxide nanoparticles and capric/caprylic triglycerides	Applied to tape-stripped and non-tape-stripped skin for 2 h		NR
Stahlman et al. (2012) [14]	17	Age: 34–77 Sex: male Occupation: NR	1.62% testosterone gel	Shoulders and upper arms	NR	5 g
Southworth et al. (2020) [15]	12	Sample size: 12 Age: 26–62 Sex: 4 females, 8 males Occupation: NR	Chemical simulant: MeS and vegetable oil, with 4 mg/mL Invisible Red S, a UV fluorescent compound	Shoulder, forearm, calf, and back	Positive displacement pipette	Shoulder, forearm, calf (volume, 21 µL), and back (volume, 200 µL)

Study characteristics		Decontamination information				Decontamination outcome	
Author (year)	Sample size	Skin residence time (min)	Washing solution	Method of washing	Analysis of decontamination	Quantification of decontamination	Corresponding decontamination outcome (CD, PD, none)
Maibach and Feldmann (1975) [13]	6	(1) 1, 5, 15, 30, 60, 120, 240, 480 (2) 240	Soap and hot water	(1) Local application for 2 min (2) Full-body shower	Liquid scintillation counting of urine samples, after dose applied to the skin, comparison to a parenteral control	(1) Penetration ranged from 0.5% to 36.3% (2) Penetration ranged from 7.2% to 41.9%	PD: 100.0% (n = 78/78)

Marquart et al. (2002) [11]	24	NR	Soap and cold tap water	As workers normally would either during their first break or after completing harvesting task	Analysis of propoxur in the washing water by high-performance liquid chromatography	Percentage washed from hands: arithmetic mean 24.5% (range, 4.8–60.2%; STD, 17.7; participants, $n = 14$) for the cutting task and arithmetic mean 50.7% (range, 17.9–103.1%; STD, 264; $n = 10$) for the sorting task	PD: 100.0% ($n = 24/24$)
	36	NR	Soap (1.5 mL) and cold water (3.0 L)	As workers normally would; washing vigour was rated on a score of 1 (superficial washing) to 4 (vigorous washing)	Analysis of chlorothalonil in washing water by high-performance liquid chromatography; analysis of mancozeb in washing water by the amount of carbon disulphide formed by acid destruction in a headspace vial	Percentage washed from hands for mancozeb, 43.5% (range, 9.0–96.1%; STD, 22.0; participants, $n = 20$); for chlorothalonil, 32.1% (range, 15.4–64.2%; STD, 14.0; participants, $n = 16$)	PD: 100.0% ($n = 36/36$)
	24	30	Soap (1.5 mL) and cold water (3.0 L)	As workers normally would; washing vigour was rated on a score of 1 (superficial washing) to 4 (vigorous washing)	As above studies	Percentage washed from hands for mancozeb, 85.7% (range, 71.3–96.2; STD, 5.3; number of measurement, 48); propoxur, 45.8% (range, 37.8–52.2%; STD, 3.4; number of measurement, 48)	PD: 100.0% ($n = 24/24$)
Curwin et al. (2003) [7]	12	Within 4 h	Soap and water	Washing hands as normal	Analysis of hand-wipe samples by gas chromatography/mass spectrometry	Decreased geometric mean (GM) acephate level by 96%, with prewash GM of 10.5 ng/cm² (range, 0.07–257 ng/cm²) and postwash GM of 0.4 ng/cm² (range, 0.04–3.7 ng/cm²)	PD: 100.0% ($n = 12/12$)

(continued)

Table 1.3 (continued)

Study characteristics		Participant characteristics	Chemical contaminant information				
Lin et al. (2012) [10]	3	NR	Soap and water	Three washes (unspecified details)	Multiphoton tomography	Significant decrease ($p < 0.01$) in positive ZnO-NP signal after one wash, with next two washes having no significant effect; positive ZnO-NP signal in furrows was significantly decreased after both one and two washes	PD: 100.0% ($n = 3/3$)
Stahlman et al. (2012) [14]	17	Gel applied daily for 7 days × 3 crossovers. Doses on Days 7, 14, and 21 were left on for 2, 6, or 10 h (120, 360, 600 min) and then washed off	Soap and water	Time: up to 10 min; other details not specified	HPLC with diode array detection of ten tape-strippings at one locations, taken on sixth day (no washing) and 30 min after washing on seventh day; LC/tandem mass spectrometry of serum samples taken at dates and times as follows: (a) baseline and Days 6, 7, 13, 14, 20, and 21, with whole blood collections at times 0, 2, 4, 6, 8, 12, 16, and 24 h; (b) predose only on Days 4, 5, 11, 12, 18, and 19; and (c) at 48, 72, and 96 h after the last dose on Day 21	Skin tape-stripping showed decontamination of at least 81% from residual skin. AUC_{0-24} decreasing mean 14% and 10% at skin residence time of 2 h and 6 h, respectively. No effect on AUC_{0-24} occurred with decontamination at skin residence time of 10 h or on C_{max} for any decontamination protocol	Minimal to no effect on systemic absorption: 100.0% ($n = 51/51$)

| Southworth et al. (2020) [15] | 12 | 15, 21 | Water (temperature, 18.5 °C; volume, 5 L) and 0.5% detergent solution | Three stages: rinsing with water, wiping with a sponge and detergent solution, and rinsing, lasting a total of 3 min | Gas chromatography/tandem mass spectrometry of skin samples, taken by tape-stripping, and urine samples; UV images were analysed for areas of fluorescence | UV analysis, simulant area and emittance significantly decreased; skin samples, MeS detected above limit of quantification (>0.23 ng/mL), significantly lower MeS recovered after decontamination; urine analysis, MeS detected above level of quantification (4.6 ng/mL) up to 8 h | PR: 100.0% ($n = 12/12$) |

CD complete decontamination, *PD* partial decontamination, *F* female, *M* male, *NR* not reported

Table 1.4 Decontamination with 10% isopropanol distilled water: study and participant characteristics, chemical contaminant and decontamination information, and outcomes

Study characteristics		Participant characteristics	Chemical contaminant information			
Author (year)	**Sample size**	**Age (years), sex (F/M), occupation**	**Chemical contaminant**	**Method of contamination**	**Location of application**	**Amount of contaminant**
Fenske and Lu (1994) [9]	12	Age: NR Sex: NR Occupation: NR	Chlorpyrifos, an organophosphorus insecticide	Contact with a test tube containing a measured amount of the pesticide on its outer surface	Hands	Skin loading levels, 3–1500 µg; contact area, 141 ± 18 cm^2
Fenske et al. (1998) [8]	15	Age: NR Sex: NR Occupation: NR	Captan, a foliar fungicide	Contact with a test tube containing a measured amount of the pesticide in a wettable formulation on its outer surface	Hands	Mean of captan spiked on test tube 6.5 mg, area density of 0.15 mg/cm^2

Study characteristics		Decontamination information			Decontamination outcome	
Author (year)	**Sample size**	**Washing solution**	**Skin residence time (min)**	**Method of washing**	**Analysis of decontamination**	**Quantification of decontamination**	**Corresponding decontamination outcome (CD, PD, none)**
Fenske and Lu (1994) [9]	12	10% isopropanol distilled water	(1) 0 (2) 60	Shaking hands in polyethylene bags containing 250 mL of the handwashing solution for 30 s	Gas chromatography and mass balance calculations of washing water	(1) 28% of chlorpyrifos was located in the handwash, 37% remained on the hands, and 35% remained on the test tube (2) 14% of chlorpyrifos was located in the handwash, 47% remained on the hands, and 39% remained on the test tube	PD: 100.0% (n = 58/58)

| Fenske et al. (1998) [8] | 15 | 10% isopropanol distilled water | (1) 0 min (n = 9/15 participants, n = 18 hands) | Shaking hands in polyethylene bags containing 250 mL of the handwashing solution for 30 s | Gas chromatography and mass balance calculations of washing water | Removal of 77.8% of captan from hands at 0 h and 68.4% at residence time of 1 h; 86.0% of captan removal occurred in the first wash, while only 14.0% occurred in the second wash | PD: 100.0% (n = 15/15) |
| | | | (2) 60 min (n = 6/15 participants, n = 12 hands) | | | | |

CD complete decontamination, *PD* partial decontamination, *F* female, *M* male, *NR* not reported

chemical/biological agent, an optical brightening powder suspended in baby oil, and a cream cleaning agent containing 10% fluorescent sodium salt.

Moffett et al. [12] decontaminated an oil-based mock chemical/biological agent and an optical brightening powder (found in commercial laundry detergents) suspended in baby oil (sample size, 20; age, not reported (NR); sex, NR; occupation, military personnel; total decontamination outcomes, 20), applied to ventral forearms by a pesticide sprayer for 3 s [12]. Skin residence time was 5 min, and then decontamination occurred by washing with warm water (temperature, 35 °C) in a shower with a hose (pressure, 60–70 psi). Decontamination was defined as absence of visible fluorescent particles on the skin from two out of three graders using an ultraviolet light source. Complete decontamination occurred in 90% (n = 18/20) of participants after 30 s of washing and in 100% (n = 20/20) at 90 s. Level of quantification was not given.

Aoki et al. [6] decontaminated a cleaning agent residue and a cream cleaning agent (0.6 g) containing 10% fluorescent sodium salt, from hair follicles (sample size, 18; age, 21–22 years; sex, male (n = 18/18); occupation, NR; total decontamination outcomes, 18), applied to hairy lower legs (radius, 3.5 cm) for 30 s by a researcher using two fingers [6]. Decontamination was completed with water (temperature, 40 °C; volume, 1 L) for 20 s, followed by gentle tapping (not wiping) five times with gauze. Decontamination was measured by the amount of fluorescence remaining on the hair root and hair bulb of three hairs from each measurement area, using a biological upright microscope, camera, and software. The intensity of fluorescence was divided by the area of hair root and bulb, respectively, to generate a "cleaning agent residual index". Median cleaning agent residual indexes of 60.9 at the hair root and 54.8 at the hair bulb were found. Level of quantification was not given.

Soap and Water Chemical Decontamination

Overall, decontamination results of chemical contaminants using soap and water achieved PD outcomes in 92.9% (n = 223/240) and minimal to no effect in 7.1% (n = 17/240). Contaminants included the pesticides acephate, azodrin, ethion, malathion, parathion, lindane, Baygon, and 2,4-D, propoxur, chlorothalonil, and mancozeb; the cosmetic agents, zinc oxide nanoparticles and capric/caprylic triglycerides; the therapeutic agent, 1.62% testosterone gel; and the chemical simulant, a 1:1 mixture of methyl salicylate (MeS) and vegetable oil.

Maibach and Feldmann [13] evaluated decontamination of pesticides labelled with radioactive carbon-14 in two studies (sample size, 6; age, NR; sex, male (n = 6/6); occupation, NR; total decontamination outcomes, 78) [13]. Contaminant was applied to the forearms, palm, or forehead with a micropipette. Decontamination was assessed using liquid scintillation counting analysis of urine samples, by comparing results of the contaminant dose applied to the skin to a parenteral control.

In the first study, the following pesticides were decontaminated with local application of soap and hot water for 2 min at skin residence time of 1, 5, 15, and/or 30 min and 1, 2, 4, 8, and/or 24 h: azodrin, ethion, malathion, parathion, lindane, Baygon, and 2,4-D (concentration, 4 $\mu g/cm^2$; location, forearm; total decontamination outcomes, 78). Additionally, parathion 4 $\mu g/cm^2$ was applied to the palm and forehead; malathion and parathion 40 $\mu g/cm^2$ and 400 $\mu g/cm^2$ were applied to the arm; and 2,4-D 40 $\mu g/cm^2$ was applied to the forearm.

Decontamination was never 100% effective. The least amount of penetration was 2,4-D 4 $\mu g/cm^2$ applied to the forearm ranging from 0.5% penetration with decontamination at skin residence time of 1 min to 5.8% penetration of skin residence time of 24 h. The most penetration was parathion 4 $\mu g/cm^2$ applied to the forehead ranging from 8.4% at skin residence time of 1 min to 36.3% at skin residence time of 24 h. See Maibach and Feldmann [13] for a full list of decontamination results.

The second study decontaminated malathion, parathion, and Baygon applied to the arm, forehead, and palm by full-body shower at skin residence time of 4 h. Penetration ranged from 7.2% to 41.9%, results being less effective as compared to local washing with soap and water. The level of quantification for both studies was not given.

Marquart et al. [11] evaluated pesticide decontamination in three studies (total decontamination outcomes, 84) [11]. The first used the contaminant propoxur (2-isopropoxyphenyl-N-methyl carbamate), applied to the hands by occupational harvesting tasks (sample size, 24; age, NR; sex, NR; occupation, NR). Dermal exposure was estimated with a model relating dislodgeable foliar residue (DFR) to exposure levels using transfer factors. Washing as workers normally would using liquid soap and cold tap water was completed either during their first break or after completing the harvesting task, with inconsistent washing times as this was left up to the individual worker, and skin residence time was not given. Decontamination was estimated by propoxur analysis in the washing water by high-performance liquid chromatography (HPLC). Limits of quantitation were 10 $\mu g/L$ for DFR solution, 0.02 $\mu g/cm^2$ for DFR, and 20 $\mu g/L$ for washing water. Recovery from DFR solution and washing water was >99%.

Mean washing efficacies (percentage washed from hands) were 24.5% (range, 4.8–60.2%; STD, 17.7; participants, $n = 14$) for the cutting task and 50.7% (range, 17.9–103.1%; STD, 264; participants, $n = 10$) for the sorting/bundling task.

The second study used chlorothalonil (2,4,5,6,-tetrachloro-1,3-benzenedi carbo-nitrile) and mancozeb ([1,2-ethanediylbis[carbamodithioato](2-)]manganese mixture with [1,2-ethanediylbis [carbamodithioato](2-)]zinc), applied during occupational harvesting tasks (sample size, 40; age, NR; sex, NR; occupation, agricultural workers) [11]. Dermal exposure was estimated as in the above study; washing occurred via a standardized water tap method using liquid soap (1.5 mL) and cold water (1.5 L), with the tap opened for 1 s initially for hand wetting, and then the soap was added, and the tap was opened for 15 s providing approximately 1.5 L of water for washing. Washing vigour was video-recorded and rated from a score of 1 (superficial washing) to 4 (vigorous washing) using a three-assessor panel. Decontamination was estimated by analysis of chlorothalonil in the washing water by HPLC with UV detector and for mancozeb by the amount of carbon disulphide formed by acid destruction in a headspace vial and analysed by gas chromatography with electron capture detection. Limits of quantitation for chlorothalonil were 0.07 $\mu g/cm^2$ for personal dislodgeable foliar residue and 15 $\mu g/cm^2$ for washing water and for mancozeb 0.7 $\mu g/cm^2$ for personal dislodgeable foliar residue and 150 $\mu g/cm^2$ for washing water. Recoveries were >80% (mancozeb) to >90% (chlorothalonil); and between-day coefficients of variations for all determinations were <5% (chlorothalonil) to <10% (mancozeb).

Mean washing efficacy of 43.5% (range, 9.0–96.1%; STD, 22.0; participants, n = 20) for mancozeb and 32.1% (range, 15.4–64.2%; STD, 14.0; participants, n = 16) for chlorothalonil were found.

The third study used mancozeb (three doses, 5, 15, and 30 mg; n = 4 participants each) and propoxur (three doses, 2.5, 5, and 7.5 mg; n = 4 participants each), applied to the hands and wrists using a pipette (sample size, 24; age, NR; sex, NR; occupation, NR). Skin residence time was 30 min, and then washing with soap and cold water occurred as in the second study, and decontamination was measured as the above studies. A panel of four assessors evaluated the videotaped washing vigour. The limits of quantitation for propoxur were 150 $\mu g/sample$ for washing water, 100 $\mu g/sample$ for control sample, and 10 $\mu g/sample$ for spill sample and for mancozeb were 150 $\mu g/sample$ for washing water, 5 $\mu g/sample$ for control sample, and 5 $\mu g/sample$ for spill sample.

Mean washing efficacy of 85.7% (range, 71.3–96.2%; STD, 5.3; number of measurements, 48) for mancozeb and 45.8% (range, 37.8–52.2%; STD, 3.4; number of measurements, 48) for propoxur were found.

Curwin et al. [7] evaluated decontamination of the pesticide, acephate (sample size, 12; age, NR; sex, 100% (n = 12/12) males; occupation, tobacco harvesters; total decontamination outcomes, 12) [7]. Contaminant was applied to the hands by occupational exposure during tobacco harvesting. Skin residence time was variable between 0 and 4 h, participants were instructed to wash their hands with soap and water as they did normally, and hand-wipe samples were collected prewash and postwash at 4-h intervals. Decontamination was determined through analysis of hand-wipe samples by gas chromatography/mass spectrometry. Limit of quantification was 50 ng/sample, and limit of detection (LOD) was 30 ng/sample. Ninety-six hand-wipe samples were collected of which three prewash and eight postwash samples (11.5%) had acephate levels below the LOD.

Handwashing with soap and water decreased the geometric mean (GM) acephate level by 96%, with a prewash GM of 10.5 ng/cm^2 (range, 0.07–257 ng/cm^2) and postwash GM of 0.4 ng/cm^2 (range, 0.04–3.7 ng/cm^2).

Lin et al. [10] evaluated decontamination of nanoparticles in a commercial product, zinc oxide nanoparticles (ZnO-NP) and capric/caprylic triglycerides vehicle (sample size, 3; age, NR; sex, NR; occupation, NR; total decontamination outcomes, 3) [10]. The contaminant was applied to tape-stripped and non-tape-stripped skin with a skin residence time of 2 h. Analysis with multiphoton tomography was used to quantify the number of particles. Level of quantification was not given.

A significant decrease ($p < 0.01$) in positive ZnO-NP signal was found after one wash, with the next two washes having no significant effect. Positive ZnO-NP signal in furrows was significantly decreased ($p < 0.01$) after both one and two washes. However, washing three times with soap and water, particles were not completely removed from the skin, especially not in furrows.

Southworth et al. [15] decontaminated the chemical simulant, a 1:1 mixture of MeS and vegetable oil, with 4 mg/mL Invisible Red S, a UV fluorescent compound, applied to the shoulder, forearm, calf (volume, 21 μL), and back (volume, 200 μL) with a positive displacement pipette (sample size, 12; age, 26–62; sex, four females, eight males; occupation, NR; total decontamination outcomes, 12) [15]. Skin residence time was 15 min, and then the skin was decontaminated in three ways using a crossover study design: dry (wiping with white tissue roll), wet (washing with water [temperature, 18.5 °C; volume, 5 L] and 0.5% detergent solution in three stages—rinsing with water, wiping with a sponge and detergent solution, and rinsing with water—lasting a total of 3 min), and combined dry and wet (where the second decontamination protocol occurred at 21 min after simulant application). Decontamination was analysed by gas chromatography/tandem mass spectrometry of skin samples, taken by tape-stripping 30 min after simulant application, and urine samples collected at baseline and each urination following simulant application for 24 h. Additionally, UV images at baseline and six time points were analysed for areas of fluorescence.

For UV image analysis, simulant area and emittance were significantly decreased across all decontamination conditions versus control, with area and emittance significantly higher on the shoulder compared to the arm and leg and on the arm compared to the leg, and pairwise comparisons confirmed that both were significantly lower for each of the three decontamination protocols. In addition, simulant area and emittance were significantly lower using the combined dry and wet decontamination compared to dry or wet decontamination alone.

For all skin sample analysis, MeS was detected above the limit of quantification (>0.23 ng/mL). Significantly lower MeS was recovered from the skin after wet decontamination (34.01 μg, SD 25.09) which was not significantly different from dry decontamination but was significantly different from dry + wet decontamination (11.22 μg, SD 11.88). As supported by UV analysis, MeS was significantly higher in the shoulder compared to the arms and legs. Urine sample analysis showed MeS detected above the level of quantification (4.6 ng/mL) for all samples ($n = 5$ participants) up to 8 h, where after negligible excretion was observed, with no significant effect of decontamination condition on MeS excreted in urine (F(3,12) = 0.87, $p = 0.467$). Decontamination did not lead to complete simulant removal.

Stahlman et al. [14] decontaminated 5 g of 1.62% testosterone gel (sample size, 17; age, 34–77; sex, male ($n = 24/24$); occupation, NR; morning serum testosterone level, <300 ng/dL; total decontamination outcomes, 51), applied to the shoulders and upper arms daily for 7 days, with a three-way crossover every 7 days [14]. Original sample size for decontamination studies was 24 with seven discontinued from the study due to non-drug ($n = 1$) and drug-related ($n = 6$) adverse event of testosterone concentration >900 ng/dL in the safety evaluation stage; despite this, an additional 16 study subjects (i.e. overall total 23/24 or 96%) had at least one observed testosterone concentration >1000 ng/dL during the decontamination studies. Decontamination for $n = 17$ was with soap and water in a shower for up to 10 min which occurred on every seventh day. Testosterone doses on Days 7, 14, and 21 were left on for 2, 6, or 10 h and then washed off. Each participant has a total of 21 days of dosing (total decontamination outcomes, 51). Decontamination was analysed by HPLC with diode array detection (HPLC-UV) of ten tape-strippings at a single location taken 30 min after washing on the seventh day and at the same time on the sixth day (no washing). Additionally, liquid chromatography/tandem mass spectrometry of serum samples was analysed for the contaminant taken at dates and times as follows: (a) baseline and Days 6, 7, 13, 14, 20, and 21, with whole blood collections at times 0, 2, 4, 6, 8, 12, 16, and 24 h; (b) predose only on Days 4, 5, 11, 12, 18, and 19; and (c) at 48, 72, and 96 h after the last dose on Day 21. Level of quantification was not given.

Pharmacokinetic assessments with C_{max}, AUC_{0-24}, and time-averaged concentration over the 24-h dosing interval were calculated. Baseline serum testosterone (24-h mean range) was 252–288 ng/dL. Mean testosterone serum concentrations were lower with decontamination on Day 7 at wash times of 2 h and 6 h as compared to Day 6 without skin washing, corresponding to a small but significant decrease in bioavailability, with AUC_{0-24} decreased by about 14% and 10%, respectively. However, decontamination at wash time of 10 h showed similar testosterone concentrations to Day 6 (no washing) and no difference in AUC_{0-24} (indicating that topical absorption has likely been completed by 10 h post-dose). Skin washing had no effect on C_{max} for any treatment time point (C_{max} likely occurred within 2 h post-dose).

Skin tape-stripping analysis showed the amount of residual testosterone recovered from the skin was reduced by at least 81% after decontamination (Day 7) compared to no skin washing (Day 6). However, since bioavailability was only reduced by 14% (2-h wash) and 10% (6-h wash), it was concluded that skin washing especially after 2 h has minimal impact on the overall absorption of applied topical testosterone for patients receiving testosterone therapy, i.e. there is little to no clinical benefit.

Chemical Decontamination with 10% Isopropanol Distilled Water

Overall, results of decontamination of chemical contaminants using 10% isopropanol distilled water achieved PD outcomes in 100.0% ($n = 73/73$) decontamination outcomes. Contaminants included the pesticides, captan and chlorpyrifos.

Fenske and Lu [9] evaluated decontamination of the pesticide, chlorpyrifos, an organophosphorus insecticide (sample size, 12 subjects [5 or 6 per protocol, providing 10 or 12 left- and right-hand independent samples]; age, NR; sex, NR; occupation, NR; total decontamination outcomes, 58) [9]. Contaminant was applied to the hands (test tube spike level, 2500, 250, 25, or 2.5 µg; skin loading levels, 0.024–12.3 µg/cm²; contact area, 141 ± 18 cm²) by grasping contact 10 times with a test tube containing a measured amount of pesticide on its outer surface while a technician twisted the tube. After contact, in order to verify skin loading levels, the test tube was eluted with solvent to determine the amount of pesticide not transferred to the hands. Washing with 10% isopropanol distilled water occurred by shaking hands in polyethylene bags containing 250 mL of the handwashing solution for 30 s and repeated with fresh handwashing solution for hands with high levels of chlorpyrifos (>1 mg). Analysis of the final handwashing solution was completed using gas chromatography and mass balance calculations. Limits of detection were 0.12 μg for elution samples and 0.50 μg for handwash samples.

For handwashing with isopropanol/water, at skin residence time of 0 h, 28% of chlorpyrifos was located in the handwash, 37% remained on the hands, and 35% remained on the test tube. At skin residence time of 1 h, 14% of chlorpyrifos was located in the handwash, 47% remained on the hands, and 39% remained on the test tube. Additionally, removal efficacy was highest at the lowest skin loading level, and at 0.1–1 μg/cm², efficacy was one half that at high skin loading levels.

Fenske et al. [8] evaluated decontamination of the pesticide, captan, a foliar fungicide (sample size, 15; age, NR; sex, NR; occupation, NR; total decontamination outcomes, 15) [8]. Contaminant was applied to the hands by contact with a test tube containing a measured amount of the pesticide in a wettable formulation on its outer surface. Handwashing procedures with 10% isopropanol distilled water at skin residence time of 0 h ($n = 9/15$ participants, $n = 18$ hands) and 1 h ($n = 6/15$ participants, $n = 12$ hands) and decontamination analysis were detailed in the above similar study by Fenske and Lu [9]. Limit of detection was 0.16 ng/μL.

Results at 0 h showed removal of 77.8% of captan from hands and at 1 h removal of 68.4%. Additionally, 86.0% of captan removal occurred in the first wash, while only 14.0% occurred in the second wash.

Discussion

This overview summarizes experimental studies reporting data on in vivo human dermal decontamination of chemical contaminants and shows that decontamination with water, soap and water, or 10% isopropanol distilled water results in incomplete removal of chemical warfare simulants and cleaning agents, cosmetic agents, and pesticides, respectively, from in vivo human skin in experimental settings. Incomplete decontamination leaves the availability for percutaneous absorption of the remaining dermal chemical materials [4].

Mass of chemical decontaminated from the skin depends on several factors including the skin residence time, chemical contaminant, decontamination solvent, amount of chemical on the skin [7], washing protocols [16], and anatomical location (Table 1.5). First, a longer skin residence time that has been associated with less effective decontamination [4, 8, 9, 17] showed decreasing decontamination at 1 h compared to 0 h. This is suggested to be as a result of increased percutaneous absorption with time and decreased availability at the surface [4, 17]. Second,

Table 1.5 Factors which may impact decontamination efficacy

Factors which may impact decontamination efficacy	Details
Chemical contaminant	Including:
	• Solubility
	• Range of molecular weights
	• Lipid and water solubilities
	• Melting points
	• Volatility
	• Hydrogen bonds
Skin residence time	Longer skin residence time associated with less effective decontamination
Decontamination solvent	Solubility
Skin loading level	Fixed amount of chemical may bind to the skin resulting in apparent decreased decontamination at lower skin loading levels as compared to higher levels *or* analyses of decontamination by identifying chemicals in washing water may be affected by a limited ability of complete dissolution of high levels of chemicals
Washing protocols	Including:
	• Number of washes
	• Washing fashion
	• Wash time
	• Water temperature
Anatomical location	Hard to reach areas may decrease decontamination efficacy
Percutaneous absorption	Affected by:
	• Varying anatomical locations (stratum corneum thickness, amount of hair and sweat glands)
	• Lipid matrix within epidermis
	• Compromised skin barriers in disease states
	• Aging
	• Concentration of applied dose
	• Surface area
	• Occlusion affecting hydration and temperature
	• Number of doses
	• Skin binding
	• Skin contact time
The "wash-in" effect	Decontamination may increase skin absorption, by washing chemical contaminants into the skin

solubility of the chemical contaminant and decontamination solvent will affect decontamination [4, 7]. Water-soluble chemicals are removed fairly equally with water-only versus soap and water solutions, as compared to lipid-soluble molecules such as organic compounds and pesticides, shown to be removed better with soap and water solutions as compared to water [4, 11, 13]. For water-soluble compounds, water is a good solvent, as compared to lipid-soluble chemicals that need the surfactant system for better decontamination [4, 11, 13]. Theoretically, the chemical and physical state of the contaminant may also affect decontamination, although limited data exists on these factors [16]. As demonstrated by Southworth et al. [15] that more contaminant remained on the shoulders as compared to both arms and legs, hard to reach areas may also decrease decontamination efficacy.

Additionally, skin loading levels affect decontamination, as seen in Fenske and Lu [9] who found that lower skin loading resulted in lower decontamination as compared with higher skin loading [9]. It is hypothesized that a fixed amount of chemical may bind to the skin, resulting in an apparent decreased decontamination at lower skin loading levels as compared to higher levels [13]. On the other hand, it has been suggested that analyses of decontamination by identifying chemicals in washing water may be affected by a limited ability of complete dissolution of high levels of chemicals [16]. Further, number of washes, washing fashion, wash time, and water temperature may be clinically relevant variables [16]. Although included studies showed great variability in skin residence times, chemical contaminants, decontamination solutions, amount of chemical contaminants, and washing protocols, the majority of studies found water-based solutions showing partial decontamination outcomes.

Similarly, factors affecting chemical percutaneous penetration may impact decontamination. These factors include varying anatomical locations (stratum corneum thickness, amount of hair and sweat glands/type of sweat glands), varying properties of the chemicals (volatility, molecular weight, pH, pKa, etc.), the lipid matrix within the epidermis, compromised skin barriers in disease states, aging, concentration of applied dose, formulation differences, surface area, occlusion affecting hydration and temperature, number of doses, skin binding, and skin contact time [13, 18–20].

Additionally, only Maibach and Feldmann [13], Stahlman et al. [14], and Southworth et al. [15] attempted to analyse the pharmacokinetics of dermal decontamination by measuring the contaminant distributed in blood samples or excreted urine. Otherwise, absorption, metabolism, distribution, and excretion of contaminants were not studied. However, none of the studies included in our review were truly mass balance studies, in which the plasma pharmacokinetics and excretion of unchanged drug and metabolites are investigated via recovery of an (often radio-labelled) dose in urine and faeces [21]. Acceptable values for recovery have been proposed to be 85% or 90% [22, 23]; however, currently acceptable recovery values are 90–95% or more. Ending data collection once the skin has been washed leads to incomplete knowledge of what may still be happening to the chemical.

We note that potential clinical toxicity should, but rarely does, include excretion kinetics from either an intravenous, intraparenteral, or intradermal dose. In the original article by Feldmann and Maibach [24], most of the percutaneous penetration data was corrected for any incomplete parenteral excretion control data.

Also of note is that there may be dose-dependent kinetics for some of the chemicals or chemical warfare simulants, if escalating doses are employed. For example, this may potentially be seen for the chemical simulant methyl salicylate. In fact, the first indication of saturation with very small doses was the observation that, as the oral dose of salicylate exceeded 300–500 mg in healthy adults, the half-life can increase from 3 h to over 20 h with increasing dose, i.e. the elimination changes from first-order to zero-order kinetics [25, 26]. A similar phenomenon may potentially be seen with percutaneous absorption of chemicals or chemical warfare simulants. If this is seen, the time needed for 90–95% recovery would be extended.

Decontamination may actually increase skin absorption, by washing chemical contaminants into the skin, a phenomenon known as the "wash-in" effect [17, 18]. The "wash-in" effect, demonstrated in animal models and in vitro human studies, may enhance both cutaneous and systemic toxicities by several likely mechanisms including the surfactant effect, hydration effect, acid/base effect, friction effect, and/or artefact effect [17]. For some chemicals, such as organophosphate pesticides and chemical warfare agents, it is possible that the resulting "wash-in" effect by decontamination could be lethal [17]. Thus, experimental data regarding the effect of decontamination on absorption and the potential for the "wash-in" effect is essential for a variety chemicals.

There are limitations to this review. First, lack of large sample sizes may limit the generalizability of our results. Second, data heterogeneity in chemical contaminants, decontamination solutions, methods of washing, and analysis of decontamination may limit the quality of our findings. Further, there may be a discrepancy between experimental data and what occurs in humans under clinical circumstances.

Additionally, our laboratory has long been interested and involved in Quantitative Structure-Activity Relationships (QSAR); unfortunately, because of highly variable experimental protocols and limited number of chemicals, this is not practical at present. We optimistically look forward to harmonized protocols and sufficient variation in physical-chemical properties to allow for such analysis in the future.

Despite these limitations, these results demonstrate that decontamination with water, soap and water, and 10% isopropanol results in incomplete removal of chemical contaminants from the skin under controlled experimental conditions. We conclude that much remains to be learned about decontamination of the large variety of chemical contaminants including a range of molecular weights, lipid and water solubilities, melting points, volatility, and hydrogen bonds, as well as clinically relevant anatomic sites. A major void exists in data confirming or denying the completeness of decontamination by measuring absorption and excretion. Further, as decontamination with soap and water, the most commonly used water-based decontamination solution, has been demonstrated to be incomplete, the development of effective decontamination solutions is of high priority. Future manuscripts will survey additional efficacy models such as in vitro, in silico, and animal assays.

Acknowledgments None.

Conflict of Interest None.

Funding Sources None.

References

1. Clarkson ED, Gordon RK. Rapid decontamination of chemical warfare agents from skin. In: Handbook of toxicology of chemical warfare agents. London: Academic Press; 2020. https://doi.org/10.1016/b978-0-12-819090-6.00073-8.
2. Etemad L, Moshiri M, Balali-Mood M. Delayed complications and long- term management of sulfur mustard poisoning: a narrative review of recent advances by Iranian researchers. Part II: Clinical management and therapy. Iranian. J Med Sci. 2018;43(3):235–47. http://www.embase.com/search/results?subaction=viewrecord&from=export&id=L621921885.
3. Brent J. Water-based solutions are the best decontaminating fluids for dermal corrosive exposures: a mini review. Clin Toxicol. 2013;51(8):731–6. https://doi.org/10.3109/15563650.2013.838628.
4. Wester RC, Maibach HI. Dermal decontamination and percutaneous absorption. Boca Raton, FL: Taylor and Francis; 2002. https://www.taylorfrancis.com/books/e/9780429186493/chapters/10.1201/9780849359033-23.
5. Moher D, Liberati A, Tetzlaff J, Altman DG, PRISMA Group. Preferred reporting items for systematic reviews and meta-analyses: the PRISMA statement. PLoS Med. 2009;6:e1000097. https://doi.org/10.1371/journal.pmed.1000097.
6. Aoki M, Ogai K, Matsumoto M, Susa H, Yamada K, Yamatake T, Kobayashi M, Sugama J. Comparison of wiping methods for the removal of cleaning agent residue from hair follicles. Skin Res Technol. 2019;25(3):355.
7. Curwin BD, Hein MJ, Sanderson WT, Nishioka M, Buhler W. Acephate exposure and decontamination on tobacco harvesters' hands. J Expo Anal Environ Epidemiol. 2003;13(3):203–10. https://doi.org/10.1038/sj.jea.7500271.
8. Fenske RA, Schulter C, Lu C, Allen EH. Incomplete removal of the pesticide captan from skin by standard handwash exposure assessment procedures. Bull Environ Contam Toxicol. 1998;61(2):194–201. https://doi.org/10.1007/s001289900748.
9. Fenske RA, Lu C. Determination of handwash removal efficiency: incomplete removal of the pesticide chlorpyrifos from skin by standard handwash techniques. Am Ind Hyg Assoc J. 1994;55(5):425–32. https://doi.org/10.1080/15428119491018862.
10. Lin L, Sundh D, Raphael AP, Roberts MS, Soyer H, Prow TW. Removing nanoparticles from human skin. Wound Repair Regen. 2012;20:A64.
11. Marquart H, Brouwer DH, Van Hemmen JJ. Removing pesticides from the hands with a simple washing procedure using soap and water. J Occup Environ Med. 2002;44(11):1075–82. https://doi.org/10.1097/00043764-200211000-00014.
12. Moffett PM, Baker BL, Kang CS, Johnson MS. Evaluation of time required for water-only decontamination of an oil-based agent. Mil Med. 2010;175(3):185–7. https://doi.org/10.7205/MILMED-D-09-00012.
13. Maibach HI, Feldmann RJ. Systemic absorption of pesticides through the skin of man. In: Report to the Federal Working Group on Pest management from the task group on occupational exposure to pesticides. Appendix B. Washington, DC: US Government Printing Office; 1975.
14. Stahlman J, Britto M, Fitzpatrick S, McWhirter C, Testino SA, Brennan JJ, Zumbrunnen TL. Effects of skin washing on systemic absorption of testosterone in hypogonadal males after administration of 1.62% testosterone gel. Curr Med Res Opin. 2012;28(2):271–9. https://doi.org/10.1185/03007995.2011.652256.
15. Southworth F, James T, Davidson L, Williams N, Finnie T, Marczylo T, Collins S, Amlôt R. A controlled cross-over study to evaluate the efficacy of improvised dry and wet emergency decontamination protocols for chemical incidents. PLoS One. 2020;15(11):e0239845. https://doi.org/10.1371/journal.pone.0239845.
16. Brouwer DH, Boeniger MF, Van Hemmen J. Hand wash and manual skin wipes. Ann Occup Hyg. 2000;44(7):501–10. https://doi.org/10.1016/S0003-4878(00)00036-3.
17. Moody RP, Maibach HI. Skin decontamination: importance of the wash-in effect. Food Chem Toxicol. 2006;44(11):1783–8. https://doi.org/10.1016/j.fct.2006.05.020.

18. Law RM, Ngo MA, Maibach HI. Twenty clinically pertinent factors/observations for percutaneous absorption in humans. Am J Clin Dermatol. 2020;21(1):85–95. https://doi.org/10.1007/s40257-019-00480-4.

19. Maibach HI, Feldmann RJ, Milby TH, Serat WF. Regional variation in percutaneous penetration in man. Arch Environ Health. 1971;23(3):208–11. https://doi.org/10.1080/00039896.1971.10665987.

20. Wester RC, Maibach HI. In vivo percutaneous absorption and decontamination of pesticides in humans. J Toxicol Environ Health. 1985;16(1):25–37. https://doi.org/10.1080/15287398509530716.

21. Bucks DAW, Guy RH, Maibach HI. Percutaneous penetration and mass balance accountability: technique and implications for dermatology. Cutan Ocul Toxicol. 1989;8(4):439–51. https://doi.org/10.3109/15569528909062949.

22. Beumer JH, Beijnen JH, Schellens JHM. Mass balance studies, with a focus on anticancer drugs. Clin Pharmacokinet. 2006;45(1):33–58. https://doi.org/10.2165/00003088-200645010-00003.

23. Sunzel MICGS. New drug development: regulatory paradigms for clinical pharmacology. London: Routledge; 2004. https://www.routledge.com/New-Drug-Development-Regulatory-Paradigms-for-Clinical-Pharmacology-and/Sahajwalla/p/book/9780824754655. Accessed 6 Jun 2021.

24. Feldmann RJ, Maibach HI. Absorption of some organic compounds through the skin in man. J investig Dermatol. 1970;54:399. https://doi.org/10.1111/1523-1747.ep12259184.

25. Davison C. Salicylate metabolism in man. Ann N Y Acad Sci. 1971;179(1):249–68. https://doi.org/10.1111/j.1749-6632.1971.tb46905.x.

26. Levy G. Drug biotransformation interactions in man: nonnarcotic analgesics. Ann N Y Acad Sci. 1971;179(1):32–42. https://doi.org/10.1111/j.1749-6632.1971.tb46889.x.

Chapter 2
Toward a Harmonized Protocol for Quantifying In Vitro Human Skin Decontamination Efficacy

Thaibinh Tran and Howard I. Maibach

Introduction

Human skin decontamination has been studied for the past century, but optimal skin decontamination metrics remain subjective. Studying skin decontamination is important for protecting military personnel and civilians from chemical warfare agents (CWAs) and industrial chemicals. Between 2012 and 2018, there have been reports of chlorine, sarin, and mustard gas being used in chemical weapon attacks against civilians by the Syrian government [1].

In addition, chemical plant workers can be exposed to dangerous chemicals during toxic industrial chemical (TIC) spills. The current popular protocol is to remove contaminated clothing and wash exposed skin thoroughly with soap and water. However, Chiang et al.'s systematic review showed that soap and water or water-only decontamination yielded partial decontamination for in vitro human skin models and that more studies are needed to evaluate the effectiveness of using soap and water as decontaminants [2]. Furthermore, Burli et al. showed using soap and water or water only resulted in incomplete decontamination in animal models [3].

Reactive skin decontamination lotion (RSDL) and Fuller's earth (FE) are widely used for skin decontamination. RSDL was developed by the Canadian Department of National Defence and is used by the military as a gold standard [4]. Although RSDL is considered as a leading decontaminant, more comparative studies about its superiority are needed [5].

Study of skin decontamination began in Belgium during WWI, but the paucity of human in vivo studies has made it difficult to quantify optimal decontamination

T. Tran (✉)
University of California, Berkeley, CA, USA

H. I. Maibach
Department of Dermatology, University of California San Francisco, San Francisco, CA, USA
e-mail: howard.maibach@ucsf.edu

A. M. Feschuk et al. (eds.), *Dermal Absorption and Decontamination*,
https://doi.org/10.1007/978-3-031-09222-0_2

techniques [6]. Chemical warfare agents and other dangerous compounds cannot be easily administered on humans for the purpose of studying decontamination for ethical/practical reasons. Therefore, the alternative modalities for assaying skin decontamination are animal models, in vitro assays, and computer modeling, through the parameters of percutaneous absorption (PA).

Measuring In Vivo Percutaneous Absorption: Animal or Man

Urine Excretion

Once a compound is absorbed through the skin, it may enter circulation and eventually be excreted through the kidneys, feces, lungs, and skin. Urine assay measures PA by quantifying the amount of chemical in urine after topical application. An advantage to urine assay is that it is minimally invasive.

A parenteral correction factor must be used since full excretion of the compound through urine is not universal. Some compounds might be stored in the body or lost through feces, exhalation, eccrine, and skin [7].

To calculate the correction factor for incomplete urinary excretion, the same amount of radiolabeled compound is injected intravenously and its urinary excretion measured for comparison. From there, dermal absorption can be approximated [8]:

$$\% \text{ dermal absorption} = \text{mass in urine} / \text{parenteral mass in urine} \times 100\%$$

Although urine assay has practical advantages, this method may underestimate absorption for compounds that are absorbed or excreted slowly [9].

Percutaneous Absorption as Sum of All Residues in Body: Animal Only

This method employs the use of urine/excretion, breath, organ tissue, and blood sampling. No correction factor is needed since this considers most routes of excretion from the body [7].

$$\% \text{ dermal absorption} = \% \text{ recovered from excreta} + \text{blood} + \text{tissues} + \text{expired air}$$

Percutaneous Absorption as Measurement of Material Lost from Skin Surface

PA can also be considered as material lost from the skin after application. A known amount of material is applied on the skin, and the amount remaining on the skin is measured and quantified as the non-absorbed dose. Problems with this method include the difficulty in quantifying the amount of material left on the skin and the fact that total recovery is not guaranteed. However, this problem can be circumvented by use of a transdermal drug delivery (TDD) device where the amount of material left on the TDD device is the amount of non-absorbed dose [7]. This method, popular to approximately the 1960s, shall be evaluated with current sensitive analytic techniques.

$$\% \text{ dermal absorption} = (\text{applied dose}-\text{non}-\text{absorbed dose}) / \text{applied dose} \times 100\%$$

Menczel raised an issue about this method by positing that certain compounds might not be absorbed but are actually bound to the stratum corneum and exfoliated later or that the compound might stay in the lower epidermis and dermis and become long-term chemical reservoirs [10]. A partial solution to validation of the method would be tape stripping followed by urine/excretion assays and blood sampling. Removal of tape from the skin acts as skin exfoliation, and the presence of the material on the piece of tape would indicate that the material was not fully absorbed.

Chemical Analytic Methods

The chemistry of decontamination studies developed with increasingly more sensitive analytical techniques. Today, high-performance liquid chromatography (HPLC) and mass spectrometry (MS) provide far greater sensitivity than earlier technology. Until the 1960s, few chemicals were believed to be absorbed in vivo in man. When radioisotope technology became available after WWII, it became apparent that many compounds penetrate human skin in vivo [8].

High-performance liquid chromatography (HPLC) and mass spectrometry (MS) may also be used to quantify percutaneous absorption. In terms of pharmacokinetics (PK), the chemicals or metabolites present in the body and/or excreta after the application of the material are measured. In terms of pharmacodynamics (PD), the body's response to the applied material is analyzed. Up until recently, decontamination studies have focused on the PD such as lethality of absorbed compounds. However, there is now increased interest in the PK of absorbed compounds, which is a more quantitative approach to PA. An advantage of studying PK over PD is that it can be studied both in vitro and in vivo.

Breath Test to Measure Percutaneous Absorption

Some chemicals are excreted via exhalation preferentially to other ways previously discussed. Poet et al. used real-time breath analysis to determine the percutaneous absorption of methyl chloroform. Human volunteers were exposed to methyl chloroform by submerging their left hand in a container with soil and methyl chloroform or soil and water. Clean air was provided via facemask, and exhaled breath was passed through a heated mixing chamber from which the mass spectrometer drew a sample every 5 s [11]. The breath test is useful because it is a noninvasive way to measure PA but is limited to compounds excreted primarily though the lungs.

Animal Models to Study Percutaneous Absorption

PA studies in animal models ideally occur when one of the two criteria is met:

1. The animal model has consistently similar PA as humans.
2. The animal model has consistently different PA as humans—but can be systematically related to man.

Optimal animal models to use for studying PA are (in order of strongest to weakest) rhesus monkeys, weanling pigs, hairless guinea pigs, and hairless rats. Mice, rabbits, and rats are less optimal for studying PA since their skin permeability is significantly different from human skin [12].

Rhesus Monkeys

Rhesus monkey skin is most similar to human skin. Wester et al. compared the permeability of hydrocortisone, testosterone, and benzoic acid and found that percutaneous absorption of these three compounds in rhesus monkeys was similar to that in humans [13]. They also compared data from Bartek et al. that compared the percutaneous absorption of testosterone (and other chemical compounds) between rats, rabbits, pigs, and humans. Among other animal models, monkeys had the closest absorption percentage to humans [14]. This could be due to the phylogenetic proximity with humans. Since both humans and monkeys have relatively hairless inner arms, legs, and trunks, those areas can be used as assay sites on monkey models [12].

Miniature Pigs

Miniature pigs are the next relevant animal model. Bartek et al. found that haloprogin, n-acetylcysteine, testosterone, cortisone, caffeine, and butter yellow had similar PA in miniature pigs as in humans [14]. Although pigs are considered as good animal models to study PA, species and seasonal differences in pigs can affect PA [15].

Hairless Guinea Pigs

Hairless guinea pigs (HGPs) have similar skin thickness and dermal vasculature as humans and appear to be a reasonable animal model to study human PA [16]. Jung et al. analyzed studies that compared HGP skin and human PA. Of the 28 compounds tested on HGP and humans, 25 had a factor of difference between 0.3 and 3 [12].

Hairless Rats

Lastly, hairless rats can also be used as animal models to study human PA. Rougier et al. concluded that hairless rats can be used when conditions are carefully controlled. In their study, three radiolabeled compounds (sodium benzoate, caffeine, and acetylsalicylic acid) were applied on the back of hairless rats and on the arms, abdomen, postauricular, and forehead of humans. Comparison of PA showed that, for both hairless rats and humans, the compounds were absorbed in this order: acetylsalicylic acid > benzoic acid > caffeine > sodium benzoate. Each of the compound's PA was different by a factor of 3 for both hairless rats and humans [17].

Studying PA Using In Vitro Models

Although in vivo human volunteers are ideal for studying PA and in vivo animal models are second best, in vitro models can be more accessible and can sidestep safety ethical concerns. However, appropriate skin type/thickness and receptor fluid must be carefully selected since in vitro assays are highly sensitive to those factors. Additionally, a direct comparison of in vitro and in vivo data can be problematic because of the variables involved [15].

Receptor Fluids

To find the appropriate receptor fluid, the solubility of the test compound in the receptor fluid must be considered [15]. Saline is often used for hydrophilic compounds and blood for lipophilic compounds. Organic solvent, bovine serum albumin (BSA), and surfactants can be added to receptor fluids to increase lipophilic compound solubility. However, this can potentially change the properties of the skin barrier and thus the PA of the compounds, e.g., de Lange et al. showed that the PA of xylene depended on the receptor fluid. Specifically, the penetration rate of xylene depended on the concentration of protein passing through the pig ear. There was an increase in penetration rate when BSA was present in the receptor fluid and a decrease when BSA was absent [18].

Human Skin Models

The different types of in vitro human skin samples are full thickness, dermatomed, and epidermal membrane and stratum corneum. Full-thickness skin contains the stratum corneum, viable epidermis, and dermis. Dermatomed skin, also known as split-thickness skin, consists of the stratum corneum, dermis, and only upper dermis. Epidermal membrane has the stratum corneum and epidermis, without the dermis [15]. Studies investigated the effect of skin thickness and PA; van de Sandt et al. compared the effects of propoxur, a pesticide, in vivo and in vitro. In vitro models included full-thickness skin membranes, non-viable epidermal membranes, and perfused pig ear model.

The absorbed dose in full-thickness skin membranes was similar to the human in vivo condition. Data generated from perfused pig ear membranes were generally in between full-thickness skin membranes and non-viable epidermal membranes. Non-viable epidermal membranes overestimated human in vivo PA by a factor of 8 [19]. Wilkinson et al. investigated the effect of skin thickness on the PA of compounds with different physiochemical properties (caffeine, testosterone, propoxur, and butoxyethanol) using skin of various thickness and found that PA of testosterone, a lipophilic compound, and butoxyethanol were reduced with full-thickness skin compared to dermatomed skin. For propoxur, PA was higher through 0.71 mm thick skin than 1.36 mm skin, but there was no difference found between 0.56 and 0.71 mm skin. For caffeine, decreasing skin thickness led to non-significant increased maximum flux. They concluded that there is a complex relationship between lipophilicity, skin thickness, and PA [20]. Jakasa et al. concluded that maximum flux of butoxyethanol in dermatomed skin correlates more closely to in vivo data than full-thickness skin [21].

Two skin models appear comparable to human skin: the HuSki model and the isolated perfused porcine skin flap (IPPSF) model. The HuSki model involves the use of human skin grafted onto a mouse. Reifenrath et al. compared how different skin models compared the human PA of caffeine, benzoic acid, N,N-diethyl-m-toluamide, three steroids, and three insecticides and showed a significant correlation in PA between the HuSki model and in vivo human model [22]. Boudry et al. compared HuSki models, in vitro skin models, and in vitro pig skin models of human in vivo PA of parathion and concluded that both human in vitro and HuSki models closely predicted the in vivo human absorption but the HuSki model allowed the analysis of the amount remaining in each skin layer after absorption [23].

IPPSF allows the study of cutaneous toxicology and pharmacology in viable skin with a normal structure and microvasculature [12]. Wester et al. compared the PA of five compounds with human skin and IPPSF and found that the absorption rate values of IPPSF were comparable to human but concluded that more studies with diverse compounds with varying physiochemical properties were needed [24].

In vitro assays have a tendency to overestimate the PA of compounds. Van de Sandt et al. compared PA of propoxur in vivo and in vitro (viable full-thickness skin and non-viable epidermal membranes) in human and rat skin; in vitro PA was often higher than in vivo with the factor of difference dependent on the type of skin membrane used. In vitro human skin values were generally higher than values from human volunteers. In vitro rat epidermal membranes had higher PA values than human epidermal membranes [19].

Using in vitro assays is a viable way to study PA when humans or animal models are not available. However, care must be taken to control the type of in vitro model (whether animal skin or human skin), skin thickness, and type of receptor fluid. Not only that, the physiochemical properties of the compound, such as particle size/molecular weight, lipophilicity, pH, pK_a, and partition coefficient, must also be taken into consideration as these can affect PA [25].

Computer Modeling

Computer modeling can also be used to predict PA. An advantage to using computer modeling to predict PA is that it considers many factors that are important in absorption such as the properties of the chemicals, solvent or formulation used, exposure scenarios, and exposure levels [26]. Despite the advantages, there isn't currently sufficient experimental data on PA of different compounds to reliably utilize computer modeling as a substitute for experimental data. For instance, Burli et al. compared the relationship between in vitro based predictive models and in vivo PA. The difference was significant with PA being either over- or underestimated by a factor of 10–100 [27].

RSDL

RSDL, a gold standard for decontamination, was developed by the Canadian government in 1991 and is now used internationally as a decontamination agent. RSDL's main active ingredient is potassium 2,3-butanedione monoximate (KBDO). RSDL degrades CWA through nucleophilic substitution between KBDO and the susceptible sites in CWA compounds [28]. The reaction starts immediately and is complete within 2 min [29].

Braue et al. compared the efficacy of RSDL, M291 SDK, 0.5% bleach, and 1% soapy water in haired guinea pigs following exposure to VX and GD in two separate studies. VX and GD are nerve agents used in chemical warfare. Haired guinea pigs were shaved, and Skin Exposure Reduction Paste Against Chemical Warfare Agents (SERPACWA) barrier cream was applied and allowed to dry. VX or GD was then applied to the guinea pigs. Decontamination followed after 2 min (or longer for delayed decontamination experiments). Guinea pigs were observed for 4 h after exposure and again at 24 h after exposure for signs of toxicity or death. RSDL was the most effective decontaminant for both VX and GD and was significantly better than the other decontamination methods [30, 31].

Fentabil et al. exposed guinea pigs to parathion and aldicarb, which were decontaminated with RSDL. For parathion, untreated guinea pigs died within 24 h and had up to 86% acetylcholinesterase (AChE) inhibition. Guinea pigs treated with RSDL showed mild signs of neurotoxicity and had 0–58% AChE inhibition. During 24-h exposure to aldicarb, untreated guinea pigs had 25–61% AChE inhibition and showed signs of severe neurotoxicity. For guinea pigs treated with RSDL, percent inhibition of AChE was 0–5% with no signs of neurotoxicity. Thus, RSDL prevented the toxic effects of organophosphate and carbamate pesticides [28].

Taysse et al. compared the efficacy of RSDL and FE in hairless mice and domestic pigs exposed to sulfur mustard (SM) and VX. In hairless mice, both RSDL and FE reduced blisters 3 days after SM exposure, but RSDL was more efficient than FE in reducing necrosis and erosion of the epidermis. In VX-exposed hairless mice, RSDL did not sufficiently prevent the inhibition of cholinesterase. Only FE significantly reduced cholinesterase inhibition [32]. In domestic pigs, RSDL significantly reduced skin injury 3 days after exposure to SM compared to FE. In VX-exposed pigs, both RSDL and FE completely prevented cholinesterase inhibition [32, 33].

Thors et al. compared the efficacy of RSDL, PS104, FE, and aqueous solution alldecontMED on the decontamination of VX through the use of a diffusion cell and dermatomed human skin. RSDL was superior in reducing penetration of VX through human skin [34]. Cao et al. compared the efficacy of RSDL and Dermal Decontamination Gel (DDGel) on diisopropyl methylphosphonate (DIMP) and 2-chloroethyl ethyl sulfide (CEES) in vitro with flow-through diffusion cells. DDGel showed significantly reduced toxicant amount and showed higher decontamination efficiency for both DIMP and CEES than RSDL [35, 36].

Feschuk et al. reviewed the available literature on RSDL efficacy and suggested that there was substantial evidence that supported RSDL superiority over other methods of decontamination. However, the lack of in vivo human studies and lack of data for different types of CWAs and TICs is an important limitation in these studies. Other shortfalls in the literature are how decontamination protocols can influence the results of studies, how RSDL can impair wound healing, and the lack of evidence of RSDL safety during pregnancy [37].

French Test Standard Method of Quantifying Decontamination Effectiveness

Having an international standard for testing decontamination is essential for gaining reliable information about effectiveness of decontamination products. Josse [6] recommends the use of FSTM (French standard test method) as a framework for international standardization of measuring decontamination effectiveness. In FSTM, decontamination effectiveness is the ability to remove contaminants from the skin surface or to neutralize the contaminant on the skin surface without exacerbating the effect of the contaminant. To evaluate the effectiveness of the decontamination method, non-decontaminated skin must be compared to decontaminated skin in the same conditions. For skin models, tests can only be performed on human volunteers if the contaminant is nontoxic. Pig skin from their abdomen or back can also be used as their skin structure and permeability are similar to humans. However, freshly excised human skin models must be used if the contaminant is significantly metabolized in the skin (more than 10% of the applied amount is degraded). Skin thickness must be less than 1 mm, and surface area must be at least 0.6 cm^2. The contaminant used for testing must be at least 95% pure and cover the entire area of the exposed skin. The contaminant can be diluted in a vehicle, but the vehicle must not affect the skin permeability or the contaminant's physicochemical properties. The amount of contaminant used must replicate real-life exposure dosages. Exposure durations are relative to the type of decontamination kits tested. For emergency decontamination kits, whose function is to reduce exposure and irritation from contaminants, exposure time must be between 5 and 30 min. For thorough decontamination kits, whose function is to prevent contamination from the skin to other surfaces, exposure times must be between 30 and 60 min. If the decontaminant is a liquid, the last step must be a drying step where a new absorbent is applied to the skin without scrubbing until the skin is dry.

An effective skin decontaminant will not increase the local and systemic effects of the contaminants. To quantify effectiveness, non-decontaminated skin and decontaminated skin will be compared where the contaminants on the skin surfaces are absorbed with a cotton ball and the skin surfaces tape stripped twice. Contaminants will be measured based on the amount extracted from the cotton ball and tape. For in vitro test models, the amount of contaminants on the skin surface, penetrating through the skin, and the rate of penetrance must be measured. In vitro test results alone can be used to evaluate skin decontamination effectiveness if the correlation between in vivo and in vitro is reliable. For in vivo animal models, the amount of contaminants eliminated from the skin surface, the amount present on the skin surface immediately after decontamination, and the amount present in the skin at the end of the experiment must be measured. In addition, lag time and maximum resorption rate should be measured when possible. For lethal agents, survival rates of the animal model will be measured. For non-lethal agents, biomarkers will be used to evaluate toxic effects on animal model (Table 2.1).

Table 2.1 Summary of FSTM

Skin models	• Abdominal or back pig skin due to structural and permeability similarities to human skin
	• Freshly excised human skin must be used if contaminant is metabolized in the skin (more than 10% of the applied contaminant is degraded)
	• Skin thickness conditions: less than 1 mm and surface area must be at least 0.6 cm²
Contaminant conditions	• Must be 95% pure and cover the entire area of the exposed skin
	• Can be diluted in a vehicle, but the vehicle must neither affect skin permeability nor the contaminant's physicochemical properties
Contaminant exposure dosage	• For emergency decontamination kits: exposure time between 5 and 30 min
	• For thorough decontamination kits: exposure times between 30 and 60 min
Liquid decontaminants	• In the last step, a new absorbent must be applied to the skin without scrubbing until the skin is dry
Quantifying effectiveness of decontamination for in vivo skin models	• Cotton balls are used to absorb contaminant on decontaminated and non-decontaminated skin. Skin surfaces will be tape stripped twice after
	• The amount of contaminant found in cotton balls and tape determines effectiveness of decontamination
Quantifying effectiveness of decontamination for in vitro test models	• The amount of contaminants on the skin surface, penetrating through the skin, and the rate of penetrance are measured
	• In vitro test results can be used to evaluate skin decontamination effectiveness if the correlation between in vivo and in vitro is reliable
Quantifying effectiveness of decontamination for in vivo animal models	• Contaminant levels are measured immediately after decontamination and at the end of the experiment
	• Lethal contaminants: survival rates of animal models are measured
	• Non-lethal contaminants: biomarkers will be used to evaluate toxicity in animal models

Conclusion

The ideal way to study decontamination is to apply the contaminant on the test model and then measure mass of the contaminant absorbed compared to the amount of contaminant absorbed with decontamination. A perfect decontaminant would result in no contaminant absorption.

An ideal test model would be human subjects; however, some compounds are extremely toxic and cannot be tested on human subjects.

The strongest model would be animals in vivo. The closest to humans (in order) are rhesus monkeys, weanling pigs, hairless guinea pigs, and hairless rats. Animal models provide some similar physiological aspects as humans. In particular, the HuSki models appear to have similar properties to human skin. Lastly, computer modeling can be used. Although computer modeling has its advantages, a limitation is the limited biologic and PK data currently available.

To assay decontamination agents on humans, the ideal way would be to measure dermal absorption as the sum recovered from expired air, blood, and urine as well as amount recovered from tape stripping (to check for reservoir effects in clinical and experimental subjects). For animals, dermal absorption should be the sum recovered from expired air, blood, urine, and tissue as well as tape stripping. Care should be taken to ensure that the area of the skin where the contaminant is applied has the same thickness as the area of human skin that is studied. For in vitro studies, penetration rate and amount should be examined when assessing decontamination methods. Skin thickness and types of receptor fluid need to be taken into consideration since these factors have an effect on the PA of a chemical. The physiochemical properties of the contaminant also need to be considered because hydrophilic and lipophilic compounds can be absorbed differently in different receptor fluids and skin thicknesses.

Moreover, a wide range of chemicals need to be tested to see how effective a decontaminating agent is. In the RSDL studies, the most widely used test contaminants were either nerve agents or vesicants; however, not all toxic chemicals fall into either of those categories. RSDL may be an ideal decontaminant for those chemicals that have similar physiochemical properties as nerve agents, but there may be better decontaminants for other chemicals. More research needs to be done in the field of percutaneous absorption and decontamination. It is important to study these due to their relevance in the daily lives of soldiers, with respect to chemical warfare agents, and in the daily lives of chemical plant workers, with respect to toxic industrial spills.

Recently, Feschuk et al. reviewed RSDL and showed that, depending on the protocol, RSDL was either more effective than control or not so. We believe that techniques summarized in their manuscript provide a systematic and harmonized approach to reliable comparative efficacy studies. In addition, we believe that Josse's recommendation of using FSTM can also be a reliable way to compare decontamination efficacy. We hope that this document will lead to an international workshop providing the first generation of such a harmonized approach.

References

1. GPPi. Nowhere to hide: the logic of chemical weapons use in Syria. n.d.. https://www.gppi.net/2019/02/17/the-logic-of-chemical-weapons-use-in-syria.
2. Chiang C, et al. Efficacy of water-only or soap and water skin decontamination of chemical warfare agents or simulants using in vitro human models: a systematic review. J Appl Toxicol. 2022;42:930. https://doi.org/10.1002/jat.4251.
3. Burli A, Kashetsky N, Feschuk A, Law RM, Maibach HI. Efficacy of soap and water based skin decontamination using in vivo animal models: a systematic review. J Toxicol Environ Health B Crit Rev. 2021;24:325–36.

4. RSDL. About RSDL. n.d.. https://www.rsdl.com/about-rsdl/.
5. Feschuk A. Comparative efficacy of reactive. In: Skin decontamination lotion (RSDL).
6. Josse D. In: Zhu H, Maibach HI, editors. Skin decontamination: a comprehensive clinical research guide. Cham: Springer International Publishing; 2020. p. 77–85. https://doi.org/10.1007/978-3-030-24009-7.
7. Ngo MA, O'Malley M, Maibach HI. Percutaneous absorption and exposure assessment of pesticides. J Appl Toxicol. 2010;30:91–114.
8. Feldmann RJ, Maibach HI. Percutaneous penetration of steroids in man*. J Investig Dermatol. 1969;52:89–94.
9. Franz TJ. Percutaneous absorption. On the relevance of in vitro data. J Investig Dermatol. 1975;64:190–5.
10. Menczel E, Maibach HI. In vitro human percutaneous penetration of benzyl alcohol and testosterone: epidermal-dermal retention. J Investig Dermatol. 1970;54:386–94.
11. Poet TS, et al. Utility of real time breath analysis and physiologically based pharmacokinetic modeling to determine the percutaneous absorption of methyl chloroform in rats and humans. Toxicol Sci. 2000;54:42–51.
12. Jung EC, Maibach HI. Animal models for percutaneous absorption. J Appl Toxicol. 2015;35:1–10.
13. Wester RC, Maibach HI. Relationship of topical dose and percutaneous absorption in rhesus monkey and man. J Investig Dermatol. 1976;67:518–20.
14. Bartek MJ, Labudde JA, Maibach HI. Skin permeability in vivo: comparison in rat, rabbit, pig and man. J Investig Dermatol. 1972;58:114–23.
15. Jakasa I, Kezic S. Evaluation of in-vivo animal and in-vitro models for prediction of dermal absorption in man. Hum Exp Toxicol. 2008;27:281–8.
16. Sueki H, Gammal C, Kudoh K, Kligman AM. Hairless guinea pig skin: anatomical basis for studies of cutaneous biology. Eur J Dermatol. 2000;10:357–64.
17. Rougier A, Lotte C, Maibach HI. The hairless rat: a relevant animal model to predict in vivo percutaneous absorption in humans? J Invest Dermatol. 1987;88:577–81.
18. Delange J, Vaneck P, Bruijnzeel PLB, Elliott GR. The rate of percutaneous permeation of xylene, measured using the 'perfused pig ear' model, is dependent on the effective protein concentration in the perfusing medium. Toxicol Appl Pharmacol. 1994;127:298–305.
19. van de Sandt JJM, Meuling WJA, Elliott GR, Cnubben NHP, Hakkert BC. Comparative in vitro–in vivo percutaneous absorption of the pesticide propoxur. Toxicol Sci. 2000;58:15–22.
20. Wilkinson SC, et al. Interactions of skin thickness and physicochemical properties of test compounds in percutaneous penetration studies. Int Arch Occup Environ Health. 2006;79:405–13.
21. Jakasa I, Mohammadi N, Krüse J, Kezic S. Percutaneous absorption of neat and aqueous solutions of 2-butoxyethanol in volunteers. Int Arch Occup Environ Health. 2004;77:79–84.
22. Reifenrath WG, Chellquist EM, Shipwash EA, Jederberg WW, Krueger GG. Percutaneous penetration in the hairless dog, weanling pig and grafted athymic nude mouse: evaluation of models for predicting skin penetration in man. Br J Dermatol. 1984;111(Suppl 27):123–35.
23. Boudry I, et al. Percutaneous penetration and absorption of parathion using human and pig skin models in vitro and human skin grafted onto nude mouse skin model in vivo. J Appl Toxicol. 2008;28:645–57.
24. Wester RC, Melendres J, Sedik L, Maibach H, Riviere JE. Percutaneous absorption of salicylic acid, theophylline, 2,4-dimethylamine, diethyl hexyl phthalic acid, and p-aminobenzoic acid in the isolated perfused porcine skin flap compared to man in vivo. Toxicol Appl Pharmacol. 1998;151:159–65.
25. Law RM, Ngo MA, Maibach HI. Twenty clinically pertinent factors/observations for percutaneous absorption in humans. Am J Clin Dermatol. 2020;21:85–95.
26. Krüse J, Verberk CWE. Modelling of systemic uptake of agrochemicals after dermal exposure; effects of formulation, application and exposure scenarios. Environmentalist. 2008;28:57–65.

27. Burli A, Law RM, Rodriguez J, Maibach HI. Organic compounds percutaneous penetration in vivo in man: relationship to mathematical predictive model. Regul Toxicol Pharmacol. 2020;112:104614.
28. Fentabil M, Gebremedhin M, Barry J, Mikler J, Cochrane L. In vivo efficacy of the Reactive Skin Decontamination Lotion (RSDL®) kit against organophosphate and carbamate pesticides. Chem Biol Interact. 2020;318:108980.
29. CHEMM. Reactive skin decontamination lotion (RSDL) - medical countermeasures database. n.d.. https://chemm.nlm.nih.gov/countermeasure_RSDL.htm.
30. Braue EH, Hanssen KA, Doxzon BF, Lumpkin HL, Clarkson ED. Evaluation of RSDL, M291 SDK, 0.5% bleach, 1% soapy water and SERPACWA. Part 1: challenge with VX. 84; 2009.
31. Braue EH, Smith KH, Doxzon BF, Lumpkin HL, Clarkson ED. Efficacy studies of reactive skin decontamination lotion, M291 skin decontamination kit, 0.5% bleach, 1% soapy water, and skin exposure reduction paste against chemical warfare agents, part 2: guinea pigs challenged with soman. Cutan Ocul Toxicol. 2011;30:29–37.
32. Taysse L, et al. Cutaneous challenge with chemical warfare agents in the SKH-1 hairless mouse (II): effects of some currently used skin decontaminants (RSDL and Fuller's earth) against liquid sulphur mustard and VX exposure. Hum Exp Toxicol. 2011;30:491–8.
33. Taysse L, Daulon S, Delamanche S, Bellier B, Breton P. Skin decontamination of mustards and organophosphates: comparative efficiency of RSDL and Fuller's earth in domestic swine. Hum Exp Toxicol. 2007;26:135–41.
34. Thors L, et al. Comparison of skin decontamination efficacy of commercial decontamination products following exposure to VX on human skin. Chem Biol Interact. 2017;273:82–9.
35. Cao Y, Hui X, Elmahdy A, Maibach H. In vitro human skin permeation and decontamination of diisopropyl methylphosphonate (DIMP) using Dermal Decontamination Gel (DDGel) and Reactive Skin Decontamination Lotion (RSDL) at different timepoints. Toxicol Lett. 2018;299:118–23.
36. Cao Y, Hui X, Zhu H, Elmahdy A, Maibach H. In vitro human skin permeation and decontamination of 2-chloroethyl ethyl sulfide (CEES) using Dermal Decontamination Gel (DDGel) and Reactive Skin Decontamination Lotion (RSDL). Toxicol Lett. 2018;291:86–91.
37. Walters TJ, Kauvar DS, Reeder J, Baer DG. Effect of reactive skin decontamination lotion on skin wound healing in laboratory rats. Mil Med. 2007;172:318–21.

Chapter 3
In Vitro Human Skin Decontamination with Water: Chemical Warfare Agents or Simulants

Chavy Chiang, Nadia Kashetsky, Aileen M. Feschuk, Anuk Burli, Rebecca M. Law, and Howard I. Maibach

Introduction

Skin decontamination is the process by which harmful substances are neutralized or removed from the skin. Cutaneous exposure to chemical contaminants can occur in various settings, including occupational exposure to pesticides and toxic industrial chemicals or military, and even civilian, exposure to chemical warfare agents (CWAs). Direct skin contact enables these chemicals to penetrate through to dermal layers, where they subsequently gain access to the circulatory system [1]. The ever-present risk of chemical contamination and targeted attacks using CWAs, as demonstrated by the use of nerve agent VX in the 2017 assassination of Kim Jong-nam and Novichok nerve agents in both the 2018 Salisbury poisonings of Sergei and Yulia Skripal and 2020 poisoning of Alexei Navalny [2], necessitate further investigation into the optimal method of decontamination.

Due to availability, timely flushing with copious amounts of water-only or water and soap is considered a preferred decontamination method [3]. This is because water flushing is thought to offer the following benefits: (1) dilution of the

C. Chiang (✉) · A. Burli
School of Medicine and Dentistry, University of Rochester, Rochester, NY, USA
e-mail: chavy_chiang@urmc.rochester.edu

N. Kashetsky
Faculty of Medicine, Memorial University, St. John's, NL, Canada

A. M. Feschuk
Faculty of Medicine, Memorial University of Newfoundland, St. John's, NL, Canada

R. M. Law
School of Pharmacy, Memorial University of Newfoundland, St. John's, NL, Canada

H. I. Maibach
Department of Dermatology, University of California San Francisco, San Francisco, CA, USA

© The Author(s), under exclusive license to Springer Nature Switzerland AG 2022
A. M. Feschuk et al. (eds.), *Dermal Absorption and Decontamination*, https://doi.org/10.1007/978-3-031-09222-0_3

contaminant, (2) rinsing of contaminant, (3) decreasing rate of chemical reaction, (4) reduction of tissue metabolism, (5) minimization of the hygroscopic effects of the chemical on the surrounding tissue, and (6) restoration of skin's physiologic pH [4]. More contemporary studies in human volunteers by Southworth et al. [5] and Chilcott et al. [6] have found that wet decontamination of methyl salicylate, a CWA simulant, from human volunteers in vivo using water-rinsing and sponge-wiping significantly reduced skin content compared to non-decontaminated controls, whereas Larner et al. [7] did not unless water-rinsing were combined with dry decontamination. Amlot et al. [8] demonstrated that 2-min rinsing with 5% soapy water followed by 1-min, water-only rinsing significantly removed more contaminant from the front and back of volunteers compared to non-decontaminated volunteers. However, quantification of total contaminant recovered in wash, remaining on the skin, or absorbing into the bloodstream was not provided in those studies. Maibach and Feldmann [9] quantified malathion and parathion percutaneous absorption over 24 h following topical administration on human volunteers and found soapy water decontamination always yielded partial decontamination, with 1.4–15.8% absorbing through the forearm into the bloodstream depending on the time of decontamination. Additionally, some absorption rates were actually higher following decontamination compared to non-decontaminated groups. This was later established and coined as the "wash-in" effect, a phenomenon in which the process of skin washing paradoxically enhances skin penetration and systemic uptake, as summarized in a review by Moody [10]. Additionally, prior reviews pending publication and conducted by Kashetsky et al. [11] and Burli et al. [12] examined the efficacy of decontamination using water-only or water and soap solutions in in vivo human and animal models, respectively, and concluded that such methods resulted in incomplete removal of contaminants in the majority of cases. Additionally, firm conclusions regarding the efficacy of soap and water decontamination could not be drawn due to lacking absorption and excretion quantification. This review summarizes data on water-only or water and soap decontamination of CWA using in vitro human skin models.

Materials and Methods

The Preferred Reporting Items for Systematic Reviews and Meta-Analysis (PRISMA) guidelines were followed [13].

Search Strategy

A search utilizing Embase, Covidence®, MEDLINE, PubMed, Web of Science, and Google Scholar databases was conducted on February 8, 2021. Search terms included "cutaneous" or "skin" or "dermal" or "percutaneous" and "decontamination" or "decontaminant" or "skin decontamination." Temporal, geographical, or language restrictions were not applied.

Eligibility

Articles were considered eligible when they are (1) experimental studies, (2) reporting chemical decontamination of the skin with water and/or soap and water solutions, (3) evaluating decontamination of CWAs/CWA simulants, (4) using in vitro human skin models, and (5) written in English.

Data Screening

Title/abstract screening was completed by two independent researchers (R.L., H.M.) with conflicts resolved by discussion with a third (N.K.). Full-text review was completed independently by two researchers (C.C., N.K.), and conflicts were resolved by a third (H.M.). Relevant article references were manually searched to identify any additional studies.

Data Extraction and Analysis

Data extraction was completed by four researchers (N.K., A.F., A.B., C.C.) and verified by two researchers (H.M., R.L.). Data on study characteristics, human skin models, chemical contaminants, and decontamination solution, method, analysis, and outcomes were extracted. Data heterogeneity among the studies prompted a descriptive analysis rather than a meta-analysis. Studies were categorized into (1) water-only decontamination, (2) soap and water decontamination, or (3) both water-only and soap and water decontamination. Decontamination outcomes were sorted into three categories: (1) no response, (2) partial decontamination, and (3) complete decontamination. "No response" was defined as a decontamination efficacy of <1%, "partial decontamination" as 1–99.4%, and "complete decontamination" as 99.5% or greater.

Results

Study Characteristics

Title and abstract screening of 3310 studies, followed by a full-text review of 61 studies, yielded seven studies that fit inclusion criteria. Details are summarized in Fig. 3.1. These seven studies collectively tested decontamination of seven chemicals classified as either CWAs or CWA simulants. VX, malathion, and methyl salicylate were the most reported contaminants of those included in this review, each

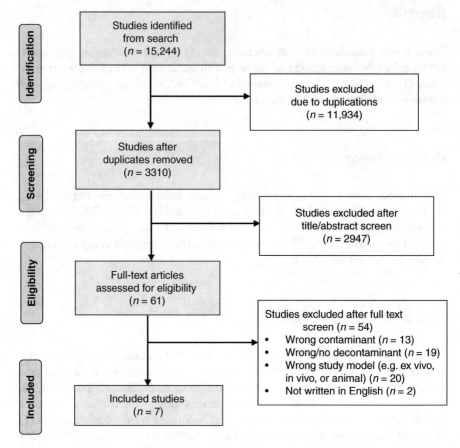

Fig. 3.1 Selection process for study inclusion

appearing in two studies (28.6%, $n = 2/7$). In vitro skin samples included those obtained from cadavers for two studies (28.6%, $n = 2/7$) or surgical waste for five studies (71.4%, $n = 5/7$). One study evaluated water-only decontamination (14.3%, $n = 1/7$), four studies evaluated water and soap decontamination (57.1%, $n = 4/7$), and the last two evaluated both water-only and soap and water decontamination (28.6%, $n = 2/7$).

Water-Only Decontamination

Thors et al. [14] studied the in vitro decontamination efficacy of water on nerve agent VX with dermatomed human skin. Abdominal skin samples were obtained from plastic surgery patients. Experiments were performed utilizing a diffusion cell containing a flow-through receptor solution, with a nominal skin diffusion area of 0.13 cm². In control samples without decontamination, an infinite dose of VX, both neat and diluted to 20% in water, was exposed on the skin throughout the complete 300-min experimental time (25 µL, equating 25.2 mg for neat VX and 5.04 mg for 20% VX). Water decontamination after 5- or 30-min exposure times to infinitely dosed VX (10 µL, equating 10.08 mg for neat VX and 2.016 mg for 20%) consisted of adding 50 µL of water onto the skin, followed by immediate vacuum suctioning, for ten repetitions (decontamination sample size, $n = 24$, 6 samples per protocol $\times$ 2 doses $\times$ 2 time points; control sample size, $n = 12$, 6 samples per protocol $\times$ 2 doses). Cumulative amounts of penetrated VX in the receptor fluid were analyzed via gas chromatography-flame photometric detector and used to determine decontamination efficacy.

Decontamination initiated at both 5 and 30 min post-exposure to neat VX significantly reduced the penetration rate compared to non-decontaminated controls ($p < 0.05$). However, decontamination at 30 min resulted in a significantly delayed reduction in penetration rate, seen at time point 250 min versus 170 min in the 5-min post-exposure group ($p < 0.05$). Cumulative amounts of 20% VX penetrating through the skin were significantly reduced when decontamination was initiated at both 5 min and 30 min post-exposure, measuring 65 ± 6 µg/cm^2 and 352 ± 33 µg/cm^2, respectively, when compared to non-decontaminated control, which measured 3622 ± 440 µg/cm^2 ($p < 0.001$). Converting penetrated amounts for each scenario to percent of applied dose penetrated for comparison purposes (by multiplying cumulative penetration by nominal diffusion area divided by applied dose) yields 0.42%, 2.3%, and 9.3% of the applied dose reaching the receptor fluid for 5-min decontamination, 30-min decontamination, and control groups, respectively. With regard to neat VX, only decontamination initiated at 5 min resulted in a significant reduction in penetrated VX ($p < 0.001$), reducing receptor fluid concentrations from 319 ± 42 µg/cm^2 in control to 140 ± 23 µg/cm^2, whereas decontamination at 30 min post-exposure did not result in a significant reduction in penetrated VX, which measured 278 ± 80 µg/cm^2, when compared to control. Similar conversion to percentage of applied dose yields 0.16%, 0.18%, and 0.35% for control, 5-min, and 30-min decontamination groups, respectively. Partial decontamination was achieved in all water-decontaminated samples, and Thors et al. concluded that decontamination efficacy is reduced with extended exposure time.

Soap and Water Decontamination

Zhu et al. [15] investigated the efficacy of 2% soapy water in decontaminating ^{14}C-labeled paraoxon. Five microliters of paraoxon, equating 0.00025 mCi (mg amount not reported), was applied to 1 cm^2 area of cadaveric abdominal skin samples in glass diffusion cells. The contaminant was in contact with the skin for 30 min before decontamination, conducted by washing once with a 2% hand soap-soaked cotton ball and twice with a cotton ball soaked in distilled deionized water and then drying (sample sizes, $n = 5$ each for decontamination and control groups). Each wet cotton ball sat on the skin for 3 min; no wiping was applied during decontamination.

Decontamination efficacy was determined by the total mass balance of ^{14}C-labeled contaminant recovery, measured using a liquid scintillation counter. Recovered percentages of the applied dose of paraoxon were $82.4 \pm 10.8\%$ in the soap-water wash, $9.8 \pm 8.7\%$ in the epidermis, and $3.1 \pm 1.2\%$ in receptor fluid. Whereas epidermal paraoxon concentration was reduced from $96.5 \pm 2.0\%$ in control to $9.2 \pm 2.5\%$ with soap-water wash, receptor fluid concentration was significantly enhanced compared to non-washed control ($p < 0.001$), which measured $1.02 \pm 0.2\%$. Therefore, while soapy water wash resulted in partial decontamination of the epidermis, it enhanced penetration into the receptor fluid, representing increased systemic paraoxon absorption. This enhanced penetration represents the "wash-in" effect, and Zhu et al. cautioned that washing could enhance toxicity.

Thors et al. [16] studied decontamination of nerve agent VX using 2% soapy water. Ten microliters of neat VX, equating 10.08 mg, was applied to a nominal skin diffusion area of 1.13 cm^2 for human Caucasian abdominal skin samples. Skin samples were mounted on in vitro diffusion cells and exposed to the nerve agent for 5 min before decontamination, executed by washing with 50 µL of soapy water instantly followed by vacuum suctioning repeatedly for ten times (sample sizes, $n = 6$ each for decontamination and control groups). Receptor solution was collected every 10 min over 300 min and decontamination efficacy determined using gas chromatography with a flame photometric detector.

Results showed that 2% soapy water significantly increased penetration of VX to the receptor fluid when compared to the non-decontaminated control, measuring 122.4 ± 22.3 µg/cm^2 and 56.0 ± 6.7 µg/cm^2, respectively. Converting receptor fluid values to percentage of applied dose (by multiplying cumulative penetrated concentration by nominal skin diffusion area and dividing by applied dose) yields 0.63% and 1.4% for control and decontaminated groups, respectively. Thors et al. emphasized the importance of keeping water content low in the decontamination of nerve agent VX due to the "wash-in" effect due to the greater-than-doubled penetration through the skin.

Moody et al. [17] studied the efficacy of skin soap washing for three warfare agent simulants: ^{14}C-radiolabeled methyl salicylate (MES), ethyl parathion (PT), and malathion (MT). Human skin was obtained from surgical waste tissue of breast origin, with the exception of one tissue sample of leg origin. Skin samples were placed in a standard Bronaugh flow-through diffusion cell system, and 0.38 cm^2 areas were incubated with contaminants at low, mid, or high doses (approximately 2, 20, and 200 mM, equating 0.0061, 0.061, and 0.61 mg for MES; 0.012, 0.1216, and 1.216 mg for PT; and 0.014, 0.14, and 1.41 mg for MT) for 390 min, with decontamination performed at 30 min (decontamination sample size, $n = 45$, 5 samples per protocol × 3 contaminants × 3 doses; control sample size, $n = 15$, 5 samples per test protocol × 3 contaminants). Decontamination involved putting 200 µL of soap wash onto the skin surface of each Bronaugh cell donor chamber. A swab was then rotated three times on the skin surface, and the tip was broken off and placed into a liquid scintillation counter (LSC) vial for analysis. The skin surface was then washed twice successively with new swabs using 200 µL of distilled water. Swabs were rotated clockwise for the soap wash and then counterclockwise and clockwise successively for the two water rinses. Researchers measured percentages recovered from soap and water wash compared to the initial amounts applied.

For MES at 2 mM, 20 mM, and 200 mM, the percentages extracted using soap and water wash were 37.3 ± 16.41%, 31.1 ± 3.78%, and 62.2 ± 5.76% of the applied dose, respectively. For PT, numbers were 45.1 ± 7.34%, 77.4 ± 11.26%, and 68.8 ± 11.26%. For MT, the soap and water wash resulted in decontamination amounts of 60.2 ± 9.08%, 85.8 ± 5.59%, and 67.4 ± 8.74%. Variable amounts recovered were explained by volatilization, especially given that the most volatile of the three, MES, demonstrated the lowest recovery in the wash. Despite achieving partial decontamination, the authors concluded that soap and water wash did not prevent substantial absorption of all three chemicals tested. Additionally, a skin depot of contaminants persisted after the experimental time of 390 min, with the largest depot seen from PT, the most lipophilic contaminant of the three.

Nielsen [18] studied the effect of skin washing with soap following 360 min of exposure to ^{14}C-radiolabeled malathion, caffeine, glyphosate, and benzoic acid. Human breast and abdominal skin samples were obtained from plastic surgery patients and mounted onto an in vitro static diffusion cell, with a median diffusion area of 2.12 cm². Malathion in aqueous solutions containing 0.9% NaCl and 2% ethanol were applied to the donor chamber at a concentration of 2 mg/mL for a total volume of 106 μL, equating 0.212 mg. At 360 min, the epidermal skin surface and donor chamber were washed in half of the groups with a neutral pH soap (pH = 7.2) and cotton swab followed by two isotonic water rinses (decontamination sample size, $n = 12$; control sample size, $n = 14$). At the end of the experimental period of 2880 min (48 h), the epidermal side of the skin was wiped four times with cotton swabs moistened with 50% acetonitrile in water and two times with dry swabs. Samples were analyzed for radioactivity using liquid scintillation counting.

Washing resulted in a significantly greater recovery amount from donor chambers, measuring 78.5 ± 1.9% of the applied dose, compared to that of the non-wash group, which measured 63.3 ± 2.4% ($p < 0.05$). Total skin deposition of malathion was also significantly lower in the decontamination group versus control group, measuring 6.0 ± 1.0% vs. 11.0 ± 2.7% of the applied dose, respectively. There was less malathion recovered in both the epidermis and dermis of the decontaminated group, although significance was only reached in the dermis ($p < 0.05$). Although partial decontamination was achieved, no significant differences were seen in receptor fluid amounts between control and decontamination. Nielsen concluded that handwashing following 360 min of skin contact time most significantly reduces the amount of residue present in the upper skin compartments and that penetrates deeper into the skin for hydrophilic substances, of which malathion is not.

Water-Only and Soap and Water Decontamination

Loke et al. [19] studied the decontamination of diethylmalonate, a simulant of the CWA soman, from human cadaver skin samples of undisclosed anatomical origin in vitro using flow-through diffusion cells. Decontamination solutions included anionic surfactant (sodium lauryl sulfate (SLS)), cationic surfactant (benzethonium chloride), nonionic surfactant (RM 21), deionized water, 0.9% saline, or 9% saline.

Skin samples containing the epidermis and uppermost layer of the dermis were placed in diffusion cells, and a diffusion area of 0.8 cm^2 was exposed to 4 μL of neat diethylmalonate, equating 4.22 mg, and perfused with saline. Decontamination with each solution was conducted 15, 30, and 60 min post-exposure by washing the epidermal surface with a flow rate of 0.5 L/min for 1 min, followed by continued incubation until 1440 min (24 h) had elapsed (decontamination sample size, $n = 54$, 3 samples per protocol × 6 decontamination solutions × 3 time points; control sample size, $n = 9$, 3 samples per protocol × 3 time points). Contaminants in wash fluid and skin samples were quantified using gas chromatography with flame ionization detection, while evaporated amounts were trapped and quantified by direct desorption. Results were compared to non-decontaminated control skin samples.

While exact decontamination efficacy values were not reported, results demonstrated no significant difference between any of the decontamination solutions. Significant differences were only reported when comparing decontamination performed between various time points, with the 15-min mark recovering the highest amount of diethylmalonate regardless of which solution was used, followed by the 30- and 60-min mark. All protocols achieved partial decontamination. Notably, decontamination at all time points except for the 15-min mark transiently enhanced percutaneous penetration of diethylmalonate for the subsequent 2 h. Enhancement rates were proportional with time delay to decontamination and dependent on solution used, with the effect observed in the following greatest-to-least order: anionic surfactant > cationic surfactant > nonionic surfactant > deionized water > 0.9% saline > saline > 9% saline. Loke et al. attributed this enhancement to be due to the hydrating properties of each solution, as they reported prior studies have noted anionic and cationic surfactants to impart the greatest skin hydration effect, while aqueous solutions with increasing salt content show a decreasing hydration effect [20]. They concluded that successful decontamination has a greater dependency on the time to decontamination rather than solution used. However, isotonic or hypertonic salt solutions impart less skin hydration and therefore reduced penetration enhancement of residual contaminant that was not washed off, making them better decontamination options for diethylmalonate.

Forsberg et al. [21] investigated decontamination efficacy of water-only and 2% soapy water against two chemical warfare agent simulants, ethyl lactate and methyl salicylate. Human skin samples from the abdominal region were exposed to 10 μL (neat) of each contaminant, equating 10.34 mg for ethyl lactate and 11.74 mg for methyl salicylate, over a 0.13 cm^2 nominal diffusion area using a flow-through diffusion cell (decontaminated sample size, $n = 48$, 6 samples per protocol × 2 contaminants × 4 time points; control sample size, $n = 12$, 6 samples per protocol × 2 contaminants). Infinite dosing was used throughout the experiments. Skin contact time with contaminants lasted either 5, 15, 45, or 120 min before decontamination. Decontamination was performed in the diffusion cell by washing with 50 μL of decontaminant solution, followed by immediate vacuum suctioning, repeated for ten times. Receptor fluid samples were collected every 10 min over 300 min, and final decontamination efficacy was determined by using gas chromatography with flame ionization detection to quantify contaminant concentration recovered in samples.

Water washing and soapy water washing significantly decreased cumulative penetration through the skin of both simulants at all time points compared to control ($p < 0.001$), with earlier decontamination yielding greater efficacy. For water-only decontamination of ethyl lactate, cumulative penetration measured 0.6 ± 0.1 µg/cm^2, 1.6 ± 0.1 µg/cm^2, 2.2 ± 0.5 µg/cm^2, and 5.5 ± 0.6 µg/cm^2 at 5 min, 15 min, 45 min, and 120 min post-exposure, respectively, compared to control, which measured 12.4 ± 1.7 µg/cm^2. Conversion of cumulative penetration to percent of applied dose (by multiplying by nominal diffusion area and dividing by initially applied dose) yields 0.016%, 0.000075%, 0.0020%, 0.0028%, and 0.0069% for control, 5 min, 15 min, 45 min, and 120 min post-exposure, respectively. Soapy water decontamination of ethyl lactate, compared to the same control of 12.4 ± 1.7 µg/cm^2, yielded cumulative penetration amounts of 0.8 ± 0.2 µg/cm^2, 1.9 ± 0.6 µg/cm^2, 2.3 ± 0.2 µg/cm^2, and 5.4 ± 0.3 µg/cm^2 for 5-min, 15-min, 45-min, and 120-min post-exposure groups, respectively. Percentage conversion for the same respective order yields 0.016%, 0.001%, 0.0024%, 0.0029%, and 0.0068% of applied dose reaching the receptor fluid. Water-only decontamination of methyl salicylate yielded penetration amounts of 2.4 ± 0.5, 2.2 ± 0.3, 3.6 ± 0.6, and 5.1 ± 0.5 µg/cm^2 at 5, 15, 45, and 120 min post-exposure, compared to the 11.8 ± 1.3 µg/cm^2 in control. Percentage conversion yields 0.013%, 0.0027%, 0.0024%, 0.0040%, and 0.0056% of applied dose for control, 5 min, 15 min, 45 min, and 120 min post-exposure, respectively. Lastly, soapy water decontamination of methyl salicylate resulted in cumulative penetration amounts measuring 1.9 ± 0.2 µg/cm^2, 2.7 ± 0.7 µg/cm^2, 4.7 ± 0.5 µg/cm^2, and 5.7 ± 0.6 µg/cm^2 for 5 min, 15 min, 45 min, and 120 min post-exposure, respectively. Conversion yields 0.0021%, 0.0030%, 0.0052%, and 0.0063% for 5 min, 15 min, 45 min, and 120 min post-exposure, respectively. All penetration rates decreased significantly following either decontamination protocol when compared to non-decontaminated control ($p < 0.05$). Methyl salicylate did, however, demonstrate a transient and slightly increased penetration rate following decontamination at the 120-min mark before trending downward again. No significant differences in cumulative amounts of penetration were seen between water wash and soapy water wash; both achieved partial decontamination. Similar to the above findings by Loke et al. [19], Forsberg et al. also concluded early decontamination to be the greatest determinant of decontamination efficacy.

Discussion

This systematic review summarizes experimental studies evaluating the decontamination efficacy of water-only or soap and water solutions on CWA or CWA simulants in in vitro human models. Table 3.1 summarizes study details. VX, its simulant malathion, and the sulfur mustard simulant methyl salicylate were the most reported contaminants in included articles, each appearing in 28.6% ($n = 2/7$) of studies. Water-only decontamination solutions, evaluated in 42.9% ($n = 3/7$) of studies, led to partial decontamination in all skin samples tested using a variety of protocols

Table 3.1 Summary of data extracted from experimental studies, including study information, contaminant information, decontaminant information, and outcomes

Study information		Contaminant information			Decontaminant information			Outcomes	
Author (year)	Sample size (per protocol)	Human in vitro model details	Contaminant (classification)	Method of contamination	Amount applied	Skin contact time (min)	Decon solution	Decon method	Analysis of decontamination	Decon quantification	Corresponding outcome (CD, PD, none)
Thors et al. (2017) [14]	6[a]	Abdomen skin samples from surgery	VX (CWA), neat and diluted to 20%	Dose applied to skin surface	25 µL in control (25.2 mg for neat and 5.04 mg for diluted) and 10 µL in test (10.08 for neat and 2.016 mg for diluted)	5, 30	Water	Wash with water followed by vacuum suctioning 10×	Gas chromatography-flame photometric detector	Decontamination factor[b] in receiver fluid ranged from 10 to 56 (20% VX) and 1–2 (neat VX) depending on time to decon[c]	PD: 100% (n = 24/24)[a]
Zhu et al. (2016) [15]	5	Abdomen skin samples from cadaver	Paraoxon (CWA simulant)	Dose applied to skin surface	5 µL (0.00025 mCi; mg amount NR)	30	2% hand soap	Wash with soap-soaked cotton ball and then 2× with water-soaked cotton ball	Liquid scintillation counter	Percent of applied dose recovered in wash was 82.4%	PD: 100% (n = 5/5) but more paraoxon reached receptor fluid
Thors et al. (2020) [16]	6	Abdomen skin samples from surgery	VX (CWA)	Dose applied to skin surface	10 µL (10.08 mg)	5	2% soapy water	50 µL soapy water washing followed by vacuum suctioning 10×	Gas chromatography-flame photometric detector	Percent of applied dose penetrating to receiver was 0.63% for control vs. 1.4% for decontaminated	PD: 100% (n = 6/6) but more VX reached receptor fluid

Moody et al. (2007) [17]	5[d]	Breast skin samples, one leg skin sample, from surgery	Methyl salicylate, parathion, malathion (all CWA simulants)	Dose applied to skin surface	2, 20, 200 mM (0.0061, 0.061, 0.61 mg for MES; 0.012, 0.12, 1.22 mg for PT; and 0.014, 0.14, 1.41 mg for MT)	30	Soap wash	200 μL soap wash placed on skin surface and removed with swab rotated three times on skin surface	Liquid scintillation counter	Percent of applied dose recovered in wash ranged from 31.1% to 62.2% for MES, 45.1–77.4% for PT, and 60.2–85.8% for MT	PD: 100% (n = 45/45)[d]
Nielsen (2010) [18]	12 (de-con) 14 (control)	Breast/abdomen skin samples from surgery	Malathion (CWA simulant)	Dose applied to skin surface	0.212 mg	180	Soap and water	Wash with soap and cotton swab, and then rinse twice with isotonic water. Wiped with cotton swabs	Liquid scintillation counter	Percent of applied dose recovered in wash was 78.5%	PD: 100% (n = 12/12)
Loke et al. (1999) [19]	3[e]	Cadaver skin samples, undisclosed region	Diethylmalonate (CWA simulant)	Dose applied to skin surface	4 μL (4.2 mg)	15, 30, 60	2% cationic, anionic, or nonionic surfactant, deionized water	Washed with 0.5 L solution over 1 min	Gas chromatography-flame ionization detection	Exact values recovered in wash NR	PD: 100% (n = 36/36)[e] but washing enhanced all penetration rates

(continued)

Table 3.1 (continued)

Study information		Contaminant information	Dose applied to skin surface		Decontaminant information			Outcomes
Forsberg et al. (2020) [21]	6[f]	Abdomen skin samples from surgery	Methyl salicylate and ethyl lactate (CWA simulants)	10 μL (11.74 mg methyl salicylate, 10.34 mg ethyl lactate)	5, 15, 45, 120	2% soapy water, 100% water	Wash with and instantly vacuum suction 50 μL for 10 times	Gas chromatography-flame ionization detection	Decontamination factor[b] for receiver fluid ranged from 2 to 23 depending on time to decontamination[c]	PD: 100% (n = 96/96)[f] but washing transiently enhanced MES penetration rates

CWA chemical warfare agent, *CD* complete decontamination, *PD* partial decontamination, *NR* not reported

[a]Protocols (sample size): neat or 20% VX with decontamination at 5 min or 30 min post-exposure (6 samples/protocol × 2 concentrations × 2 time points = 24)

[b]Decontamination factor is the ratio of contaminant concentration penetrating through without decontamination to contaminant concentration penetrating through with decontamination

[c]In studies reporting various decontamination factor values, all variables were held constant except for time to decontamination. Earlier decontamination yielded higher decontamination factor values, which is consistent with a better outcome due to reduced contaminant penetration

[d]Protocols (sample size): methyl salicylate, parathion, or malathion dosed at either 2, 20, or 200 mM (5 samples/protocol × 3 contaminants × 3 doses = 45)

[e]Protocols (sample size): decontamination performed with 2% cationic, anionic, or nonionic surfactant and deionized water at 15, 30, or 60 min post-exposure (3 samples/protocol × 4 decon solutions × 3 time points = 36)

[f]Protocols (sample size): methyl salicylate or ethyl lactate decontaminated with 2% soapy water or 100% water at 5, 15, 45, or 120 min post-exposure (6 samples/protocol × 2 contaminants × 2 decon solutions × 4 time points = 96)

(100%, $n = 81/81$). Soap and water decontamination, evaluated in 85.7% ($n = 6/7$) of studies, also led to partial decontamination in all (100%, $n = 143/143$) skin samples. Given these findings, a more efficacious method of decontamination is needed, as residual contaminants left behind have potential to be absorbed. Contemporary human volunteer studies recommend pairing water or soapy water decontamination (wet decontamination) with dry decontamination, which will be discussed later, to achieve best outcomes [7, 22]. This review's findings support those recommendations by highlighting the insufficiency of water or soapy water decontamination alone.

Decontamination outcomes were grouped into three categories of efficacy according to the semiquantitative scale introduced in the "Methods" section. This grouping method was chosen to highlight the completeness of using either water or soap and water as sole decontamination solutions for a variety of contaminants. Alternative methods of grouping decontamination efficacy are certainly acceptable, for example, utilizing <1% as no response, 1–33.33% as a poor response, 33.34–66.66% as a moderate response, 66.67–99.5% as a good response, and 99.5+% as complete response, since not all contaminants are potent enough to require complete decontamination for favorable clinical outcomes. However, a scale with narrower categories as presented in the example is better used in scenarios where the evaluated contaminants share similar potencies, which was not the case for this review, since removing 33.33% of high-potency VX may be considered a poor response, but the same removal quantity of low-potency malathion may be clinically sufficient.

Varying efficacy rates for decontamination can be partly explained by physicochemical properties of each contaminant, such as hydrophobicity, molecular size, and volatility, which all affect skin penetration rates [23]. Higher penetration enables contaminants to partition into the stratum corneum, where they are no longer amenable to being washed off. Thus, chemical properties favoring penetration will hamper decontamination efficacy. Patel et al. [24] analyzed data for 158 chemicals penetrating through excised human skin in vitro and found that the key determinants of penetration are hydrophobicity and low molecular size. A parabolic relationship is seen between skin penetration and hydrophobicity [25], expressed as the logarithm of its octanol/water partition coefficient (log $P_{o/w}$), in which the two increase proportionally up to a peak, after which highly lipophilic chemicals (log $P_{o/w} > 3.87$) face decreasing penetration [26]. Higher volatility reduces absorption rates due to the chemical's oppositional desires to evaporate from or penetrate into the skin [27, 28].

Forsberg et al. [21] found acrylonitrile to have the highest penetration rate and tributylamine the lowest out of five chemicals, attributing this to acrylonitrile having the lowest molecular weight, measuring 53.06 g/mol, and tributylamine the highest, measuring 185.36 g/mol. Secondly, Moody et al. [17] compared parathion, methyl salicylate, and malathion penetration at three doses, 2, 20, and 200 mM. Malathion always penetrated the least, which might be explained by its greatest molecular weight. Interestingly, despite methyl salicylate having the lowest molecular weight, parathion penetrated in greatest amounts more frequently. This is likely explained by the higher lipophilicity of parathion compared to methyl salicylate, whose log $P_{o/w}$ values are 3.83 and 2.55, respectively. Additionally, methyl salicylate is more volatile and has a slightly over 10^6-fold higher vapor pressure of 1 mmHg versus 6.68×10^{-6}. Whenever cumulatively penetrated amounts were higher, decontamination efficacy was lower. Other factors known to govern penetration rates include dose of contaminant, size of contaminated surface area, anatomical region, occlusion, single-dose versus repeated-dose contamination, and healthy versus impaired skin barrier [29].

Skin contact time is yet another governing factor for decontamination efficacy. Four studies evaluated decontamination efficacies at different time points. All four noted that a shorter time to decontamination significantly improved decontamination efficacy [14, 17, 19, 21]. This can be explained by Wester and Maibach's [29] observation that decreased contact time reduces skin absorption. Less absorption also results in higher surface concentrations available for decontamination.

While none of the in vitro studies directly compared a water or soapy water decontamination protocol with a washing aid versus that of one without, Amlot et al. [8] demonstrated in vivo on human volunteers that using a washcloth in addition to a 3-min shower significantly increased decontamination efficacy by 20% when compared to those who had only showered for the same duration. Conversely, Thors et al. [14] found that Reactive Skin Decontamination Lotion® (RSDL®)-impregnated sponges used to scrub VX-contaminated skin samples for 2 min performed worse than if RSDL® was allowed to sit on the skin for 30 min. However, RSDL® contains VX-degrading components, and increased efficacy was concluded to be due to the increased skin contact time with RSDL® when it was allowed to sit. Additionally, a subsequent experiment by Thors et al. [16] showed that scrubbing twice with an RSDL®-infused sponge for 2 min each yielded greater decontamination efficacy than scrubbing once. It is thus likely that the use of washing aids such as the cotton balls or swabs used by Moody et al. [17], Nielsen [18], and Zhu et al. [15] to mechanically wipe or swab skin samples also affected decontamination outcomes.

In addition to incomplete removal of contaminants, water-only or water and soap decontamination may be limited by the "wash-in" effect, which paradoxically enhances cumulative amounts of contaminant penetrating through the skin. In vivo, Maibach and Feldmann [9] showed malathion applied to volunteers' forearms and decontaminated at 2 and 4 h yielded greater percutaneous absorption than non-decontaminated controls over a 24-h experimental period, as did parathion decontaminated at 8 h post-exposure. In vitro, "washing in" was readily observed in two studies referenced [15, 16], with another two demonstrating transiently enhanced penetration rates, but no overall increase in cumulative amounts penetrated [19, 21]. The "wash-in" effect is thought to occur for several reasons, chief of which is that hydration of the stratum corneum mobilizes skin depot residues [10]. Additionally, when surfactant systems are incorporated, as in the case of soapy water, they tend to impart a surfactant effect which promotes percutaneous penetration [10, 30], perhaps by damaging the stratum corneum and disrupting its barrier function [31]. Moody [10] also reports a friction effect, acid/base effect, and artifact effect as potential contributors to the "wash-in" phenomenon. Overall, the "wash-in" effect of water or soap and water decontamination may be a significant limitation that deserves considerable attention, as a circulatory "burst" in pesticide or CWA concentrations could result in devastating clinical consequences. More in vivo studies monitoring excreted and/or serum contaminant, metabolite, or radiolabel concentrations following decontamination are needed to confirm or refute this phenomenon, since in vivo decontamination more frequently resulted in reduced organophosphate pesticide absorption in Maibach and Feldmann's data.

Considering the potential for the "wash-in" effect of wet decontamination, both the USA's Primary Response Incident Scene Management (PRISM) and the UK's Initial Operational Response (IOR) guidelines recommend dry decontamination be performed as the default response to non-corrosive liquid chemical incidents while waiting for emergency services to arrive [32]. This recommendation comes from ex vivo and in vivo studies that have demonstrated blotting and rubbing with absorbent materials such as wound dressings, incontinence pads, and tissue paper (or "blue roll") effectively decontaminates methyl salicylate from the skin [33, 34]. Other potential benefits of dry over wet decontamination include the prevention of transferring contaminant from clothing to the skin and generating large volumes of contaminated effluent [35]. It should be emphasized that dry decontamination, along with immediate disrobing, is simply the first step to a comprehensive decontamination protocol that is followed up with, upon arrival of rescue personnel, gross decontamination by water rinsing using a ladder pipe system, active drying with a towel, and, finally, technical decontamination, involving disrobing and thorough body surface cleansing under the optimal parameters of a 90-s shower duration, with 0.5% (v/v) detergent, at a water temperature of 35 °C, and with a cotton washcloth, followed by re-robing for optimal outcomes [36].

Conversely, water and soap and water have the advantage of being easily accessible resources when compared to specialized decontamination kits. This allows for an earlier time to decontamination, which has been highly established as a key factor for decontamination success. Accessibility is of relevance given its potential mass need. This is contrasted with decontaminating agents such as RSDL®, which has been shown to be effective but lacking in availability and affordability. Additionally, RSDL® decontamination applied directly to open wounds delays wound healing in in vivo pig models [37]. Water-only or water and soap solutions in contact with wounds have not been shown to delay wound healing in a Cochrane review [38]. This is of relevance considering the high likelihood of obtaining cutaneous wounds in the event of chemical warfare.

It is worth exploring the clinical relevance of residual contaminant concentrations observed in the experimental studies. VX was chosen because of its potency [39], with an estimated median lethal dose (LD_{50}) of 10 mg for a 70 kg man when contacting bare skin in liquid form [40]. When Thors et al. [16] applied 10 mg VX to 1.13 cm^2 human skin samples in vitro, they found on average that the total amount of VX penetrating through to the receptor fluid was 56 $\mu g/cm^2$ over a 5-h period, or a total absorbed dose of 63.28 μg. It is possible that this 63.28 μg could be extrapolated to represent the LD_{50} of *absorbed* VX, but it is impossible to make any definitive conclusion. Kimura et al. [41] reported that a VX dose of 0.04 $\mu g/kg$ injected intravenously (IV) over 30 s resulted in headaches 45 min afterward, but no other symptoms. Injecting 0.225 µg/kg over 30 s, they noted increased respiratory minute volume, mild pupillary dilation, red blood cell cholinesterase dropping to 63% of baseline levels, complaints of heat, and headaches of self-limited nature in the subject. Out of four subjects infused 1 µg/kg over 4 h and two subjects infused over 1.75 and 2.5 h, only one experienced headache, while the others were asymptomatic. 2.12 µg/kg administered over 5.5 h appeared to be the maximum tolerable intravenous dose without necessitating atropine, oxime, or resuscitation. When Thors et al. [16] decontaminated the skin with soapy water, 122.4 µg/cm^2 penetrated to the receptor fluid. When Thors et al. [14] decontaminated the skin 5 min or 30 min post-exposure to VX, receptor fluid amounts measured 140 µg/cm^2 and 278 µg/cm^2, respectively. All of these "absorbed" contaminant concentrations greatly surpassed the 0.225 µg/kg limit necessary to induce symptoms in a 70 kg man, measuring 1.75, 2, and 3.97 µg/kg, and likely represent dangerous doses that were reached despite/because of water or soapy water decontamination. This implies that water or soapy water decontamination of VX could still yield dangerous outcomes that would require additional medical treatment to manage. However, it is likely that soapy water decontamination would result in lower amounts of VX being absorbed over a longer period, thus improving patient recovery long term. Moreover, an in vivo study demonstrated that soapy water decontamination of swine dosed with five times the LD$_{50}$ of VX 30 min post-exposure protected against mortality and signs of poisoning, whereas most non-decontaminated controls died [42]. Thus, while an initial, short-term spike in blood concentrations might occur with soapy water decontamination, this study demonstrated benefits of survival and reduced toxicity, favoring decontamination.

A major limitation to this review is that in vitro data is unable to fully replicate and account for the physiological processes that occur in in vivo settings [43], such as active metabolism and circulatory perfusion, making it challenging to extrapolate these findings. Very few in vivo data assessing percutaneous absorption and decontamination of topically applied CWAs or their simulants exist, but a comparison will be made between in vitro data presented here and existing in vivo data.

First, Maibach and Feldmann [9] documented the in vivo absorption rates of topically applied and decontaminated [^{14}C]-labeled malathion and parathion in human volunteers by comparing urine excretion of carbon-14 label from a topical dose to that from a parenteral dose. When 4 µg/cm^2, 40 µg/cm^2, and 400 µg/cm^2 malathion were applied to the forearm and subsequently decontaminated using hot soapy water at 15 min post-exposure, 4.3%, 4.7%, and 1.4% of the respectively applied dose were absorbed over a 24-h period. Moody et al. [17] found 11.6%, 3%, and 0.7% of topically applied malathion at respective concentrations of 37, 370, and 3700 µg/cm^2 reached the receptor fluid over 6.5 h in breast/leg skin samples decontaminated after 30 min of exposure. Only the 11.6% absorption rate is far off from the in vivo values observed by Maibach and Feldmann, while the others are relatively close. However, in vitro findings made by Nielsen [18] applying 100 µg/cm^2 of malathion to breast and abdomen skin samples before decontaminating with soap and water at 180 min post-exposure yielded an even greater discrepancy with an

18.3% absorption rate over 42 h, perhaps due to the longer exposure and experimental times.

For parathion, in vivo and in vitro absorption rates were quite similar. When $4 \mu g/cm^2$, $40 \mu g/cm^2$, and $400 \mu g/cm^2$ concentrations were applied by Maibach and Feldmann [9] on the forearm and decontaminated with soapy water 15 min afterward, 6.7%, 3.1%, and 2.2% of the topically applied doses were respectively absorbed over 24 h. Moody et al. [17] found 7.1%, 1.9%, and 0.7% of topically applied parathion reached the receptor fluid respective to an initial dose of 32, 320, and 3200 $\mu g/cm^2$. It should be noted that various parameters between the above referenced experiments examining malathion and parathion were different, including initial dose, exposure times, experimental times, and anatomical region evaluated, which may limit comparability.

One study making a direct in vivo and in vitro comparison of percutaneous arsenic absorption and decontamination between rhesus monkeys and human skin samples under otherwise identical conditions showed similarities and discrepancies as well [44]. In vivo percutaneous absorption of low-dose arsenic by rhesus monkeys, applied as water or soil mixtures, measured 6.4% and 4.5%, respectively, while in vitro amounts reaching receptor fluid through human skin samples mounted in diffusion cells were 0.93% and 0.43% for water and soil, or 1.91% and 0.76% if arsenic content within the skin was also counted. Either method of quantification is quite different from in vivo values. Soap and water decontamination of low-dose water and soil mixtures in rhesus monkeys recovered 76.3% and 68.8% of arsenic in the wash, respectively, while 69.8% and 99.2% were recovered in human skin samples. Although soil mixture recoveries were highly variable, water mixture recoveries were quite similar between the two models. Existing literatures that compare in vivo versus in vitro percutaneous absorption and decontamination efficacy thus demonstrate conflicting data, in which some scenarios yield outcomes that are relatively close to the other, while others vary widely. Whenever possible, in vitro findings should therefore be validated via comparison with in vivo experiments.

Other limitations of this systematic review include small sample sizes that limit the reliability of this data. Additionally, the heterogeneity of data between each experimental study, including contaminants, anatomical region evaluated, concentrations, exposure time, method of application and decontamination, and analysis of endpoints, limits interstudy comparisons to understand when water and soap and water are best used.

Despite being widely recommended as decontaminating solutions, in vitro human experiments summarized here demonstrate that both water-only and water and soap always led to partial decontamination for various CWA/CWA simulants. There is thus a need for the development of a more efficacious decontaminating agent. There is also potential for these solutions to incite a "wash-in" effect in vitro, resulting in a sudden rise in penetration rates and systemic uptake of contaminants. In the case of CWAs, this would hasten lethality without additional medical intervention given their potencies at low doses. However, in vitro findings do not always reliably translate to an in vivo context, and more in vivo studies are needed to validate in vitro decontamination outcomes, including efficacy rates and the "wash-in" effect. Additionally, gaps in understanding when to use water or soapy water or what the ideal decontaminants are for various CWAs persist. This requires great insight into the physicochemical properties of contaminants to model their percutaneous behaviors as well as how they interact with decontaminants, and more studies are needed to fill this gap. Future studies attempting to understand when water or soapy water, or any other decontaminating agent, is best used should utilize a harmonized efficacy protocol, largely standardized by factoring in contaminant properties and concentration, application method, skin sample characteristics and anatomical region, contaminated surface area, exposure time, decontaminant used, method of decontamination, and analysis. Slight variations can be made in the setup to study the effect of a specific parameter, as needed. Such a harmonized efficacy protocol would enhance inter-experimental comparison between international labs, thereby hastening our understanding of which decontaminants are best suited for which contaminants. Additional details on decontamination science are found in *Skin Decontamination: A Comprehensive Research Guide* [45].

References

1. Blickenstaff NR, Coman G, Blattner CM, Andersen R, Maibach HI. Biology of percutaneous penetration. Rev Environ Health. 2014;29(3):145–55. https://doi.org/10.1515/reveh-2014-0052.
2. Greathouse B, Zahra F, Brady MF. Acetylcholinesterase inhibitors toxicity. In: StatPearls. Treasure Island, FL: StatPearls Publishing LLC.; 2021.
3. Houston M, Hendrickson RG. Decontamination. Crit Care Clin. 2005;21(4):653–72, v. https://doi.org/10.1016/j.ccc.2005.06.001.
4. Bromberg BE, Song IC, Walden RH. Hydrotherapy of chemical burns. Plast Reconstr Surg. 1965;35:85–95. https://doi.org/10.1097/00006534-196501000-00010.
5. Southworth F, James T, Davidson L, Williams N, Finnie T, Marczylo T, Collins S, Amlôt R. A controlled cross-over study to evaluate the efficacy of improvised dry and wet emergency decontamination protocols for chemical incidents. PLoS One. 2020;15(11):e0239845. https://doi.org/10.1371/journal.pone.0239845.
6. Chilcott RP, Mitchell H, Matar H. Optimization of nonambulant mass casualty decontamination protocols as part of an initial or specialist operational response to chemical incidents. Prehosp Emerg Care. 2019c;23(1):32–43. https://doi.org/10.1080/10903127.2018.1469705.
7. Larner J, Durrant A, Hughes P, Mahalingam D, Rivers S, Matar H, Thomas E, Barrett M, Pinhal A, Amer N, Hall C, Jackson T, Catalani V, Chilcott RP. Efficacy of different hair and skin decontamination strategies with identification of associated hazards to first responders. Prehosp Emerg Care. 2020;24(3):355–68. https://doi.org/10.1080/10903127.2019.1636912.
8. Amlot R, Larner J, Matar H, Jones DR, Carter H, Turner EA, Price SC, Chilcott RP. Comparative analysis of showering protocols for mass-casualty decontamination. Prehosp Disast Med. 2010;25(5):435–9. https://doi.org/10.1017/s1049023x00008529.
9. Maibach H, Feldmann R. Systemic absorption of pesticides through the skin of man. Occupational Exposure to Pesticides. In: Report to the Federal Working Group on Pest Management from the Task Group on Occupational exposure to pesticides. Washington, DC: Federal Working Group on Pest Management; 1974. p. 120–7.
10. Moody RP, Maibach HI. Skin decontamination: importance of the wash-in effect. Food Chem Toxicol. 2006;44(11):1783–8. https://doi.org/10.1016/j.fct.2006.05.020.

11. Kashetsky N, Law RM, Maibach HI. Efficacy of water skin decontamination in vivo in humans: a systematic review. J Appl Toxicol. 2021;42:346. https://doi.org/10.1002/jat.4230.

12. Burli A, Kashetsky N, Feschuk A, Law RM, Maibach HI. Efficacy of soap and water based skin decontamination using in vivo animal models: a systematic review. J Toxicol Environ Health B Crit Rev. 2021;24:325–36. https://doi.org/10.1080/10937404.2021.1943087.

13. Moher D, Liberati A, Tetzlaff J, Altman DG. Preferred reporting items for systematic reviews and meta-analyses: the PRISMA statement. BMJ. 2009;339:b2535. https://doi.org/10.1136/bmj.b2535.

14. Thors L, Koch M, Wigenstam E, Koch B, Hägglund L, Bucht A. Comparison of skin decontamination efficacy of commercial decontamination products following exposure to VX on human skin. Chem Biol Interact. 2017;273:82–9. https://doi.org/10.1016/j.cbi.2017.06.002.

15. Zhu H, Jung EC, Phuong C, Hui X, Maibach H. Effects of soap-water wash on human epidermal penetration. J Appl Toxicol. 2016;36(8):997–1002. https://doi.org/10.1002/jat.3258.

16. Thors L, Wigenstam E, Qvarnström J, Hägglund L, Bucht A. Improved skin decontamination efficacy for the nerve agent VX. Chem Biol Interact. 2020;325:109135. https://doi.org/10.1016/j.cbi.2020.109135.

17. Moody RP, Akram M, Dickson E, Chu I. In vitro dermal absorption of methyl salicylate, ethyl parathion, and malathion: first responder safety. J Toxicol Environ Health A. 2007;70(12):985–99. https://doi.org/10.1080/15287390600870874.

18. Nielsen JB. Efficacy of skin wash on dermal absorption: an in vitro study on four model compounds of varying solubility. Int Arch Occup Environ Health. 2010;83(6):683–90. https://doi.org/10.1007/s00420-010-0546-y.

19. Loke WK, U SH, Lau SK, Lim JS, Tay GS, Koh CH. Wet decontamination-induced stratum corneum hydration--effects on the skin barrier function to diethylmalonate. J Appl Toxicol. 1999;19(4):285–90. https://doi.org/10.1002/(sici)1099-1263(199907/08)19:4<285::aid-jat580>3.0.co;2-x.

20. Wilhelm KP, Cua AB, Wolff HH, Maibach HI. Surfactant-induced stratum corneum hydration in vivo: prediction of the irritation potential of anionic surfactants. J Investig Dermatol. 1993;101(3):310–5. https://doi.org/10.1111/1523-1747.ep12365467.

21. Forsberg E, Öberg L, Artursson E, Wigenstam E, Bucht A, Thors L. Decontamination efficacy of soapy water and water washing following exposure of toxic chemicals on human skin. Cutan Ocul Toxicol. 2020;39(2):134–42. https://doi.org/10.1080/15569527.2020.1748046.

22. Chilcott RP, Larner J, Durrant A, Hughes P, Mahalingam D, Rivers S, Thomas E, Amer N, Barrett M, Matar H, Pinhal A, Jackson T, McCarthy-Barnett K, Reppucci J. Evaluation of US Federal Guidelines (Primary Response Incident Scene Management [PRISM]) for mass decontamination of casualties during the initial operational response to a chemical incident. Ann Emerg Med. 2019a;73(6):671–84. https://doi.org/10.1016/j.annemergmed.2018.06.042.

23. Law RM, Ngo MA, Maibach HI. Twenty clinically pertinent factors/observations for percutaneous absorption in humans. Am J Clin Dermatol. 2020;21(1):85–95. https://doi.org/10.1007/s40257-019-00480-4.

24. Patel H, Berge WT, Cronin MTD. Quantitative structure–activity relationships (QSARs) for the prediction of skin permeation of exogenous chemicals. Chemosphere. 2002;48(6):603–13. https://doi.org/10.1016/S0045-6535(02)00114-5.

25. Grice JE, Moghimi HR, Ryan E, Zhang Q, Haridass I, Mohammed Y, Roberts MS. Non-formulation parameters that affect penetrant-skin-vehicle interactions and percutaneous absorption. In: Percutaneous penetration enhancers drug penetration into/through the skin. Berlin: Springer; 2017. p. 45–75.

26. Ngo MA, O'Malley M, Maibach HI. Percutaneous absorption and exposure assessment of pesticides. J Appl Toxicol. 2010;30(2):91–114. https://doi.org/10.1002/jat.1505.

27. Bronaugh RL, Stewart RF, Wester RC, Bucks D, Mailbach HI, Anderson J. Comparison of percutaneous absorption of fragrances by humans and monkeys. Food Chem Toxicol. 1985;23(1):111–4. https://doi.org/10.1016/0278-6915(85)90228-5.

28. Bronaugh RL, Wester RC, Bucks D, Maibach HI, Sarason R. In vivo percutaneous absorption of fragrance ingredients in rhesus monkeys and humans. Food Chem Toxicol. 1990;28(5):369–73. https://doi.org/10.1016/0278-6915(90)90111-y.
29. Wester RC, Maibach HI. In vivo percutaneous absorption and decontamination of pesticides in humans. J Toxicol Environ Health. 1985;16(1):25–37. https://doi.org/10.1080/15287398509530716.
30. Bettley FR, Donoghue E. Effect of soap on the diffusion of water through isolated human epidermis. Nature. 1960;185:17–20. https://doi.org/10.1038/185017a0.
31. Ashton P, Hadgraft J, Walters KA. Effects of surfactants in percutaneous absorption. Pharm Acta Helv. 1986;61(8):228–35.
32. Collins S, James T, Carter H, Symons C, Southworth F, Foxall K, Marczylo T, Amlôt R. Mass casualty decontamination for chemical incidents: research outcomes and future priorities. Int J Environ Res Public Health. 2021;18(6):3079. https://doi.org/10.3390/ijerph18063079.
33. Amlôt R, Carter H, Riddle L, Larner J, Chilcott RP. Volunteer trials of a novel improvised dry decontamination protocol for use during mass casualty incidents as part of the UK'S Initial Operational Response (IOR). PLoS One. 2017;12(6):e0179309. https://doi.org/10.1371/journal.pone.0179309.
34. Kassouf N, Syed S, Larner J, Amlôt R, Chilcott RP. Evaluation of absorbent materials for use as ad hoc dry decontaminants during mass casualty incidents as part of the UK's Initial Operational Response (IOR). PLoS One. 2017;12(2):e0170966. https://doi.org/10.1371/journal.pone.0170966.
35. Chilcott RP, Larner J, Matar H. UK's initial operational response and specialist operational response to CBRN and HazMat incidents: a primer on decontamination protocols for healthcare professionals. Emerg Med J. 2019b;36(2):117–23. https://doi.org/10.1136/emermed-2018-207562.
36. Chilcott RP, Amlôt R. Primary Response Incident Scene Management (PRISM) guidance for chemical incidents. 2015. https://www.medicalcountermeasures.gov/media/36872/prism-volume-1.pdf.
37. Connolly JM, Stevenson RS, Railer RF, Clark OE, Whitten KA, Lee-Stubbs RB, Anderson DR. Impairment of wound healing by reactive skin decontamination lotion (RSDL®) in a Göttingen minipig® model. Cutan Ocul Toxicol. 2020;39(2):143–57. https://doi.org/10.1080/15569527.2020.1751183.
38. Fernandez R, Griffiths R. Water for wound cleansing. Cochrane Database Syst Rev. 2008;(1):CD003861. https://doi.org/10.1002/14651858.CD003861.pub2.
39. CDC. Facts about VX. 2018. https://emergency.cdc.gov/agent/vx/basics/facts.asp.
40. National Research Council US Committee on Toxicology. Review of acute human-toxicity estimates for VX. Review of acute human-toxicity estimates for selected chemical-warfare agents. Washington, DC: National Academies Press; 1997. https://www.ncbi.nlm.nih.gov/books/NBK233724/.
41. Kimura KK, McNamara BP, Sim VM. Intravenous administration of VX in man. 1960. https://apps.dtic.mil/sti/pdfs/AD1028432.pdf.
42. Bjarnason S, Mikler J, Hill I, Tenn C, Garrett M, Caddy N, Sawyer TW. Comparison of selected skin decontaminant products and regimens against VX in domestic swine. Hum Exp Toxicol. 2008;27(3):253–61. https://doi.org/10.1177/0960327108090269.
43. Blaauboer BJ. Biokinetic modeling and in vitro-in vivo extrapolations. J Toxicol Environ Health B Crit Rev. 2010;13(2-4):242–52. https://doi.org/10.1080/10937404.2010.483940.
44. Wester RC, Maibach HI, Sedik L, Melendres J, Wade M. In vivo and in vitro percutaneous absorption and skin decontamination of arsenic from water and soil. Fundam Appl Toxicol. 1993;20(3):336–40. https://doi.org/10.1006/faat.1993.1043.
45. Zhu H, Maibach HI. Skin decontamination: a comprehensive clinical research guide. Berlin: Springer; 2020.

Chapter 4
In Vitro Human Skin Decontamination with Water: Occupational Contaminants

Chavy Chiang, Nadia Kashetsky, Aileen M. Feschuk, Anuk Burli, Rebecca M. Law, and Howard I. Maibach

Introduction

Dermal decontamination is the process of removing harmful substances from the external surfaces of the body [1]. Skin exposure to contaminants might occur in various settings, including military or occupational settings, after which chemicals are capable of diffusing through the stratum corneum to the dermal layers, where these substances can then access the circulatory system [2]. Skin decontamination is a primary intervention that mitigates chemical absorption through the skin and minimizes its potentially toxic sequelae [3]. Although the incidence of occupational illnesses secondary to percutaneous absorption is unknown, Leigh et al. [4] suggested that even if a small fraction of the annual 2.8 million nonfatal occupational injuries occurring in 2019 in the United States [5] were attributed to skin exposure, this would still amount to a significant number of cases. This warrants further investigation into the decontamination of occupational contaminants.

C. Chiang (✉) · A. Burli
School of Medicine and Dentistry, University of Rochester, Rochester, NY, USA
e-mail: chavy_chiang@urmc.rochester.edu

N. Kashetsky
Faculty of Medicine, Memorial University, St. John's, NL, Canada

A. M. Feschuk
Faculty of Medicine, Memorial University of Newfoundland, St. John's, NL, Canada

R. M. Law
School of Pharmacy, Memorial University of Newfoundland, St. John's, NL, Canada

H. I. Maibach
Department of Dermatology, University of California San Francisco, San Francisco, CA, USA

© The Author(s), under exclusive license to Springer Nature Switzerland AG 2022
A. M. Feschuk et al. (eds.), *Dermal Absorption and Decontamination*,
https://doi.org/10.1007/978-3-031-09222-0_4

Flushing with water or soapy water is considered the cornerstone of decontamination due to availability [3, 6, 7] and is recommended by the Canadian Centre for Occupational Health and Safety [8] and the National Institute for Occupational Safety and Health's [9] Pocket Guide to Chemical Hazards in response to skin exposure to a chemical. Whereas neutralization may seem logical, it is not recommended due to (1) lack of clear benefit over water irrigation, (2) potential for delayed decontamination when searching for contaminant-appropriate neutralizing agents, and (3) possible thermal burns arising from exothermic acid-base reactions [8]. Further, although some studies demonstrate that flushing with other agents may offer better contaminant-specific outcomes than water or soapy water, such as the case of using corn oil or propylene glycol instead to remove lipophilic methylene bisphenyl isocyanate [10], sufficient data is lacking to recommend these alternative agents on a larger scale, thus maintaining water or soapy water flushes as the current gold standard. Water flushing dilutes the contaminant, rinses it off, decreases chemical reaction rates, reduces tissue metabolism and consequent inflammation, minimizes the chemical's hygroscopic effects on surrounding tissue, and restores skin's pH [11]. Surfactant-containing soaps may be added to improve the solubility of lipophilic compounds.

In the United States, the Occupational Safety and Health Administration (OSHA) mandates the provision of "suitable facilities" for flushing the eyes and body wherever injurious corrosive materials are handled under standard 29 CFR 1910.151(c). This has led to the installation of emergency showers and eyewash stations throughout the nation in workplaces that handle hazardous materials. Little direction is provided for installation and performance requirements of these safety showers, and OSHA has rather referred employers to follow the American National Standard for Emergency Eyewash and Shower Equipment (ANSI Z358.1), put forth by the American National Standards Institute. Approved in January 2015, the latest edition, ANSI/ISEA Z358.1-2014, requires emergency showers to deliver, at a temperature of 16–38 °C, 20 gallons of flushing fluid per min for a minimum of 15 min, a flushing fluid column of 208.3 cm in height, and a spray pattern diameter of 50.8 cm, among other maintenance, testing, and performance requirements, where flushing fluid is defined as potable water, preserved water, preserved buffered saline solution, or other medically acceptable solution manufactured and labeled in accordance with applicable government regulations [12]. Eyewash equipment contains a separate set of requirements. While ANSI Z358.1 is commonly referred to by OSHA, it is not adopted as law. Nonetheless, knowledge of ANSI Z358.1 provides an understanding of the minimum capabilities of most, if not all, flushing fluid systems designed to address occupational skin exposure to chemicals.

Although water flushing is a widely recommended first aid practice, multiple in vitro percutaneous studies of pesticides demonstrated cleansing with soapy water to induce a "wash-in" effect, in which decontamination itself enhances percutaneous penetration and/or systemic absorption [13]. In addition, a prior systematic review evaluating the efficacy of water-only or soap and water decontamination in in vivo human volunteers as well as in vivo animal models concluded that both solutions achieved incomplete decontamination in most cases and therefore recommended the development of a more effective decontaminating solution priority [6, 14]. This systematic review summarizes available efficacy data on water-only or water and soap decontamination of occupational contaminants, including industrial chemicals, pesticides, and pharmaceutical drugs, in in vitro human models.

Materials and Methods

The Preferred Reporting Items for Systematic Reviews and Meta-Analysis (PRISMA) guidelines were followed [15].

Search Strategy

Embase, MEDLINE, PubMed, Web of Science, and Google Scholar databases were searched on February 8, 2021, using the terms "skin" or "cutaneous" or "dermal" or "percutaneous" and "decontaminant" or "decontamination" or "skin decontamination." No time, geographical, or language restrictions were applied.

Eligibility

Articles were included if they were (1) experimental studies, (2) reporting chemical decontamination of the skin with water-only and/or soap and water solutions, (3) evaluating decontamination of occupational contaminants, (4) using in vitro human skin models, and (5) written in English. A prior systematic review of studies evaluating the decontamination of chemical warfare agents and their simulants using water-only or soap and water solutions was conducted separately and was therefore excluded [16].

Data Screening

Title/abstract screening was completed by two independent researchers (R.L., H.M.) with conflicts resolved by discussion with a third (N.K.). Full-text review was completed independently by two researchers (C.C., N.K.), and conflicts were resolved by a fifth (H.M.). Article references were manually searched to identify any additional, relevant studies.

Data Extraction and Analysis

Four independent researchers completed data extraction (N.K., A.F., A.B., C.C.), which was then verified by two independent researchers (H.M., R.L.). Data were extracted on study characteristics, human skin model details, contaminants, and decontamination agents, methods, analyses, and outcomes. Due to data heterogeneity between the included investigations, a descriptive analysis was conducted rather than a meta-analysis. Studies were categorized into (1) water-only decontamination, (2) soap and water decontamination, or (3) both water-only and soap and water decontamination groups. Decontamination outcomes were sorted into three categories, (1) no response, (2) partial decontamination, and (3) complete decontamination, where "no response" was defined as a decontamination efficacy of <1%, "partial decontamination" as 1–99.4%, and "complete decontamination" as 99.5% or greater. This grouping method was selected to highlight the completeness of water or soapy water as sole decontaminating agents for a variety of chemicals.

Results

Study Characteristics

After title/abstract screening of 3310 studies and full-text review of 61 studies, we identified 15 studies that fit our inclusion criteria (Fig. 4.1). These investigations collectively evaluated 21 occupational contaminants, further classified as 13 industrial chemicals, five drugs, and three pesticides. In vitro human skin samples included those obtained from cadavers in six studies (40.0%, $n = 6/15$), surgical waste in eight studies (53.3%, $n = 8/15$), and a reconstructed 3D skin model in one study (6.67%, $n = 1/15$). Three studies evaluated water-only decontamination (20.0%, $n = 3/15$), seven studies evaluated soap and water decontamination (46.7%, $n = 7/15$), and five studies evaluated both water-only and soap and water decontamination (33.3%, $n = 5/15$) (Table 4.1).

Water-Only Decontamination

Zhai et al. [17] studied decontamination of formaldehyde, an industrial chemical, from human cadaver skin samples of undisclosed anatomic region using tap water (sample size per protocol, $n = 5$; decontamination protocols, $n = 3$). Skin samples were dosed with 10 μL aliquots (approximately 0.25 μg) of [^{14}C]-formaldehyde by high-performance liquid chromatography (HPLC) syringe onto 3 cm^2 of the skin. Decontamination occurred at 1, 3, or 30 min post-exposure by washing the epidermal surface three times with 4 mL solution (12 mL total for each skin sample).

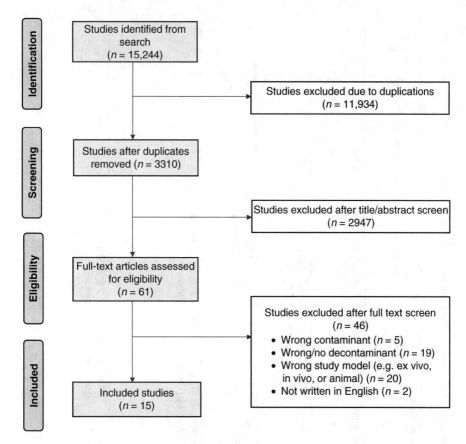

Fig. 4.1 Selection process for study inclusion

Liquid scintillation counting was used to determine the amount of formaldehyde recovered from washing solutions, two tape strips taken at the end, receptor fluid, and the remaining skin samples. Results found that percent decontaminated at 1 min post-exposure by tap water was 82.6%, at 3 min was 62.6%, and at 30 min was 41.7%, leading to partial decontamination in all protocols ($n = 15/15$).

Zhai et al. [18] measured decontamination of radiolabeled [^{14}C]-glyphosate, a pesticide, from human cadaver skin samples of undisclosed anatomic region (decontamination sample size per protocol, $n = 6$; protocols, $n = 3$) using tap water. Skin samples were dosed with 10 μL aliquots of radiolabeled [^{14}C]-glyphosate, approximately 375 μg, by HPLC syringe onto each skin surface, measuring 3 cm^2. Decontamination was conducted 1, 3, or 30 min post-exposure by washing the epidermal surface three times with 4 mL each solution (12 mL total), followed by scrubbing with a scrubber for 15 s after each wash. Liquid scintillation counting was used to determine the amount of glyphosate decontaminated from washing solutions, two tape strips taken at the end, receptor fluid, and the remaining skin. Data showed that percent decontaminated at 1 min post-exposure by tap water was

Table 4.1 Study information, contaminant information, decontaminant information, and outcomes in included studies on human in vitro decontamination of occupational chemicals

Study information			Contaminant information			
Author (year)	Sample size per protocol (no. of protocols)	Human in vitro model details	Contaminant (classification)	Method of contamination	Amount applied	Skin contact time (min)
Zhai et al. (2007) [17]	5 (3)	Cadaver skin samples of undisclosed origin	Formaldehyde (industrial chemical)	Dose applied to the skin using syringe	10 µL (approximately 0.25 µg)	1, 3, 30
Zhai et al. (2008) [18]	6 (3)	Cadaver skin samples of undisclosed origin	Glyphosate (pesticide)	Dose applied to the skin using syringe	10 µL (approximately 375 µg)	1, 3, 30
Fosse et al. (2010) [19]	NR	Reconstructed 3D skin model, EpiSkin	Tetramethylammonium hydroxide (TMAH; industrial chemical)	Dose applied to the skin	60 µL of 25% TMAH in aqueous solution (mg NR)	0.17, 0.5
Weber et al. (1992) [20]	3 (2)	Cadaver skin samples of undisclosed origin, tape-stripped or not prior to exposure	2,3,7,8-Tetrachlorodibenzo-p-dioxin (TCDD; industrial chemical)	Dose applied to the skin	40 µL (approximately 2500 ng)	100
Larese Filon et al. (2008) [21]	Decontaminated: 32 (1) Control: 48 (1) Blank control: 2 (1)	Abdomen skin samples from surgery	Chromium powder (industrial chemical)	Dose applied to the skin	2.5 g in 50 mL synthetic sweat	30

Zhu et al. (2016) [22]	Hydroquinone and clonidine, each: 8 (1) Benzoic acid: 4 (1)	Abdomen skin samples from cadavers	Hydroquinone (drug), clonidine (drug), benzoic acid (industrial chemical)	Dose applied to the skin	5 μL (equating 0.00025 mCi; mg NR)	30
Hui et al. (2012) [23]	8 (2)	Abdomen or thigh skin samples from cadavers	3,5-Dichloro-2,4,6-trifluoropyridine (DCTFP; pesticide)	Dose applied to the skin with syringe	10 μL of 2% solution	10, 30
Debouzy et al. (2002) [24]	8 (1)	Abdomen skin samples from surgery	Radioactive cobalt chloride (industrial chemical)	Dose applied to the skin	20 μL (equating 10.806 kBq; mg NR)	120
Filon et al. (2006) [25]	NR	Abdomen skin samples from surgery	Lead oxide (industrial chemical)	Dose applied to the skin	5 mg/cm^2 (equating 80 mg)	30
Nielsen (2010) [26]	Benzoic acid and caffeine, decontaminated, each: 12 (1) Glyphosate, decontaminated: 13 (1) Control for all chemicals, each: 14 (1)	Abdomen and breast skin samples from surgery	Benzoic acid (industrial chemical), caffeine (drug), glyphosate (pesticide)	Dose applied to the skin	424 μg	360

(continued)

Table 4.1 (continued)

Study information			Contaminant information			
Thors et al. (2020) [27]	5–6	Abdomen skin samples from surgery	Fentanyl, in hydrochloride or free base forms, in solution or dry powder (drug)	Dose applied to the skin	100 µL (equating 500 µg) for solution; 106 or 134 mg for powder	5
Noury et al. (2014) [30]	3 (12)	Abdomen skin samples from surgery	Salicylic acid, aminophylline (both drugs)	Dose applied to the skin	20 µL (mg NR)	5, 30, 60
Wester et al. (1990) [28]	1 (12)	Powdered stratum corneum from cadavers	Polychlorinated biphenyls dissolved in mineral oil (PCBs; industrial chemical)	Mixed with powdered stratum corneum	2 µg/4 mL	15
Hewitt et al. (1994) [31]	4–10 (12)	Breast skin samples from surgery	MbOCA, MDA (both industrial chemicals)	Dose applied to the skin under occlusion or not	5 µL (yielding 9.7–17.7 µg/cm² for MbOCA or 17.6–21.6 µg/cm² for MDA)	4320
Forsberg et al. (2020) [29]	6 (20)	Abdomen skin samples from surgery	Acrylonitrile, 2-butoxyethanol, tributylamine (all industrial chemicals)	Dose applied to the skin	10 µL (8.1 mg for acrylonitrile, 9.02 mg for 2-butoxyethanol, and 7.8 mg for tributylamine)	5, 15, 45, 120

CD complete decontamination, *PD* partial decontamination, *NR* not reported

98.7%, at 3 min 95.6%, and at 30 min 79.0%, achieving partial decontamination in all scenarios ($n = 18/18$).

Fosse et al. [19] studied decontamination of tetramethylammonium hydroxide (TMAH), an industrial chemical, from reconstructed three-dimensional human skin model samples (EpiSkin, SkinEthic Laboratories, Nice, France) with a surface area of 0.33 cm² and supplied on 24-well high-throughput screening plates (sample size, NR). Decontamination solutions included tap water or Diphoterine®. EpiSkin specimens were exposed to 60 µL 25% TMAH aqueous solution in a preliminary test for 30 or 60 s, prior to tap water rinsing, and then for a separate skin protection assay for 10 and 30 s prior to tap water or Diphoterine® rinsing. Decontamination for the latter occurred immediately post-exposure by flushing samples with 150 µL either tap water or Diphoterine® 20 times for a total of 7.5 min. Decontamination was assessed by cell survival using MTT (3-(4,5-dimethylthiazol-2-yl)-2,5-diphenyltetrazolium bromide) cell viability assay.

Preliminary study results found that cell viability percent (standard deviation) after the 30-s TMAH exposure was 34.3% (18.2%) and after the 60-s exposure was 10.7% (17.6%). Tap water decontamination yielded a cell viability of 87.8% (2.3%) and 33.8% (6.5%) after 10 s and 30 s of TMAH exposure, respectively. Results from the Diphoterine® skin protection assay demonstrated cell viability to be 98.7% (1.6%) and 66.5% (8.5%) after 10- and 30-s TMAH exposure, respectively. Fosse et al. concluded that water sometimes displays a limited action on major corrosive chemical splashes, making Diphoterine® a potentially better agent for decontamination of TMAH. Decontamination outcomes could not be determined due to their experimental approach.

Soap and Water Decontamination

Weber et al. [20] evaluated the in vitro decontamination of cadaveric human skin samples (undisclosed anatomic region) exposed to 2,3,7,8-tetrachlorodibenzo-p-dioxin (TCDD), an industrial chemical, using soap (decontamination sample size per protocol, $n = 3$, protocols, $n = 2$; control sample size per protocol, $n = 3$, protocols, $n = 2$). Half of the skin samples were tape-stripped to remove the stratum corneum prior to TCDD exposure to simulate wounded skin. Carbon-14-radiolabeled TCDD was dissolved in acetone at 62.5 ng/µL and applied to a 3.8 cm² circular area of the skin at 650 ng/cm². Contaminated skin samples were then placed on top of saline-soaked gauze pads inside a petri dish and incubated for 100 min, after which samples were decontaminated by wiping four times using water-soaked cotton balls rubbed on a soap bar. Decontaminated skin samples then continued to be incubated until 300 min elapsed. Control skin samples from stripped and non-stripped groups were wiped with four dry cotton balls 300 min post-exposure. Intact skin samples were then tape-stripped, and tape strips plus remaining skin samples were analyzed via liquid scintillation counting to quantify TCDD concentrations.

For both tape-stripped and non-tape-stripped samples prior to contamination, soapy water-wiping significantly reduced TCDD concentrations in all skin layers when compared to control. In the stratum corneum, epidermis, and dermis of skin samples that were not tape-stripped prior to exposure, 43.7%, 4.06%, and 2.14% were recovered from each respective layer in the control versus 22.3%, 2.17%, and 0.91% in the soapy water-wipe group. For skin samples tape-stripped prior to exposure, and therefore lacking stratum corneum, higher amounts of TCDD were found in all viable cell layers. In the epidermis and upper dermis, 37.5% and 4.19% were recovered from each respective layer in the control group versus 4.19% and 1.36% from each respective layer in soapy water-wipe groups. Weber et al. reported enhanced penetration was not noted in the present study, unlike other investigations employing rinse-based protocols, likely due to reduced skin hydration from the presented decontamination protocols. All decontaminated skin samples achieved partial decontamination ($n = 6/6$), and evidence indicated that water and soap-soaked cotton balls were effective agents for TCDD decontamination.

Larese Filon et al. [21] examined decontamination of chromium (Cr) powder, an industrial chemical, from human skin samples of abdominal origin in Franz diffusion cells using liquid soap (decontaminated sample sizes per protocol, $n = 32$; control sample sizes per protocol, $n = 48$; protocols, $n = 1$ for both). Skin samples were exposed to 2.5 g Cr powder in 50 mL synthetic sweat, comprised of 0.5% w/v sodium chloride, 0.1% w/v urea, and 0.1% w/v lactic acid in water, at pH 4.5 in exposure chambers. Decontamination occurred at 30 min post-exposure by cleaning of skin samples with three cotton balls wetted with soap. Decontamination analysis was conducted via inductively coupled plasma atomic emission spectroscopy (ICP-AES) after 24 h elapsed.

Results showed that mean Cr skin content was significantly higher in decontaminated samples versus non-decontaminated control samples, measuring 5.46 µg/cm^2 versus 3.19 µg/cm^2, respectively, indicating decontamination at 30 min did not reduce percutaneous penetration of Cr but rather enhanced absorption, illustrating the "wash-in" effect. However, the receiving phase of decontaminated samples demonstrated lower mean Cr content beneath the limit of detection (LOD), whereas values in controls measured 0.016 µg/cm^2. Larese Filon et al. [21] attributed this to SLS interfering with the stratum corneum's structure and thus enhancing Cr binding capacity to the skin, which elevated skin content while diminishing penetration rates. Partial decontamination was seen in all skin samples ($n = 32/32$).

Zhu et al. [22] investigated in vitro efficacy of 2% soapy water in decontaminating ^{14}C-labeled drugs, hydroquinone (decontaminated sample size, $n = 8$; control sample size, $n = 4$) and clonidine (decontaminated sample size, $n = 8$; control sample size, $n = 8$), and the industrial chemical benzoic acid (decontaminated sample size, $n = 4$; control sample size, $n = 4$). Five microliter 0.05 mCi/mL solutions of each contaminant were applied to cadaveric abdominal skin samples in glass diffusion cells and maintained skin contact for 30 min before decontamination, performed by washing once with a 2% soap-soaked cotton ball and twice with a distilled deionized water-soaked cotton ball and then drying. Wet cotton balls sat on the skin for 3 min, and no wiping was applied during decontamination.

Decontamination efficacy was determined by the total mass balance of ^{14}C-labeled contaminant recovery, measured using a liquid scintillation counter.

Recovered percent of applied dose in the soapy water wash were 82.3% benzoic acid, 83.0% hydroquinone, and 89.0% clonidine, yielding partial decontamination in all experiments. Importantly, decontamination significantly reduced penetration of hydroquinone into the receptor fluid, representative of the circulatory system, compared to non-decontaminated controls, measuring 0.5% and 1.4%, respectively. Although no marked differences were noted in the receptor fluids of control versus decontaminated groups for clonidine or benzoic acid, Zhu et al. [22] reported that decontamination transiently enhanced benzoic acid penetration rates to surpass that of non-decontaminated control samples, before returning to levels below them, indicative of the "wash-in" effect. Zhu et al. [22] concluded that although soapy water decontamination removed the majority of surface contaminants and may be beneficial in the long term, considerable amounts remained in the epidermis despite skin cleansing, yielding partial decontamination in all samples ($n = 20/20$). In addition, these investigators underscored the potential risk for enhanced toxicity by "washing-in" certain contaminants.

Hui et al. [23] documented the decontamination efficacy of 10% soapy water on 2% ^{14}C-labeled 3,5-dichloro-2,4,6-trifluoropyridine (DCTFP), a pesticide, in N-methyl-2-pyrrolidinone (decontaminated sample sizes per protocol, $n = 8$, protocols, $n = 2$). Abdomen or thigh skin samples from human cadavers were clamped onto glass scintillation vials. Ten microliter aliquots of 2% solution were then applied to a 1 cm^2 area of the skin using a syringe. Decontamination was performed at either 10 or 30 min post-exposure by washing with the following five cotton-tipped swabs: (1) tip wetted with liquid soap water, (2) dry tip to remove residue, (3) tip wetted with liquid soap water, (4) dry tip to remove residue, and (5) dry tip to dry surface. Skin samples were then transferred to continuous flow-through diffusion cells and incubated for 24 h, after which ten consecutive D-Squame tape strips were performed on all skin samples. Radioactivity was measured with liquid scintillation spectrometry for decontamination analysis.

Results showed that percent pesticide successfully recovered from tape strips, skin samples, receptor fluid, and wash was 30.58% in total for the 10-min exposure group, with 30.17% found in wash, and 10.48% in total for the 30-min exposure group, with 9.68% found in wash. A separate volatility test demonstrated that the majority of DCTFP was lost to evaporation, with only 27% and 5% remaining at 10 min and 30 min, partially explaining the low recovery rates. All protocols achieved partial decontamination in all skin samples ($n = 16/16$). Hui et al. [23] noted that the small amounts penetrated and recovered were predominantly due to rapid evaporation, emphasizing that factors contributing to decontamination efficacy include the contaminant's physicochemical properties, such as volatility, solubility, and molecular weight, as well as skin contact time and anatomic site of the skin.

Debouzy et al. [24] investigated the decontamination of radiocontaminating agent cobalt chloride (CoCl$_2$) using soap solution (decontamination sample sizes per protocol, $n = 8$; control sample sizes per protocol, $n = 8$; protocols, $n = 1$ for both). Human skin samples from abdominal surgery were placed in Franz diffusion cells and exposed to a 20 μL droplet of cobalt solution (540.3 kBq/mL in HCl) for 2 h. Decontamination was then conducted by applying 0.5 mL of soap solution to the skin sample, allowing it to sit for 1 min, and then removing it with 0.5 mL of a 0.9% NaCl isotonic solution. Decontamination efficacy was determined by radioactivity measurements recorded on a Compugamma gamma counter with a thallium-doped sodium iodide pit probe. It was found that 79.7% of the contaminant was recovered in soapy water wash, indicating partial decontamination of $CoCl_2$ from skin samples ($n = 8/8$).

Filon et al. [25] assessed the in vitro penetration and rapid decontamination of lead oxide (PbO) powder on human abdominal skin samples placed in Franz diffusion cells using liquid soap (sample sizes not reported). Skin samples of 16 cm^2 were exposed to 5 mg PbO/cm^2 and 2 mL of synthetic sweat at pH 5. Decontamination was performed 30 min post-exposure by cleansing the skin with a cotton ball soaked in soap, rinsing under running water for 30 s, and wiping with three dry cotton balls for 10 s each. Skin samples then had another 2 mL synthetic sweat reapplied and continued incubating until 24 h elapsed. Positive control samples exposed to PbO powder were incubated for the full 24 h, without decontamination performed at the 30-min mark, followed by 30 s of rinsing and wiping with three dry cotton balls. Negative controls mirrored each experimental condition without the addition of PbO powder. These experiments were repeated with the skin abraded with a 19-gauge needle tip drawn across the surface 20 times in one direction and another 20 times perpendicular. Skin samples and receiver solutions were all collected at the end to quantify Pb content using electrothermal atomic absorption spectrometry.

Median penetration concentrations of Pb into the skin and through the skin into the receiver were reported, as well as adjusted median values calculated by subtracting blank cell median values. Blank-adjusted median values of Pb recovered in the receiving cells of unabraded skin samples were 2.9 ng/cm^2 and 23.6 ng/cm^2 for positive control and decontamination with soap, respectively. Blank-adjusted median Pb content found in the skin for the same samples measured 321.3 and 19.7, respectively. While decontamination significantly reduced Pb content penetrating into the skin when compared to positive control, it also significantly increased the amount penetrating into the receiving solutions over the 24-h period. In abraded skin, decontamination significantly enhanced penetration into the receiving cells, from 26.8 ng/cm^2 in control to 100.2 ng/cm^2 Pb while reducing skin penetration from 296.9 in control to 135.6 ng/cm^2. Partial decontamination was achieved, and Filon et al. [25] concluded that decontamination of lead 30 min post-exposure with a common cleanser significantly elevated metal penetration into receiving cells in vitro.

Nielsen [26] examined the effect of skin washing with soap following 6-h exposure to ^{14}C-radiolabeled benzoic acid (industrial chemical; decontaminated sample size, $n = 12$; control sample size, $n = 14$), glyphosate (pesticide; decontaminated sample size, $n = 13$; control sample size, $n = 14$), and caffeine (drug; decontaminated sample size, $n = 12$; control sample size, $n = 14$). Human breast and abdominal skin samples from plastic surgery patients were mounted onto in vitro static diffusion cells. The model compounds in aqueous solutions, containing 0.9% NaCl and 2% ethanol, were applied to the donor chamber in concentrations of 4 mg/mL for a total volume of 106 µL. Decontamination was conducted 6 h post-exposure by washing skin surfaces with soap and a cotton swab, followed by two washing steps in isotonic water without swabs. After 48 h, the epidermis of both groups was wiped four times with swabs wetted with 50% acetonitrile in water and two times with dry swabs to remove remaining contaminant. Radioactivity in samples was quantified with liquid scintillation counting.

Glyphosate recovery from donor chambers in the decontaminated group was significantly more than from control, measuring 99.8% and 79%, respectively. Further, less glyphosate concentrations were found in the epidermis, dermis, and receptor fluid for decontaminated groups compared to non-decontaminated groups, although significance was only reached in the epidermis. Caffeine recovery from donor chambers in the decontaminated group was significantly more than from control, measuring 90.1% and 67.4%, respectively ($p < 0.05$). Deposition in both skin layers and receptor fluid was significantly reduced in decontaminated groups compared to control. Benzoic acid recovery from donor chambers of the decontaminated group was also significantly more than control, measuring 10.2% versus 3.1%, respectively, and significantly lower in the skin and receptor fluid when compared to control. Soap wash achieved complete decontamination of glyphosate-contaminated skin samples ($n = 13/37$) and partial decontamination of the remaining skin samples contaminated with benzoic acid or caffeine ($n = 24/37$). Nielsen [26] concluded that handwashing following 6-h dermal exposure decreased not only the amount of residue present in the upper skin compartments but also the quantity subsequently penetrating the skin, particularly for hydrophilic compounds.

Water-Only and Soap and Water Decontamination

Thors et al. [27] determined the efficacy of water and soapy water decontamination for human skin exposed to fentanyl (decontaminated and control sample size per protocol, $n = 5$–6 for both; protocols, $n = 4$ for both). Abdominal skin samples obtained from plastic surgery were mounted in vitro on a flow-through diffusion cell. The skin was exposed to the free base or the hydrochloride salt of fentanyl in 2% isopropyl alcohol solution or as dry powder and incubated for 24 h. One hundred microliliter fentanyl of both forms suspended in 2% isopropyl alcohol solution, 106 mg of dry powder in salt form, or 134 mg of dry powder in free base form was exposed on the skin for 5 min prior to decontamination. Powder applications were dosed with artificial sweat, an industry-designed solution formulated to mimic human sweat. Water or 2% soapy water was then used for decontamination by adding 50 µL solution onto the skin, instantly followed by vacuum suctioning, repeated ten times. Lipochromatography-mass spectrometry was performed for analysis.

Both decontamination procedures significantly decreased the cumulative amount of fentanyl of both forms penetrating through the skin during the 24-h experimental period, except for free base, powdered fentanyl decontaminated with water. For fentanyl hydrochloride in solution, decontamination significantly lowered mean cumulative penetration from 10.3 µg/cm^2 in control down to 0.4 µg/cm^2 and 0.3 µg/cm^2 in water-only and 2% soapy water groups, respectively. In powder form, decontamination of fentanyl hydrochloride applied to sweaty skin diminished mean concentrations from 7.4 µg/cm^2 in control to 1.4 µg/cm^2 and 0.8 µg/cm^2 in water-only and soapy water wash groups, respectively. Mean cumulative amounts of free base fentanyl in solution penetrating through the skin decreased from 18.5 µg/cm^2 in control to 2.3 µg/cm^2 and 0.9 µg/cm^2 in water-only and soapy water samples, respectively. In powder form on sweaty skin, free base fentanyl decontamination reduced mean concentrations from 8.5 µg/cm^2 to 5.8 µg/cm^2 and 1.6 µg/cm^2 for water (not significantly) and soapy water groups (significantly), respectively. All protocols achieved partial decontamination (total sample sizes excluded due to ambiguous reporting), and Thors et al. [27] concluded that washing with soap and water is a sufficient decontamination procedure for fentanyl.

Noury et al. [30] studied in vitro decontamination of two radiolabeled pharmaceutical drugs, salicylic acid and aminophylline, from human abdominal skin samples in static diffusion cells, using distilled water or 10% Softsoap® Aloe vera in water (decontaminated sample size per protocol, $n = 3$; protocols, $n = 12$). Twenty microliter of contaminants was applied to the surface of the skin with a syringe. Decontamination occurred at 5, 30, and 60 min post-exposure by rinsing the skin three times with 1 mL solution and applying three pieces of cotton on the skin to absorb the washing solution. Skin samples were then tape-stripped. Liquid scintillation counting was used to quantify contaminant concentration in washing solutions extracted from cotton, tape strips, receptor fluid, and remaining skin.

Data demonstrated that the majority of total contaminant recovery was from washing solution, measuring 73% or higher for all protocols, except for aminophylline at 60 min, which recovered only 42.5%. Percutaneous penetration increased with time, suggesting shorter skin contact times are associated with better decontamination outcomes. All solutions yielded partial decontamination in contaminated skin samples ($n = 36/36$). Noury et al. [30] concluded that washing with water only and soap and water are appropriate choices, since both solutions exhibited similar efficacy at removing lipophilic (salicylic acid) and hydrophilic (aminophylline) chemicals from the skin. In addition, the skin needs to be decontaminated as soon as possible to circumvent the observed diminishing efficacy of decontamination with prolonged contact time.

Wester et al. [28] determined in vitro decontamination of polychlorinated biphenyls (PCBs), a group of industrial chemicals, from powdered human stratum corneum using water only or soap and water (decontaminated sample size per protocol, $n = 1$; protocols, $n = 12$). Callus was obtained from adult soles of cadavers, ground with dry ice, and freeze-dried to form a stratum corneum powder. ^{14}C-radiolabeled PCBs dissolved in a mineral oil vehicle of 2 µg PCB/4 mL were added to 2 mg of powdered callus for 15 min prior to 1 mL decontaminant addition and mixing. The decontaminant-containing mixture then sat for 0, 1, 10, 60, 240, or 480 min before centrifugation and removal of decontaminant for ^{14}C measurement.

Water-only decontaminant removed the least PCBs, totaling <1% of PCBs recovered from powdered stratum corneum regardless of contact time, yielding no response ($n = 6/12$). Soap and water removed 33.3% PCBs on average across all contact times, yielding partial response ($n = 6/12$). Soap and water demonstrated a trend of increasing contact times correlating with enhanced decontamination, which Wester et al. [28] reported was due to stratum corneum lipids containing PCBs leaching into the decontaminants. Interestingly, in vitro soap and water decontamination findings did not correlate with their in vivo findings conducted in rhesus monkeys, which demonstrated soap and water to be an effective decontaminant, removing 93% of PCBs. Thus, Wester et al. [28] concluded the in vitro model used here to be of limited applicability.

Hewitt et al. [31] examined the decontamination of industrial chemicals 4,4′-methylenebis[2-chloroaniline] (MbOCA) and 4,4′-methylenedianiline (MDA) from fresh human breast skin samples, obtained from surgery, in vitro using flow-through diffusion cells (decontamination sample size per protocol, $n = 4$–10; protocols, $n = 12$). Decontaminant solutions tested included 100% water, 1% soap, and 10% soap. Five microliter aliquots of ^{14}C-MbOCA (9.7–17.7 µg/cm^2 in ethanol) or ^{14}C-MDA (17.6–21.6 µg/cm^2) were applied to the skin in diffusion cells left open to the environment (unoccluded) or closed with a Teflon cap (occluded). After 72 h post-exposure, decontamination was performed by rubbing the skin samples with lint swabs soaked in 100% water, 1% soap, or 10% soap for 10 s. Contaminants in receptor fluid, on swabs, and in the skin were quantified using liquid scintillation spectrometry. A separate time course study looking at the effects of delay to decontamination on penetration of MbOCA and MBA was also conducted, in which 100% ethanol-soaked swabs were used to decontaminate the skin surface after 3-min, 30-min, 1-h, 2-h, 4-h, or 6-h exposure, followed by continued incubation until 72 h in total elapsed.

For MbOCA and MDA, no marked difference was noted in decontamination efficacy between swabs soaked with 100% water, 1% soap aqueous solution, or 10% soap aqueous solution, regardless of occlusion status. Specifically, 33.3–42.8% MbOCA was recovered from unoccluded samples and 24.6–29.9% from occluded samples. MDA recovery ranged from 43.7% to 47% for unoccluded skin and 22.9–30.7% for occluded skin. Time course studies demonstrated that decontamination at 3 and 30 min post-exposure significantly reduced MbOCA and MDA penetration into the skin and through the skin into the receptor fluid. Significance was not achieved when decontamination was performed at later time points, demonstrating a critical time window. All protocols achieved partial decontamination in contaminated skin samples ($n = 84/84$), and Hewitt et al. [31] concluded that solution of choice did not matter as much as decontaminating skin within the critical window of 30 min post-exposure.

Forsberg et al. [29] evaluated the decontamination efficacy of water only and 2% soapy water against three toxic industrial chemicals: acrylonitrile, 2-butoxyethanol, and tributylamine (decontamination sample size per protocol, $n = 6$, protocols, $n = 20$; control sample size per protocol, $n = 6$, protocols, $n = 10$). Abdominal skin samples from surgery were exposed to 10 µL (neat) of each contaminant using a flow-through diffusion cell. Infinite dosing was used throughout the experiments, except for those with acrylonitrile. Skin contact time lasted 5, 15, 45, or 120 min before decontamination, except for acrylonitrile, lasting only 5 or 15 min due to its high volatility. Decontamination was conducted by washing with 50 μL solution followed by its immediate removal using vacuum suctioning, repeated ten times. Decontamination efficacy was determined 5 h post-exposure using liquid chromatography with UV/visible spectroscopy for acrylonitrile and liquid chromatography with triple quadrupole mass spectrometry for 2-butoxyethanol and tributylamine.

Data showed that both water-only and soapy water decontamination significantly reduced skin penetration of all chemicals compared to non-decontaminated controls at 5, 15, and 45 min post-exposure. At 120 min, only tributylamine continued to demonstrate significantly less skin penetration than non-decontaminated control in both decontamination groups. Soapy water decontamination conducted at 120 min post-exposure transiently enhanced penetration rate of 2-butoxyethanol above that of control prior to returning to levels below it, perhaps representing a temporary "wash-in" effect. No marked differences were noted in cumulative amounts penetrating through the skin in water-only versus soapy water decontamination groups, and all protocols yielded a partial response in tested skin samples ($n = 120/120$). Forsberg et al. [29] concluded that early decontamination is paramount for maximizing contaminant removal.

Discussion

This systematic review summarizes experimental studies examining decontamination of occupational chemicals using water-only or soap and water solutions in in vitro human skin models. Water-only decontamination was assessed in 53.3% of studies ($n = 8/15$) and yielded partial decontamination in 95.7% ($n = 134/140$) and no response in 4.3% ($n = 6/140$) of protocols. Soap and water decontamination was evaluated in 80% of studies ($n = 12/15$) and yielded complete decontamination in 4.9% ($n = 13/264$) and partial decontamination in 95.1% ($n = 251/264$) of protocols. Prior reviews evaluating water or soapy water decontamination in vivo and in vitro also mostly reported partial decontamination outcomes [6, 14, 16]. Outcomes yielding no response or partial decontamination leave residual contaminants behind on or within the skin, which then possess potential to be absorbed [32].

While percent applied dose recovered in wash was used to determine decontamination efficacy rates, this does not provide information on the quantity of the absorbed dose in control samples that was prevented from being absorbed in decontaminated samples. Given that the primary goal of dermal decontamination is to minimize toxicity by interrupting skin uptake of harmful substances, an alternative definition of decontamination efficacy that quantifies this blockade may more accurately capture decontamination objectives. Such an "efficacy of interrupting absorption" would require calculating the amount of absorbed dose in non-decontaminated samples which was blocked from absorption in decontaminated samples due to decontamination and may serve as a more reliable marker of decontamination efficacy. This would be calculated as follows:

$$\left(1-\frac{\begin{array}{c}\text{percent absorbed in decontaminated samples at end of study}\\ -\text{percent absorbed at time of decontamination}\end{array}}{\begin{array}{c}\text{percent absorbed in nondecontaminated samples at end of study}\\ -\text{percent absorbed at time of decontamination}\end{array}}\right)\times100\%$$

The mass balance accountability technique introduced by Bucks et al. [33], paired with the use of radiolabeled contaminants quantified by liquid scintillation spectrometry, may be used to account for contaminant concentrations in the skin sample, donor chamber, wash, and receptor fluid of a diffusion cell at various time points to calculate these values. Mass balance accounting would need to be performed on several skin samples at multiple time points: (1) a non-decontaminated control sample at the time of decontamination to assess how much contaminant would have already been absorbed into the skin from the time of contaminant application to the time of decontamination, and (2) another non-decontaminated control sample at the end of the study to determine the amount of contaminant that would have absorbed at that time point, and (3) a decontaminated skin sample at the end of the study to assess the quantity that would have been absorbed in decontaminated skin samples. Amounts absorbed in the contaminated and decontaminated skin samples at the end of the study might then be subtracted by the amount absorbed at the time of decontamination to calculate percent absorbed between those time points. The resultant percent absorbed in decontaminated controls divided by the resultant percent absorbed in non-decontaminated controls would then yield the fraction of *absorbed* contaminant in decontaminated to non-decontaminated samples. Subtracting one by this fraction and then multiplying by 100% to convert to percentage would then yield the percent applied dose of the contaminant that was *interrupted from absorption*. Not only might this efficacy rate better represent decontamination objectives, but it is also unaffected by chemicals that rapidly penetrate the skin and are no longer accessible for rinsing, unlike wash recovery rates (discussed below).

Although various factors impact decontamination efficacy, time to decontamination is critical, as shorter durations are known to maximize decontamination efficacy [1]. Wester and Maibach [34] reported that increased skin contact times resulted in greater percutaneous absorption. Greater percutaneous absorption presumably reduces the amount of contaminant on the skin surface available for decontamination, hindering decontamination efficacy. Our results support this hypothesis, as the seven studies evaluating decontamination at varying time points all yielded better decontamination efficacy or less tissue damage when cleansing was performed sooner rather than later, regardless of the varying decontamination methods and solutions employed [17–19, 23, 29–31]. Minimizing skin contact time should thus be prioritized whenever hazardous spills or splashes occur in the workplace and partly explains the varying efficacy rates observed.

Certain chemicals were found to rapidly "lock in" to the stratum corneum and subsequently enter the bloodstream despite immediate decontamination. For example, immediate decontamination of the pesticide malathion did not prevent 9.6% of the applied dose from absorbing through dermal routes in vivo in humans [34]. This rapid absorption through the skin may partly explain the low rates of complete decontamination seen in experimental studies, as, again, penetration through the skin might inhibit water or soapy water solutions from reaching the contaminants, ultimately rendering surface decontamination less effective.

In addition to skin contact time, the physicochemical properties of a contaminant, such as molecular weight and lipophilicity, are also known to affect decontamination efficacy [32]. Generally, compounds with smaller molecular weights tend to penetrate the skin more readily, as do increasingly lipophilic compounds, up to an extent when assessed by the log of their octanol/water partition coefficient (log $P_{o/w}$) [35], due to the hydrophobic nature of stratum corneum [36]. Five experimental investigations evaluated the decontamination of varying chemicals with different physicochemical properties. Two of these demonstrated clear patterns in how these properties affected contaminant concentrations penetrating the skin and recovered in wash. When Nielsen [26] examined glyphosate, caffeine, and benzoic acid, data demonstrated that the compound with the highest lipophilicity, benzoic acid (log $P_{o/w}$ = 1.83), penetrated the most and had the lowest recovery amount in wash, whereas the least lipophilic compound, glyphosate (log $P_{o/w}$ = −1.7), penetrated the least and exhibited the highest recovery amount in wash. Forsberg et al. [29] found that the compound with greatest skin penetration was that with the lowest molecular weight, acrylonitrile (53.06 g/mol), and the compound with the highest molecular weight displayed the lowest skin penetration, which was tributylamine (185.36 g/mol). Conversely, Hewitt et al. [31], Noury et al. [30], and Zhu et al. [22] all found similar concentrations recovered in wash and/or penetrating skin between multiple contaminants despite varying molecular weights and lipophilicities. This discrepancy is potentially attributed to the different vehicles in which contaminants were dissolved in, as vehicles influence in vitro percutaneous absorption through human skin [37]. Nielsen [26] used mostly water with 2% ethanol and 0.9% NaCl; Forsberg et al. [29] employed neat solutions, whereas Zhu et al. [22] and Hewitt et al. [31] both used pure ethanol vehicles. Fifty percent ethanol was found to enhance penetration through the skin [38], thus potentially masking contaminant penetration differences arising from lipophilicity and molecular weight. Noury et al. [30] assessed salicylic acid in a solvent comprised of a 2:8 ratio of ethanol to water and aminophylline dissolved in a 2:8 ratio of contaminant to water. The different vehicles within the same study may have negated the influence of physicochemical properties on penetration, as a contaminant's solubility within a vehicle versus that of the skin might also modify its ability to partition out of vehicle and into the skin [39]. Despite these differences, it is apparent that when contaminant properties favor higher percutaneous penetration, decontamination efficacy is reduced.

Other factors known to affect decontamination efficacy include (1) total contaminant dose; (2) anatomic site of contamination; (3) duration of decontamination; (4) hydrodynamics such as flow rate, pressure, and temperature of water; (5) use of physical washing aids; and (6) spread of involved skin surface [1, 32], many of which varied in the included experimental studies.

Finally, water-only or soap and water decontamination may enhance percutaneous penetration via the "wash-in" effect, which was observed in four experimental studies. Two investigators found increased cumulative amounts of PbO or Cr powder penetrating in decontaminated groups compared to control [21, 25], while another two reported decontamination transiently enhanced penetration rates for benzoic acid or 2-butoxyethanol, surpassing that of controls [22, 29]. The "wash-in" effect is suggested to occur predominantly due to hydration and surfactant effects of decontamination [13]. Firstly, increased skin hydration is thought to mobilize and activate the diffusion of residue that has accumulated in the stratum corneum [13]. Interestingly, Zhu et al. [22] investigated the effects of rising stratum corneum hydration levels and noted that doing so enhanced benzoic acid penetration rates, experimentally confirming the contribution of hydration effect. However, hydroquinone and clonidine demonstrated decreasing penetration rates with increasing stratum corneum hydration, indicating the hydration effect to be chemical-dependent. Secondly, introducing surfactants results in potential delipidation, membrane fluidization, or skin irritation that compromises stratum corneum integrity [13] and promotes percutaneous penetration [40]. A friction effect from rubbing the skin, acid/base effect from skin interaction with solutions of varying pH levels, and artifact effect from experimental setup were also suggested to be potential, although less likely, contributors [13]. Of the remaining 11 studies evaluated, eight did not include control groups to assess for the presence of a "wash-in" effect, and three did not report one when comparing data from decontaminated versus control groups. Weber et al. [20] attributed this absence to be due to their decontamination method, which was minimally hydrating. Nielsen [26] also assessed benzoic acid but, unlike Zhu et al. [22], did not observe elevated penetration rates or concentrations upon decontamination, which might also be explained by their varying decontamination methods. Zhu et al. [22] allowed one soap-soaked and two water-soaked cotton balls to sit on the skin for 3 min each, while Nielsen [26] cotton-swabbed skin with soap followed by water rinsing. Lastly, Thors et al. [27] only reported data on cumulatively penetrated amounts, whereas the "wash-in" effect is sometimes only captured by transiently elevated penetration rates rather than total concentration penetrating the skin [22, 29, 41]. In vivo investigations monitoring the urinary excretion and/or systemic absorption of contaminants following water or soapy water decontamination are desperately needed to confirm or refute this phenomenon, as it has potential to acutely enhance toxicity depending on the contaminant in question. Enhanced penetration of the potent nerve agent VX does lead to lethality, whereas benzoic acid exposure might be relatively uneventful [42].

A list of the following contaminants that have exhibited increased penetration following water and/or soapy water decontamination in in vitro human skin studies was compiled: benzo[a]pyrene, 2,4-D acid, 2,4-D amine, DDT, DEET, diazinon (see references in [13]), Cr powder [21], PbO [25], VX, and paraoxon [22]. The following contaminants transiently exhibited enhanced penetration rates, but no overall rise in cumulative amounts penetrated: diethylmalonate [41], benzoic acid [22],

2-butoxyethanol, and methyl salicylate [29]. It is important to recognize that these in vitro investigations do not necessarily contraindicate water decontamination for their respective chemicals, since in vitro findings do not always correlate with in vivo results. An in vivo study of swine topically exposed to fivefold higher than the median lethal dose of VX demonstrated that those decontaminated with soapy water 30 min post-exposure survived with minimal signs of toxicity compared to most non-decontaminated controls that died [43]. Thus, while it is possible that a temporary spike in VX blood concentrations may have initially occurred, the choice to decontaminate conferred protection overall. Therefore, in vitro findings alone are insufficient for determining contraindications but require in vivo confirmation to understand the true risks, if any, of the "wash-in" effect.

Limitations to this review include small sample sizes, which limit data reliability. Further, variation in contaminants, dosage, anatomic skin sites, skin contact times, decontamination solutions and methods, and endpoint analyses limits comparisons between studies. This variation and the in vitro model's inability to fully capture the processes occurring within the internal milieu of living organisms [44] also limit the applicability of these findings. Finally, percutaneous toxicity of each contaminant was not analyzed due to a lack of data and feasibility. This limits our understanding of the clinical relevance of partial decontamination outcomes and whether complete decontamination of a given contaminant is necessary for best clinical outcomes.

Despite these limitations, the widely recommended decontaminating agents, water or soap and water, were noted to almost always yield partial decontamination of various occupational contaminants, including industrial chemicals, pesticides, and drugs. Many factors contribute to efficacy rates, including skin contact time, loading dose, anatomic site, surface area affected, duration of decontamination, and contaminant physicochemical properties, among others [1, 32]. Given each contaminant's unique properties, it is unlikely that water or soap and water are capable of universally decontaminating all occupational chemicals, and it remains unclear which contaminants they best remove. In addition, they may precipitate a "wash-in" effect that enhances a contaminant's penetration rate or concentration, potentially exacerbating its deleterious effects. Further investigation is needed to understand when water or soap and water needs to be used as decontaminating agents of choice in the workplace and to confirm or deny the in vivo existence of the "wash-in" phenomenon. Standardization of methodologies (e.g., contaminant dose, surface area involved, etc.) within future experimental studies, by utilizing a similar contaminant dose, vehicle, application method, skin sample, anatomic region, surface area involved, exposure time, method of decontamination, decontaminant used, and analysis, would greatly assist with interstudy comparisons to elucidate the most appropriate decontaminants. It is noteworthy that variations may be made in the setup to study the effect of a specific parameter, as needed. Zhu and Maibach [45] provide additional decontamination details in *Skin Decontamination: A Comprehensive Research Guide*.

Taken together, with the limited in vitro and in vivo available data, key points for future exploration include categorizing which physicochemical properties of a toxicant do or do not favor use of water alone or water and soap for acute decontamination (0–4 min) versus that for delayed decontamination (>30 min) and development of more effective decontaminating agents while also considering the potential for the "wash-in" effect.

Acknowledgments   The authors received no financial support for the research, authorship, and/or publication of this article.

The authors of this chapter would like to acknowledge the original source of publication, Taylor & Francis Online, whose website can be accessed via the following link: https://www.tandfonline.com/. The original publication of this chapter can be found via the following link: https://doi.org/10.1080/10937404.2021.1957048.

Declaration of Interest   The authors report no conflict of interest.

References

1. Chilcott RP. Mitigating dermal exposure to agrochemicals. In: Shah VP, Maibach HI, et al., editors. Topical drug bioavailability, bioequivalence, and penetration. New York, NY: Springer; 2015. p. 41–57.
2. Blickenstaff NR, Coman G, Blattner CM, Andersen R, Maibach HI. Biology of percutaneous penetration. Rev Environ Health. 2014;29:145–55. https://doi.org/10.1515/reveh-2014-0052.
3. Levitin HW, Siegelson HJ, Dickinson S, Halpern P, Haraguchi Y, Nocera A, Turineck D. Decontamination of mass casualties--re-evaluating existing dogma. Prehosp Disast Med. 2003;18:200–7. https://doi.org/10.1017/s1049023x00001060.
4. Leigh JP, Markowitz SB, Fahs M, Shin C, Landrigan PJ. Occupational injury and illness in the United States. Estimates of costs, morbidity, and mortality. Arch Intern Med. 1997;157:1557–68.
5. Bureau of Labor Statistics. U.S. Department of Labor 2020. Employer-reported workplace injuries and illnesses [Press release]. 2019. https://www.bls.gov/iif/soii-data.htm.
6. Burli A, Kashetsky N, Feschuk A, Law RM, Maibaich HI. Efficacy of soap and water based skin decontamination using in vivo animal models: systematic review. J Toxicol Environ Health B Crit Rev. 2021;24(7):325.
7. Houston M, Hendrickson RG. Decontamination. Crit Care Clin. 2005;21(653-672):v. https://doi.org/10.1016/j.ccc.2005.06.001.
8. Canadian Centre for Occupational Health and Safety. The safety data sheet: a guide to first-aid recommendations. 2012. https://www.ccohs.ca/products/publications/firstaid/#chap3.
9. National Institute for Occupational Safety and Health. Pocket guide to chemical hazards. Atlanta, GA: CDC; 2007. https://www.cdc.gov/niosh/docs/2005-149/pdfs/2005-149.pdf.
10. Wester RC, Hui X, Landry T, Maibach HI. In vivo skin decontamination of methylene bisphenyl isocyanate (MDI): soap and water ineffective compared to polypropylene glycol, polyglycol-based cleanser, and corn oil. Toxicol Sci. 1999;48:1–4. https://doi.org/10.1093/oxfordjournals.toxsci.a034663.
11. Bromberg BE, Song IC, Walden RH. Hydrotherapy of chemical burns. Plast Reconstr Surg. 1965;35:85–95. https://doi.org/10.1097/00006534-196501000-00010.
12. American National Standards Institute. American National Standard for emergency showers and eyewash equipment. ANSI/ISEA Z358.1-2014. Arlington, VA: International Safety Equipment Association; 2015. Approved 8 Jan 2015.
13. Moody RP, Maibach HI. Skin decontamination: importance of the wash-in effect. Food Chem Toxicol. 2006;44:1783–8. https://doi.org/10.1016/j.fct.2006.05.020.

14. Kashetsky N, Law RM, Maibach HI. Efficacy of water skin decontamination in vivo in humans: a systematic review. Personal communication. 2021.

15. Moher D, Liberati A, Tetzlaff J, Altman DG. Preferred reporting items for systematic reviews and meta-analyses: the PRISMA statement. Br Med J. 2009;339:b2535. https://doi.org/10.1136/bmj.b2535.

16. Chiang C, Kashetsky N, Feschuk A, Burli A, Law RM, Maibach HI. Efficacy of water-only or soap and water skin decontamination of chemical warfare agents using in vitro human models: a systematic review. Personal communication. 2021.

17. Zhai H, Barbadillo S, Hui X, Maibach HI. In vitro model for decontamination of human skin: formaldehyde. Food Chem Toxicol. 2007;45:618–21. https://doi.org/10.1016/j.fct.2006.10.007.

18. Zhai H, Chan HP, Hui X, Maibach HI. Skin decontamination of glyphosate from human skin in vitro. Food Chem Toxicol. 2008;46:2258–60. https://doi.org/10.1016/j.fct.2008.03.001.

19. Fosse C, Mathieu L, Hall AH, Bocchietto E, Burgher F, Fischbach M, Maibach HI. Decontamination of tetramethylammonium hydroxide (TMAH) splashes: promising results with Diphoterine in vitro. Cutan Ocul Toxicol. 2010;29:110–5. https://doi.org/10.3109/15569521003661288.

20. Weber LW, Zesch A, Rozman K. Decontamination of human skin exposed to 2,3,7,8-tetrachlorodibenzo-p-dioxin (TCDD) in vitro. Arch Environ Health. 1992;47:302–8. https://doi.org/10.1080/00039896.1992.9938366.

21. Larese Filon F, D'Agostin F, Crosera M, Adami G, Bovenzi M, Maina G. In vitro percutaneous absorption of chromium powder and the effect of skin cleanser. Toxicol in Vitro. 2008;22:1562–7. https://doi.org/10.1016/j.tiv.2008.06.006.

22. Zhu H, Jung EC, Phuong C, Hui X, Maibach H. Effects of soap-water wash on human epidermal penetration. J Appl Toxicol. 2016;36:997–1002. https://doi.org/10.1002/jat.3258.

23. Hui X, Domoradzki JY, Maibach HC. In vitro study to determine decontamination of 3,5-dichloro-2,4,6-trifluoropyridine (DCTFP) from human skin. Food Chem Toxicol. 2012;50:2496–502. https://doi.org/10.1016/j.fct.2012.03.069.

24. Debouzy J-C, Tymen H, Gall B, Fauvelle F, Martel B, Gadelle T, Gadelle A. First evaluation of per(3,6-anhydro, 2-O-carboxymethyl)α-cyclodextrin for biological decontamination of cobalt. S.T.P. Pharma Sci. 2002;12:397–402.

25. Filon FL, Boeniger M, Maina G, Adami G, Spinelli P, Damian A. Skin absorption of inorganic lead (PbO) and the effect of skin cleansers. J Occup Environ Med. 2006;48:692–9. https://doi.org/10.1097/01.jom.0000214474.61563.1c.

26. Nielsen JB. Efficacy of skin wash on dermal absorption: an in vitro study on four model compounds of varying solubility. Int Arch Occup Environ Health. 2010;83:683–90. https://doi.org/10.1007/s00420-010-0546-y.

27. Thors L, Öberg L, Forsberg E, Wigenstam E, Larsson A, Bucht A. Skin penetration and decontamination efficacy following human skin exposure to fentanyl. Toxicol in Vitro. 2020;67:104914. https://doi.org/10.1016/j.tiv.2020.104914.

28. Wester RC, Maibach HI, Bucks DA, McMaster J, Mobayen M, Sarason R, Moore A. Percutaneous absorption and skin decontamination of PCBs: in vitro studies with human skin and in vivo studies in the rhesus monkey. J Toxicol Environ Health. 1990;31:235–46. https://doi.org/10.1080/15287399009531453.

29. Forsberg E, Öberg L, Artursson E, Wigenstam E, Bucht A, Thors L. Decontamination efficacy of soapy water and water washing following exposure of toxic chemicals on human skin. Cutan Ocul Toxicol. 2020;39:134–42. https://doi.org/10.1080/15569527.2020.1748046.

30. Noury B, Coman G, Blickenstaff N, Maibach H. In vitro skin decontamination model: comparison of salicylic acid and aminophylline. Cutan Ocul Toxicol. 2015;34:124–31. https://doi.org/10.3109/15569527.2014.913061.

31. Hewitt PG, Hotchkiss SA, Caldwell J. Decontamination procedures after in vitro topical exposure of human and rat skin to 4,4'-methylenebis[2-chloroaniline] and 4,4'-methylenedianiline. Fundam Appl Toxicol. 1995;26:91–8. https://doi.org/10.1006/faat.1995.1078.

32. Chan HP, Zhai H, Hui X, Maibach HI. Skin decontamination: principles and perspectives. Toxicol Ind Health. 2013;29:955–68. https://doi.org/10.1177/0748233712448112.
33. Bucks DAW, Guy RH, Maibach HI. Percutaneous penetration and mass balance accountability: technique and implications for dermatology. J Toxicol Cutan Ocul Toxicol. 1989;8:439–51. https://doi.org/10.3109/15569528909062949.
34. Wester RC, Maibach HI. In vivo percutaneous absorption and decontamination of pesticides in humans. J Toxicol Environ Health. 1985;16:25–37. https://doi.org/10.1080/15287398509530716.
35. Grice JE, Moghimi HR, Ryan E, Zhang Q, Haridass I, Mohammed Y, Roberts MS. Non-formulation parameters that affect penetrant-skin-vehicle interactions and percutaneous absorption. In: Percutaneous penetration enhancers drug penetration into/through the skin. Berlin: Springer; 2017. p. 45–75.
36. Bos JD, Meinardi MM. The 500 Dalton rule for the skin penetration of chemical compounds and drugs. Exp Dermatol. 2000;9:165–9. https://doi.org/10.1034/j.1600-0625.2000.009003165.x.
37. Hilton J, Woollen BH, Scott RC, Auton TR, Trebilcock KL, Wilks MF. Vehicle effects on in vitro percutaneous absorption through rat and human skin. Pharm Res. 1994;11:1396–400. https://doi.org/10.1023/a:1018931503784.
38. Nielsen JB. Effects of four detergents on the in-vitro barrier function of human skin. Int J Occup Environ Health. 2000;6:143–7. https://doi.org/10.1179/oeh.2000.6.2.143.
39. Ngo MA, Maibach HI. 15 Factors of percutaneous penetration of pesticides. In: Parameters for pesticide QSAR and PBPK/PD models for human risk assessment, vol. 1099. Washington, DC: American Chemical Society; 2012. p. 67–86.
40. Bettley FR, Donoghue E. Effect of soap on the diffusion of water through isolated human epidermis. Nature. 1960;185:17–20. https://doi.org/10.1038/185017a0.
41. Loke WK, U SH, Lau SK, Lim JS, Tay GS, Koh CH. Wet decontamination-induced stratum corneum hydration--effects on the skin barrier function to diethylmalonate. J Appl Toxicol. 1999;19:285–90. https://doi.org/10.1002/(sici)1099-1263(199907/08)19:4<285::aid-jat580>3.0.co;2-x.
42. Johnson W, Bergfeld WF, Belsito DV, Hill RA, Klaassen CD, Liebler DC, Marks JG, Shank RC, Slaga TJ, Snyder PW, Andersen FA. Safety assessment of benzyl alcohol, benzoic acid and its salts, and benzyl benzoate. Int J Toxicol. 2017;36(3 Suppl):5S–30S. https://doi.org/10.1177/1091581817728996.
43. Bjarnason S, Mikler J, Hill I, Tenn C, Garrett M, Caddy N, Sawyer TW. Comparison of selected skin decontaminant products and regimens against VX in domestic swine. Hum Exp Toxicol. 2008;27:253–61. https://doi.org/10.1177/0960327108090269.
44. Blaauboer BJ. Biokinetic modeling and in vitro-in vivo extrapolations. J Toxicol Environ Health B. 2010;13:242–52. https://doi.org/10.1080/10937404.2010.483940.
45. Zhu H, Maibach HI. Skin decontamination: a comprehensive clinical research guide. Berlin: Springer; 2020. https://doi.org/10.1007/978-3-030-24009-7.

Chapter 5
Skin Decontamination with Water: Evidence from In Vivo Animal Models

Anuk Burli, Nadia Kashetsky, Aileen M. Feschuk, Rebecca M. Law, and Howard I. Maibach

Introduction

Chemical dermal decontamination is defined as removal or neutralization of chemical contaminants from the skin [1]. Chemical contamination may occur from occupational exposure to toxic industrial chemicals (TICs) such as pesticides or exposure to chemical warfare agents (CWAs) first introduced in World War I and remaining a potential threat to society today [2]. Given these potential threats, determining the most effective and efficient decontamination strategies is vital to decrease morbidity and mortality in the event of exposure to TICs or CWAs.

A commonly accepted decontamination strategy includes the use of water or soap and water. Flushing with water is thought to work by diluting the contaminant, washing off the contaminant, decreasing the chemical reaction rate, decreasing tissue metabolism and inflammation, minimizing the chemical's hygroscopic effects of chemicals, and restoring the skin's normal pH [3]. The addition of soap, a metallic salt of a higher fatty acid, is recommended to assist decontamination of oily or lipophilic substances, as soap has both non-polar and polar molecules making it an

A. Burli (✉)
Faculty of Medicine and Dentistry, University of Rochester, Rochester, NY, USA
e-mail: anuk_burli@urmc.rochester.edu

N. Kashetsky
Faculty of Medicine, Memorial University, St. John's, NL, Canada

A. M. Feschuk
Faculty of Medicine, Memorial University of Newfoundland, St. John's, NL, Canada

R. M. Law
School of Pharmacy, Memorial University of Newfoundland, St. John's, NL, Canada

H. I. Maibach
Department of Dermatology, University of California San Francisco, San Francisco, CA, USA

© The Author(s), under exclusive license to Springer Nature
Switzerland AG 2022
A. M. Feschuk et al. (eds.), *Dermal Absorption and Decontamination*,
https://doi.org/10.1007/978-3-031-09222-0_5

emulsifier, capable of helping water mix with unmixable liquids [4, 5]. However, recent textbooks suggest that decontamination with soap and water may be incomplete (Wester et al. 2002). In fact, water washing may actually increase percutaneous penetration of chemical contaminants by a phenomenon known as the "wash-in effect," which therefore suggests washing may also increase systemic toxicity (Wester et al. 2002; [6]). Additionally, literature evaluating efficacy of decontamination using soap and water relies largely on in vitro experimentation. However, the applicability of in vitro experiments to in vivo situations is limited by in vitro skin structural changes and absence of blood flow, artificially affecting the rate of percutaneous penetration as well as difficulty of determining the effect of anatomical location [7].

Brent [8] summarized human clinical data on decontamination of corrosive dermal exposure and concluded that aggressive water lavage was associated with the best clinical outcomes, including decreased mortality and decreased tissue destruction [8]. However, the data included in the review was limited. Additionally, a systematic review by Kashetsky et al. [9] summarized the data on efficacy of water skin decontamination in vivo in human and concluded that a major void exists in in vivo human data confirming or denying the efficacy of decontamination with water [9]. Due to the limited availability of data involving clinical studies and human volunteer studies, studies utilizing animal models are next on the hierarchy of methodological approaches [8]. Hence, this systematic review summarizes animal in vivo experimental studies reporting decontamination with water and soap and water-based solutions.

Methods

The Preferred Reporting Items for Systematic Reviews and Meta-Analysis (PRISMA) guidelines were followed [10].

Search Strategy

On February 8, 2021, a literature search was conducted utilizing Covidence, Embase, MEDLINE, PubMed, Web of Science, and Google Scholar databases. Search terms included "cutaneous" or "skin" or "dermal" or "percutaneous" and "decontamination" or "decontaminant" or "skin decontamination." Date, geographical, or language restrictions were not used.

Eligibility

Articles were considered eligible if they were (1) experimental studies, (2) reporting chemical decontamination of the skin with water and/or soap and water solutions, (3) using in vivo animal subjects, and (4) reporting data in English language.

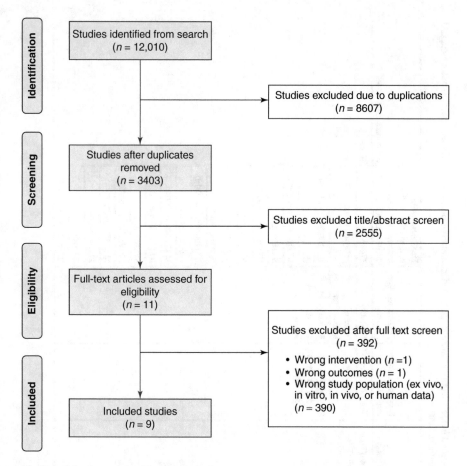

Fig. 5.1 Selection process for study inclusion

Data Screening

Title/abstract screening was completed by two independent researchers (R.L. and H.M.) with conflicts resolved by discussion with a third (A.B.). Full-text review was completed independently by two researchers (A.B. and N.K.), and conflicts were resolved by a third (A.F.). Relevant article references were manually searched to identify any additional studies.

Figure 5.1 demonstrates the data screening process.

Data Extraction and Analysis

Data extraction was completed by three independent researchers (N.K., A.B., A.F.) and verified by two independent researchers (H.M., R.L.). Data on study characteristics, animal models, chemical contaminants, decontamination, decontamination

Table 5.1 Decontamination category, paper, contaminant, animal model, decontamination method, decontamination analysis, decontamination outcomes, and additional conclusions of each paper included in this systematic review

Decontamination category	Paper	Contaminant	Animal model	Decontamination method	Decontamination analysis	Decontamination outcomes (mortality, incomplete, complete decontamination)	Additional conclusions
Water-only decontamination	Brown et al. [11]	Phenol, cumene hydroperoxide, phenol/acetone cleavage product, sodium hydroxide 45%, and sulfuric acid	Cartworth Form E rats (*n* = 10 each procedure)	Spraying water	Mortality	*Phenol*	None
				Quick wiping	Signs of intoxication	Spraying water:	
				Swabbing water 10, 20, 30, 45, 60, 90, and 120 s	Formation of necrotic areas/burns	ID (100.0%, *n* = 10/10)	
						Quick wiping:	
						ID (100.0%, *n* = 10/10)	
						Swabbing:	
						ID (98.6%, *n* = 69/70)	
						M (1.4%, *n* = 1/70)	
						Cumene hydroperoxide	
						Spraying water:	
						ID (100.0%, *n* = 10/10)	
						Quick wiping:	
						M (80.0%, *n* = 8/10)	
						ID (20.0%, *n* = 2/10)	
						Swabbing:	
						ID (95.7%, *n* = 67/70)	
						M (4.3%, *n* = 3/70)	
						Phenol/acetone	
						Spraying water:	
						ID (100.0%, *n* = 10/10)	

Quick wiping:			
M (90.0%, $n = 9/10$)			
ID (10.0%, $n = 1/10$)			
Swabbing:			
ID (82.9%, $n = 58/70$)			
M (17.1%, $n = 12/70$)			
Sodium hydroxide			
Spraying water:			
CD (70.0%, $n = 7/10$)			
ID (30.0%, $n = 3/10$)			
Quick wiping:			
CD (50.0%, $n = 5/10$)			
ID (50.0%, $n = 5/10$)			
Swabbing:			
ID $n = $ (94.3%, $n = 66/70$)			
CD (5.7%, $n = 4/70$)			
Sulfuric acid			
Spraying water:			
ID (100.0%, $n = 10/10$)			
Quick wiping:			
ID (100.0%, $n = 10/10$)			
Swabbing:			
ID (100.0%, $n = 70/70$)			

(continued)

Table 1.3 (continued)

Decontamination category	Paper	Contaminant	Animal model	Decontamination method	Decontamination analysis	Decontamination outcomes (mortality, incomplete, complete decontamination)	Additional conclusions
	Pullin et al. [12]	Phenol	Mixed breed swine (n = 4)	Plain-water shower	Concentration of blood plasma phenol	ID (100.0%, n = 4/4)	Although ID, authors concluded that "phenol concentration and retention time values substantially lower than corresponding values for the control group"
	Höjer et al. [13]	Hydrofluoric acid	Sprague-Dawley rats (n = 10)	Soap and water washing	Scoring severity of burns from 0 (no visible injury) to 5 (necrotic wounds covering the whole burn surface) daily for 5 days	ID (100.0%, n = 10/10)	Although ID, it was superior to the control (Statistical analysis not performed for controls)
Soap and water	Wester et al. [14]	Polychlorinated biphenyl: [14C]Aroclor 1242 in trichlorobenzene or mineral oil vehicle	Rhesus monkeys (n = 4)	Soap and water washes (13 protocols)	Carbon-14 analysis done by scintillation counting	CD (15.4%, n = 8/52), ID (84.5%, n = 44/52)	Decontamination is time-dependent with percutaneous absorption increasing and decontamination ability decreasing with time
	Bjarnason et al. [15]	VX	York-Landrace cross pigs (n = 4 each protocol)	Soapy water wash	Signs of poisoning; Mortality	30 min PE; CD (100.0%, n = 4/4); 45 min PE; ID (25.0%, n = 1/4); M (75.0%, n = 3/4)	Decontamination is time-dependent

Soap and water versus only water							
	Pelletier et al. [16]	2,4-Dichlorophenoxy-acetic acid dimethylamine salt	Fischer 344 rats (n = 4 each protocol)	Water washes (4 time intervals) Soap and water washes (four time intervals)	Blood samples Urinary excretion	Water-only: ID (100.0%, n = 16/16) Soap and water: ID (100.0%, n = 16/16)	No difference between soap and water and water
	Wester et al. [17]	Alachlor	Rhesus monkeys (n = 4 each protocol)	Soap and water Water	Scintillation counting	Water-only: ID (100.0%, n = 4/4) Soap and water: ID (100.0%, n = 4/4)	Authors concluded that "Decontamination with only water was less effective than with soap and water"
	Wester et al. [18]	Methylene bisphenyl isocyanate	Rhesus monkeys (n = 4 each protocol)	Soap and water (5% and 50%) or water (four time intervals each)	Scintillation counting	Soap and water: ID (100.0%, n = 32/32) Water-only: ID (100.0%, n = 16/16)	Statistical significance that 5% and 50% soapy water was better than water at 4 and 8 h No statistical difference between 5% and 50% soapy water at 4 and 8 h
	Monteiro-Riviere et al. [19]	Phenol	Yorkshire pigs (n = 6)	Water wash (1, 5, 15, or 30 min) Soap and water wash	Draize scoring system (including erythema and edema)	Water washes: ID (100.0%, n = 24/24) Soap and water: ID (100.0%, n = 6/6)	No significant difference was seen in mean erythema scores between treatments or sites Edema in the 1- and 5-min water wash was significantly less ($p < 0.05$) than the 30-min water wash

CD complete decontamination, *ID* incomplete decontamination, *M* mortality, *PE* post-exposure

analysis, and outcomes was extracted. Due to data heterogeneity, only a descriptive analysis was completed, and a meta-analysis was not performed. Data was categorized into studies using (1) water-only decontamination, (2) soap and water decontamination, and (3) both water-only and soap and water decontamination. Decontamination outcomes were sorted into three categories: (1) mortality, (2) incomplete decontamination, and (3) complete decontamination. Incomplete versus complete decontamination status was determined based on criteria established by individual studies.

Results

Study Characteristics

After title and abstract screening of 3310 studies and full-text review of 755 studies, nine studies met eligibility criteria. Collectively, these nine studies reported on 11 chemical contaminants and three animal models (Fig. 5.1, Table 5.1). Animal models included rhesus monkey, rat, and swine in 30.0% ($n = 3/9$) of studies each. Three studies included water-only decontamination data (33.3%, $n = 3/9$), two included soap and water decontamination data (22.2%, $n = 2/9$), and four included both water-only and soap and water protocol data (44.4%, $n = 4/9$). Table 5.1 summarizes the main characteristics of each study.

Water-Only Chemical Decontamination

Brown et al. [11] investigated decontamination of phenol, cumene hydroperoxide, a phenol/acetone cleavage product, sodium hydroxide 45%, and sulfuric acid from the skin of Cartworth Farm "E" strain rats ($n = 10$ each protocol) [11]. Contaminant was applied to the abdomen for 1 min before immediate decontamination by either spraying water over the contaminated area for 45 s, quick wiping, or swabbing for 10, 20, 30, 45, 60, 90, or 120 s using gauze or cotton tissue saturated with water. Decontamination was measured by monitoring symptoms including mortality, hematuria, convulsions, conditions of the skin, and miscellaneous symptoms. For phenol, spraying water achieved incomplete decontamination in $n = 10/10$ rats (hematuria, convulsions, and moderate burns), and quick wiping achieved incomplete decontamination in $n = 10/10$ (hematuria, convulsions, and severe black burns). Swabbing methods led to incomplete decontamination in $n = 69/70$ rats (convulsions, all protocols; hematuria, 10- to 45-s protocols; mild burns in the 120-s protocol to black severe burns in the 10-s swab). One mortality occurred in the 30-s swabbing method ($n = 1/50$). For cumene hydroperoxide, spraying with water had incomplete decontamination in $n = 10/10$ rats (mild burns, no hematuria, no convulsions). Quick wiping had mortality in $n = 8/10$ rats and incomplete decontamination in $n = 2/10$ (severe black burns, no convulsions, no hematuria). Swabbing methods achieved incomplete decontamination in $n = 67/70$ rats (mild to moderate burns, no hematuria, and no convulsions) and mortality in $n = 3/70$. For phenol/acetone, spraying with water achieved incomplete decontamination in $n = 10/10$ rats (mild burns, no mortality, no hematuria, no convulsions). Quick wiping resulted in mortality in $n = 9/10$ rats and incomplete decontamination in $n = 1/10$ (severe black burns, hematuria, convulsions). Swabbing methods achieved incomplete decontamination in $n = 58/70$ rats (hematuria, convulsions, and mild to severe burns) and mortality in $n = 12/70$. For sodium hydroxide and sulfuric acid, hematuria, convulsions, and mortality were not reported. For sodium hydroxide, as compared to control who had severe burns in $n = 10/10$ rats, spraying achieved no burns in $n = 7/10$ and mild burns in $n = 3/7$. Quick wiping resulted in severe burns in $n = 2/10$ rats, mild burns in $n = 3/10$, and no burns in $n = 5/5$. Swabbing methods between 10 s and 30 s had no burns in $n = 26/30$ rats and mild burns in $n = 4/30$ and between 45 s and 120 s had no burns in $n = 40/40$. Finally, for sulfuric acid recipients, when compared to the control (severe necrotic burns in $n = 10/10$ rats), the quick wipe and 10-s swab had severe burns in $n = 20/20$; the spray and the 20- to 45-s swabs had moderate burns in $n = 40/40$; and the 60- to 120-s swab had mild burns in $n = 30/30$.

Höjer et al. [13] decontaminated 50% hydrofluoric acid (HF) from the skin of Sprague-Dawley rats ($n = 10$), applied to the back with standard filter paper soaked in the contaminant (dose, 0.1 mL) for 3 min [13]. At 30 s post-exposure, the skin was rinsed with 500 mL of water for 3 min. Decontamination was analyzed by scoring burn severity from 0 (no visible injury) to 5 (necrotic wounds covering the whole burn surface) daily for 5 days. After decontamination, the highest and lowest mean severity of burn scores were 2.90 at Day 2 and 2.40 at Day 5 (two, distinct erythema; three, distinct erythema plus wounds of discolored spots). In comparison, the control group ($n = 5$) had daily mean severity of burn scores of 5. Although decontamination was incomplete, it was concluded that washing HF from the skin as quickly as possible is of utmost importance, evident by comparison between water decontamination as compared to the control.

Pullin et al. [12] decontaminated phenol from the skin of mixed breed swine ($n = 4$), applied to 35–40% body surface area (dose, 500 mg/kg) [12]. After 1 min, decontamination for 15 min using a plain-water shower (volume flow rate, 100 L/min; temperature, room temperature) was completed in $n = 4$ swine. Three swine were designated controls and did not receive decontamination. Decontamination was analyzed by concentration of blood plasma phenol measured using gas chromatography. Dermal and systemic effects including tremors, twitching, dilated pupils, salivation, nasal discharge, dyspnea, convulsions, coma, cyanosis, number of deaths/number of animals, dermal necrosis, and recovery time were also recorded. Immediately after decontamination, all animals ($n = 4$) showed immediate signs of toxicity, including muscular twitching and tremors. At 2–3 h after exposure, animals began to recover and at 24 h were functioning normally. No skin discoloration was noted, and dermal necrosis was slight to moderate. No animals in the water decontamination group died, whereas two out of three of the control animals did. The peak phenol plasma concentration was 24.2 ppm at 15 min post-exposure. However, mean plasma phenol concentration in the decontamination group was significantly lower than the control group. The control group hit a peak plasma phenol concentration of approximately 55 ppm at approximately 2 h post-exposure. Pullin concluded that decontamination was incomplete as phenol was absorbed rapidly.

Soap and Water

Wester et al. [14] decontaminated polychlorinated biphenyls (PCBs) from the skin of adult female rhesus monkeys (n = 4) [14]. The contaminant, [^{14}C]Aroclor 1242 in trichlorobenzene or mineral oil, was applied to abdominal skin (dose, 2 μL vehicle/cm containing 4 μg/cm^2 PCBs; area, 1 cm^2). At 0, 10, and 15 min and 1, 3, 6, and 24 h, the skin was washed five times using soap (20% v/v Ivory liquid soap/water) and water washing. Decontamination efficacy was measured with carbon-14 analysis by scintillation counting. For the trichlorobenzene vehicle, no difference in decontamination occurred between 0 and 1 h with percent applied dose removed ranging from 92 ± 8% to 102 ± 7%. However, the applied dose removed decreased at 3 h to 74 ± 12% and continued to decrease until only 25 ± 19% was removed at 24 h. For the mineral oil vehicle, no difference in decontamination occurred between 0 and 1 h with percent applied dose removed ranging from 63 ± 4% to 72 ± 8%. Applied dose removed also decreased at 3 h to 49 ± 3% and continued to decrease until only 26 ± 7% was removed at 24 h. Wester concluded that soap and water washing was remarkably effective at removing PCBs from the skin. Additionally, the authors concluded that chemical removal is time-dependent with irreversibility increasing with time due to increased percutaneous absorption with time.

Bjarnason et al. [15] decontaminated the chemical warfare agent, VX, from the skin of York-Landrace cross pigs (n = 4), applied to the ventral ear (dose, 5× the median lethal dose) [15]. At 30 and 45 min, decontamination with soapy water (25 oz. of Dawn™ in 32 gallons of distilled water) was completed by rubbing decontaminant infused into foam pads over the contaminated site for 10 s. Decontamination was assessed by reduction in sign of poisoning and mortality. Soapy water was effective in decontaminating 5× LD50 VX at 30 min post-exposure, and the test animals displayed few signs of serious poisoning. However, soapy water was ineffective in decontamination of 5× LD50 VX at 45 min post-exposure. Three of the four animals in this test group died. Additionally, by termination of the experimental period (6 h post-exposure), the fourth animal appeared to be near death. Bjarnason et al. concluded that using soap and water as a decontaminant against VX is time-dependent, as it was effective in preventing mortality when applied 30 min post-exposure, but not when applied 45 min post-exposure.

Soap and Water Versus Water

Pelletier et al. [16] decontaminated 2,4-dichlorophenoxyacetic acid dimethylamine salt (2,4-D amine) from the skin of Fischer 344 rats ($n = 4$), applied to the mid-dorsal area [16]. At 7, 8, 23, and 24 h, decontamination with either soap and water (0.25% Ivory soap) or water-only occurred. Decontamination was measured by analysis of ^{14}C-labelled 2,4-D amine in skin samples, blood samples, and urinary excretion. Skin sample, blood sample, and urinary excretion analysis showed statistical insignificance between soap and water and water-only methods. Blood sample analysis at 8 h showed a mean 2,4-D amine concentration of 0.019 ± 0.004% with soap and water methods versus 0.020 ± 0.003% with water-only. Urinary excretion analysis at 8 h showed the percent of 2,4-D amine dose was 8.8 ± 2.0% vs. 12.1 ± 1.3%. There were no significant differences between soap and water and water-only with regard to blood and urinary concentration.

Wester et al. [17] decontaminated alachlor from the skin of rhesus monkeys ($n = 4$), applied to the abdomen [17]. Alachlor was applied either in Lasso® (a brand of alachlor made by Monsanto) diluted 1:20 with water or in Lasso® diluted 1:29 with water. At 12 h, decontamination occurred with three successive soap and water washes (10% Ivory liquid 1:1 v/v with water) or water-only washes. Decontamination was analyzed by the amount of alachlor removed from the skin measured by scintillation counting. The first soap and water wash removed 73.2 ± 15.8% from the abdomen, with a total of 82.3 ± 14.8% removed after three washes. In contrast, water-only performed significantly inferior to soap and water, removing 36.6 ± 12.3% on the first wash and a total of 56.0 ± 14.0 after three washes. Both soap and water and water-only methods resulted in incomplete alachlor decontamination. However, soap and water was significantly ($p < 0.01$) more effective than water-only decontamination.

Similarly, Wester et al. [18] decontaminated methylene bisphenyl isocyanate (MDI) from the skin of rhesus monkeys ($n = 4$), applied to the abdomen [18]. At designated times (5 min, 1 h, 4 h, and 8 h post-exposure), decontamination occurred with five washes of either water-only, 5% soap in water, or 50% soap in water and a cotton applicator. Decontamination was analyzed by scintillation counting and by examining removal of contaminant with ten successive tape strips following skin washes. At 5 min, water-only decontamination removed 60 ± 11.1% of contaminant, 5% soap in water removed 71.2 ± 5.2%, and 50% soap in water removed 67.3 ± 9.6%. At 8 h of exposure, only 29.2 ± 9.7%, 36.6 ± 12.8%, and 45.7 ± 6.6% were removed, respectively. For tape strip analysis, after washing with water at 5 min versus 8 h, recovery of mean ^{14}C-MDI radioactivity increased from 18.2 ± 9.5% to 56.3 ± 9.3%. After 5% soap and water washing, recovery increased from 11.9 ± 5.9% to 36.8 ± 7.0%, and after 50% soap and water washing, recovery increased from 3.6 ± 2.4% to 24.4 ± 10.4%. Wester concluded skin residence time is an important factor for decontamination and it is best to wash the skin as soon as decontamination occurs. In addition, although soap and water and water-only decontamination was incomplete, soap and water was more effective than water-only decontamination ($p < 0.05$). The 50% soap wash was more effective initially than 5% soap ($p < 0.05$).

Monteiro-Riviere et al. [19] decontaminated 89% aqueous phenol from Yorkshire pigs ($n = 6$), applied to the dorsum using Hill Top® chambers at ten sites for 1 min (dose, 400 μL) [19]. Decontamination occurred immediately with either a 1-, 5-, 15-, or 30-min water wash or a 1-min water, 1-min soap (Ivory soap), or 4-min water wash (3×). Decontamination was assessed using the Draize scoring system based on erythema and edema pre-phenol exposure, post-phenol exposure, and post-decontamination and at 1, 3, 5, and 8 h [20]. The 8-h mean erythema values were designated to represent effectiveness of decontamination protocols. Mean erythema values ± standard error of the mean (SEM) were 3.0 ± 0.3, 3.3 ± 0.2, 3.0 ± 0.0, 3.2 ± 0.2, and 2.7 ± 0.3 for 1-min, 5-min, 15-min, and 30-min water washes and the soap and water wash, respectively (two, well-defined erythema; three, moderate to severe erythema). There were no significant differences in mean erythema score between treatments or sites. Mean edema ± SEM values were 0.0 ± 0.0, 0.0 ± 0.0, 0.7 ± 0.2, 0.8 ± 0.3, and 0.7 ± 0.2 for the 1-min, 5-min, 15-min, and 30-min water washes and the soap and water wash, respectively (one, very slight edema; two, slight edema with raised margin). Edema in the 1- and 5-min water wash was significantly less ($p < 0.05$) than the 30-min water wash. Additionally, biopsy specimens showed the following morphological features after all water-only washes, "mild to severe intracellular epidermal edema, mild intercellular epidermal edema, mild papillary dermal edema, mild to moderate perivascular infiltrates, moderate to severe numbers of basal pyknotic cells, and focal epidermal–dermal separation," and water-only washes except the 30-min water wash showed epidermal and collagen necrosis. Sites treated with soap and water showed "severe intracellular epidermal edema, mild intercellular edema, moderate perivascular cellular infiltrate, moderate to high numbers of basal pyknotic cells, and occasional focal epidermal–dermal separation" [19]. Monteiro-Riviere et al. concluded that the decontamination protocols reduced but did not eliminate the systemic phenol exposure.

Discussion

This systematic review summarizes experimental studies reporting decontamination data with water-only and soap and water solutions in in vivo animal studies. Phenol was the most commonly reported contaminant in 33.3% ($n = 3/9$) of studies. Water-only decontamination solutions led to complete decontamination in 3.1% ($n = 16/524$) of protocols, incomplete decontamination in 90.6% ($n = 475/524$) of protocols, and mortality in 6.3% ($n = 33/524$) of protocols; and soap and water decontamination solutions led to complete decontamination in 6.9% ($n = 8/116$) of protocols, incomplete decontamination in 92.2% ($n = 107/116$) of protocols, and mortality in 6.9% ($n = 8/116$) of protocols. Incomplete decontamination increases the possibility of percutaneous penetration and systemic exposure of toxic dermal chemicals.

There has been recent research regarding the potential mechanisms behind each decontamination agent. Decontamination using water is thought to be effective via one or more mechanisms including (1) diluting the chemical or toxic agent, (2) rinsing off the chemical agent, (3) decreasing the rate of chemical reaction, (4) decreasing tissue metabolism and inflammation, (5) minimizing the ability of the toxin to remove moisture, and (6) restoring normal skin pH [21]. The ideal decontamination agent should be sterile to avoid infection, hypertonic to avoid tissue damage, amphoteric to neutralize acidic or basic chemicals, water-soluble, and non-toxic [21]. Soap is often added to this decontamination method because of its ability to solubilize lipophilic substances through the formation of micelles, which engulf lipophilic substances and are then washed away by water. Water and soap satisfy many criteria listed above, but it is important to ensure that the water is non-toxic [21].

Efficacy of decontamination using soap and water depends upon the properties of the specific contaminant. This review studied nine publications that collectively studied various toxins. The most studied was phenol ($n = 3/9$). The other toxins tested were VX, phenol/acetone, cumene hydroperoxide, sodium hydroxide, sulfuric acid, polychlorinated biphenyls, 2,4-dichlorophenoxyacetic acid dimethylamine salt, alachlor, methylene bisphenyl isocyanate, and hydrofluoric acid, each in one study. Sodium hydroxide had the smallest molecular weight (39.997 g/mol) and polychlorinated biphenyl the largest molecular weight (326.4 g/mol). VX had the lowest melting point (−38.02 °F) and sodium hydroxide the highest (604.4 °F). Decontamination of VX was time-dependent, and PCB was able to be completely decontaminated, but still in a time-dependent fashion. Some studies showed water achieved complete decontamination, while others found water-only able to achieve incomplete sodium hydroxide decontamination. Further research must be done to examine how molecular weight, hydrogen bonds, volatility, and melting point of the contaminant affect the choice of decontamination agent and method.

Additionally, water-soluble chemicals were removed at the same rate with both water and water with soap, whereas lipid-soluble molecules were better removed by soap and water (Wester et al. 2002). Four articles compared water-only versus soap and water decontamination efficacy of alachlor, 2,4-dichlorophenoxyacetic acid, and methylene bisphenyl isocyanate, which all have minimal water solubility. However, soap and water were significantly better in the decontamination of alachlor and methylene bisphenyl isocyanate.

Conversely, no significant difference was found between soap and water and just water in the decontamination of 2,4-dichlorophenoxyacetic acid. A possible explanation for this includes that the experimental protocol in the Brown et al. [11] study did not include both the "rubbing" and "solvent" action, which affects the decontamination efficacy of soap and water [11]. Furthermore, studies involving alachlor and methylene bisphenyl isocyanate focused on rhesus monkey, an animal model with arguably greater applicability to human in vivo studies than rats, which were used in Brown et al. [11]. It is possible that by using a rat model, tissue metabolism differs greatly from human tissue, thereby affecting the decontamination ability of soap and water. However, soap and water and just water were equally effective in phenol decontamination, which is water-soluble. Additionally, incomplete decontamination using water-only and soap and water for phenol occurs as phenol forms a coagulated protein layer which can interfere with the ability of other liquids to penetrate the skin [22].

Many studies showed that efficacy of decontamination depends on chemical contaminant skin residence time. The longer a chemical or toxin remains on the skin, the more likely percutaneous penetration will begin, allowing the substance to be absorbed into the skin and reach systemic circulation [6]. At this point, decontamination removal plateaus [23]. Only some in vivo studies regarding decontamination efficacy have compared immediate versus delayed decontamination [24]. By studying decontamination efficacy after an extended time period, soap and water would be at a limited decontaminating capacity and no longer be able to effectively remove toxins. Furthermore, decreased availability of the contaminating agent at the surface leads to further decrease in decontaminating agent effectiveness. Additionally, only some studies included both a "rubbing" component and a "solvent" component, helping facilitate desquamation of the stratum corneum, especially with cells undergoing exfoliation, washing away the toxin with it [14]. In addition, increasing the soap concentration and the length of cleansing time can affect decontamination [23].

The heterogeneity of articles included here is an important limitation of determining efficacy of water-only and soap and water decontamination. Firstly, the way in which water-only and soap and water was used as a decontaminating agent was not standardized between articles. The number of washes, washing fashion, washing time, and water temperature are potentially clinically relevant variables [25]. Another inconsistency between articles includes the use of different animal models. Several factors that can affect percutaneous penetration, and therefore, decontamination, differ between animal species. Each animal has different stratum corneum thickness, amount of hair, and number and composure of sweat glands. Furthermore, the relative age, or the point in the animals' life span when tested, was not standardized between studies. Relative age has an effect on skin barrier function involved in percutaneous penetration [23]. Finally, some studies utilized tape stripping, which can disrupt the epidermal barrier, which enhances the delivery of drugs and various decontamination agents. This is an inconsistency between studies that can lead to differential decontamination outcomes [26].

Furthermore, only Pullin et al. [12], Pelletier et al. [16], and Wester et al. [14] analyzed the pharmacokinetics of dermal decontamination by measuring the amount of contaminant in blood and/or excreted urine samples [12, 16, 27]. Other studies did not observe absorption, metabolism, distribution, and excretion of toxins and contaminants. Water and soap work by influencing metabolism and affecting chemical reactions [21]. Therefore, it is imperative to include this information to find the best decontaminating agent for each toxin.

The field of dermal decontamination is relatively new and ever evolving. Despite this, this review investigated studies dating back 46 years, namely, Brown et al. [11] studied the use of swabbing vs. spraying for decontamination [11]. A more contemporary article proposed a triple decontamination method using various chemicals and rubbing, similar to the swabbing method. Both these approaches require contemporary follow-up [28].

Several additional limitations of this review must be considered. Firstly, small sample sizes increase the influence of confounding variables and outliers. Secondly, as described above, data heterogeneity in contaminants, methods of applications and location of application, decontamination solutions, animal models, washing techniques, and analysis of pharmacokinetics must be considered. Thirdly, the applicability of each animal model to humans differs. No in vivo animal model can be fully representative of human physiology and pharmacokinetics. Therefore, data collected through in vivo animal model studies can be extrapolated to make generalization about in vivo effects in humans but should never be considered fully conclusive. The rhesus monkey is the preferred animal model, followed by pigs and finally by guinea pigs and mice [29].

Previous manuscripts have discussed the comparison of in vitro mathematical models to estimate percutaneous penetration of various compounds using the widely used Potts and Guy model to in vitro laboratory data [30]. Currently, there is a lack of available in vivo human laboratory data for stimulants for chemical warfare agents. We hope that this manuscript encourages further investigation in this area.

Regulatory agencies who monitor decontamination efficacy of various agents have particular interest in the "parallelogram" approach which includes in vitro data to estimate human dermal absorption. The "parallelogram" approach focuses on the area under the curve of a genotoxic metabolite in human, which is challenging to measure. This can be obtained by extrapolating from measured protein adduct levels of that toxic metabolite formed in mice and rat models in addition with comparison of in vitro formation/elimination of the metabolite in humans and the studied rodent model [31, 32]. Further research should be conducted using this approach for chemical warfare agents discussed in this manuscript.

Conclusion

Water-only and soap and water are considered a gold standard for decontamination due to their availability and low cost. However, this study found that the majority of data on in vivo animal data shows decontamination with water-only and/or soap and water is incomplete, and a major gap in data on decontamination using soap and water still exists. As shown in this manuscript, there is room for considerable improvement for research regarding advanced efficacy of decontamination protocols. In order to determine the most effective decontaminant for occupational safety, research involving in vitro data, in silico assays, and systematic reviews focusing on each widely used decontaminating agent must be conducted. Furthermore, more in vivo studies using humans, when feasible, must be conducted, as there are limitations which hinder the applicability of conclusions formed using in vivo animal studies and in vitro data. Although the field of dermal decontamination is moving rapidly, we have insufficient data for standard decontamination protocols to produce various mathematical models (QSAR). We believe that developing standardized protocols that will allow comparison from one laboratory to another will greatly accelerate the development of mathematical models. Furthermore, it is highly unlikely that there will be sufficient human volunteers, nor ethical approval, for studies regarding highly potent chemical warfare agents, and hence, we will depend on the simulants for chemical warfare agents.

Additionally, much more is to be learned about the wide variety of contaminants and their chemical properties. It is reasonable that there may be a generally useful decontamination system. However, it is also likely that certain chemicals such as hydrofluoric acid might require a special decontamination system. We believe that the decontamination scenario will be different for those situations in which one can get immediate decontamination, but we need to evaluate efficacy for the common circumstance where decontamination is delayed. Finally, more data assessing pharmacokinetic parameters such as absorption, metabolism, distribution, and excretion is of utmost importance in the field of occupational dermatology and toxicology.

Acknowledgments We thank Dr. Howard I. Maibach and Dr. Rebecca M. Law for all their coaching throughout this project.

The authors of this chapter would like to acknowledge the original source of publication, Taylor & Francis Online, whose website can be accessed via the following link: https://www.tandfonline.com/. The original publication of this chapter can be found via the following link: https://doi.org/10.1080/10937404.2021.1943087.

Funding None.

Declaration of Interest Statement The authors declare that they have no known competing financial interests or personal relationships that could have appeared to influence the work reported in this paper.

References

1. Clarkson ED, Gordon RK. Rapid decontamination of chemical warfare agents from skin. In: Handbook of toxicology of chemical warfare agents. London: Academic Press; 2020. https://doi.org/10.1016/b978-0-12-819090-6.00073-8.
2. RSDL. About RSDL. 2021. https://www.rsdl.com/about-rsdl/#history. Accessed 26 Feb 2021.
3. Bromberg BE, Song IC, Walden RH. Hydrotherapy of chemical burns. Plast Reconstr Surg. 1965;35(1):85–95. https://doi.org/10.1097/00006534-196501000-00010.
4. Chilcott RP, Larner J, Matar H. UK's initial operational response and specialist operational response to CBRN and HazMat incidents: a primer on decontamination protocols for healthcare professionals. Emerg Med J. 2019;36(2):117–23. https://doi.org/10.1136/emermed-2018-207562.
5. Jordon JW, Dolce FA, Osborne ED. Dermatitis of the hands in housewives. J Am Med Assoc. 1940;115(12):1001–6. https://doi.org/10.1001/jama.1940.02810380031007.
6. Moody RP, Maibach HI. Skin decontamination: importance of the wash-in effect. Food Chem Toxicol. 2006;44(11):1783–8. https://doi.org/10.1016/j.fct.2006.05.020.

7. Joosen MJA, van den Berg RM, de Jong AL, van der Schans MJ, Noort D, Langenberg JP. The impact of skin decontamination on the time window for effective treatment of percutaneous VX exposure. Chem Biol Interact. 2017;267(SI):48–56. https://doi.org/10.1016/j.cbi.2016.02.001.
8. Brent J. Water-based solutions are the best decontaminating fluids for dermal corrosive exposures: a mini review. Clin Toxicol. 2013;51(8):731–6. https://doi.org/10.3109/1556365 0.2013.838628.
9. Kashetsky N, Law RM, Maibach HI. Efficacy of water skin decontamination in vivo in humans: a systematic review. J Appl Toxicol. 2022;42(3):346.
10. Moher D, Liberati A, Tetzlaff J, et al. Preferred reporting items for systematic reviews and meta-analyses: the PRISMA statement. PLoS Med. 2009;6(7):e1000097. https://doi.org/10.1371/journal.pmed.1000097.
11. Brown VKH, Box VL, Simpson BJ. Decontamination procedures for skin exposed to phenolic substances. Arch Environ Health. 1975;30(1):1–6. https://doi.org/10.1080/00039896.197 5.10666623.
12. Pullin TG, Pinkerton MN, Johnston RV, Kilian DJ. Decontamination of skin of swine following phenol exposure - comparison of relative efficacy of water versus polyethylene glycol-industrial methylated spirits. Toxicol Appl Pharmacol. 1978;43(1):199–206. https://doi.org/10.1016/S0041-008X(78)80044-1.
13. Höjer J, Personne M, Hultén P, Ludwigs U. Topical treatments for hydrofluoric acid burns: a blind controlled experimental study. J Toxicol Clin Toxicol. 2002;40(7):861–6. https://doi.org/10.1081/CLT-120016957.
14. Wester RC, Maibach HI, Bucks DAW, et al. Percutaneous absorption and skin decontamination of pcbs: in vitro studies with human skin and in vivo studies in the rhesus monkey. J Toxicol Environ Health. 1990;31(4):235–46. https://doi.org/10.1080/15287399009531453.
15. Bjarnason S, Mikler J, Hill I, et al. Comparison of selected skin decontaminant products and regimens against VX in domestic swine. Hum Exp Toxicol. 2008;27(3):253–61. https://doi.org/10.1177/0960327108090269.
16. Pelletier O, Ritter L, Caron J. Effects of skin preapplication treatments and postapplication cleansing agents on dermal absorption of 2, 4-dichlorophenoxyacetic acid dimethylamine by fischer 344 rats. J Toxicol Environ Health. 1990;31(4):247–60. https://doi.org/10.1080/15287399009531454.
17. Wester RC, Melendres J, Maibach HI. In vivo percutaneous absorption and skin decontamination of alachlor in rhesus monkey. J Toxicol Environ Health. 1992;36(1):01–12. https://doi.org/10.1080/15287399209531619.
18. Wester RC, Hui XY, Landry T, Maibach HI. In vivo skin decontamination of methylene bisphenyl isocyanate (MDI): soap and water ineffective compared to polypropylene glycol, polyglycol-based cleanser, and corn oil. Toxicol Sci. 1999;48(1):1–4.
19. Monteiro-Riviere NA, Inman AO, Jackson H, Dunn B, Dimond S. Efficacy of topical phenol decontamination strategies on severity of acute phenol chemical burns and dermal absorption: in vitro and in vivo studies in pig skin. Toxicol Ind Health. 2001;17(4):95–104. https://doi.org/10.1191/0748233701th095oa.
20. Draize JH, Woodard G, Calvery HO. Methods for the study of irritation and toxicity of substances applied topically to the skin and mucous membranes. J Pharmacol Exp Ther. 1944;82:377–90.
21. Hall AH, Maibach HI. Water decontamination of chemical skin/eye splashes: a critical review. Cutan Ocul Toxicol. 2006;25(2):67–83. https://doi.org/10.1080/15569520600695520.
22. Conning DM, Hayes MJ. The dermal toxicity of phenol: an investigation of the most effective first-aid measures. Br J Ind Med. 1970;27(2):155–9. https://doi.org/10.1136/oem.27.2.155.
23. Maibach HI, Wester RC. Percutaneous absorption: in vivo methods in humans and animals. J Am Coll Toxicol. 1989;8(5):803–13. https://doi.org/10.3109/10915818909018039.

24. Braue EH Jr, Smith KH, Doxzon BF, Lumpkin HL, Clarkson ED. Efficacy studies of reactive skin decontamination lotion, M291 skin decontamination kit, 0.5% bleach, 1% soapy water, and skin exposure reduction paste against chemical warfare agents, Part 2: Guinea pigs challenged with soman. Cutan Ocul Toxicol. 2011;30(1):29–37. https://doi.org/10.3109/15569527.2010.515281.
25. Brouwer DH, Boeniger MF, Van Hemmen J. Hand wash and manual skin wipes. Ann Occup Hyg. 2000;44(7):501–10. https://doi.org/10.1093/annhyg/44.7.501.
26. Choi MJ, Zhai H, Löffler H, Dreher F, Maibach HI. Effect of tape stripping on percutaneous penetration and topical vaccination. Exog Dermatol. 2003;2:262–9. https://doi.org/10.1159/000078695.
27. Wester RC, Maibach HI. Dermal decontamination and percutaneous absorption. Boca Raton, FL: Taylor and Francis Inc.; 2002. https://www.taylorfrancis.com/books/e/9780429186493/chapters/10.1201/9780849359033-23. Accessed 11 Dec 2020.
28. Elmahdy A, Cao Y, Hui X, Maibach H. Follicular pathway role in chemical warfare simulants percutaneous penetration. J Appl Toxicol. 2020;41:964. https://doi.org/10.1002/jat.4081.
29. Bronaugh RL, Maibach HI. Percutaneous absorption: drugs, cosmetics, mechanisms, methods. 4th ed. London: Routledge; 2005. https://www.routledge.com/Percutaneous-Absorption-Drugs-Cosmetics-Mechanisms-Methods/Bronaugh-Dragicevic-Maibach/p/book/9781574448696. Accessed 26 Feb 2021.
30. Burli A, Law RM, Rodriguez J, Maibach HI. Organic compounds percutaneous penetration in vivo in man: relationship to mathematical predictive model. Regul Toxicol Pharmacol. 2020;112:104614. https://doi.org/10.1016/j.yrtph.2020.104614.
31. Allen DG, Rooney J, Kleinstreuer N, Lowit A, Perron M. Retrospective analysis of dermal absorption triple pack data. ALTEX. 2021;38:463. https://doi.org/10.14573/altex.2101121.
32. Motwani HV, Frostne C, Törnqvist M. Parallelogram based approach for in vivo dose estimation of genotoxic metabolites in humans with relevance to reduction of animal experiments. Sci Rep. 2017;7:17560. https://doi.org/10.1038/s41598-017-17692-5.

Chapter 6
Skin Decontamination with Water: Evidence from In Vitro Animal Models

Maxwell Green, Nadia Kashetsky, Aileen M. Feschuk, and Howard I. Maibach

Introduction

Chemical dermal decontamination is defined as removal or neutralization of chemical contaminants from the skin [1]. Skin contamination can occur from various chemical exposures, including exposures at the workplace or from chemical warfare. Chemical warfare continues to be of increasing concern as terrorist groups have the potential to misuse these compounds worldwide [2]. With ever-growing concerns, it is important to identify the best strategies for both rapid and effective dermal decontamination. The current PRISMA guidance for dermal decontamination outlines a protocol in which anyone contaminated should immediately evacuate the scene, disrobe all clothes, and be sprayed by a "ladder pipe system" made of two fire pumps that rinse them with large amounts of water [3].

As many as 20 clinically relevant factors have been identified in affecting percutaneous absorption that are important to consider in decontamination strategies [4]. However, the most conventional strategy for decontamination, though, still remains washing with water and/or soap and water. This strategy, however, may actually increase percutaneous absorption of chemicals through the "wash-in effect" and thus cause increased systemic effects [5]. Water and/or soap and water may then result in incomplete decontamination and decontamination inferior to that of other methods. Regardless of decontamination method used, many studies, including that

M. Green (✉)
Tulane University School of Medicine, New Orleans, LA, USA
e-mail: mgreen15@tulane.edu

N. Kashetsky · A. M. Feschuk
Faculty of Medicine, Memorial University of Newfoundland, St. John's, NL, Canada

H. I. Maibach
Department of Dermatology, University of California San Francisco, San Francisco, CA, USA

© The Author(s), under exclusive license to Springer Nature Switzerland AG 2022
A. M. Feschuk et al. (eds.), *Dermal Absorption and Decontamination*,
https://doi.org/10.1007/978-3-031-09222-0_6

conducted by Magnano et al. [6], have suggested that the most efficient way to reduce intoxication by dermal contamination is by incorporating rapid decontamination strategies [6].

Experimental studies comparing water and/or soap and water to other decontamination methods using in vitro animal models have been limited. Brent [7] concluded through their review of clinical studies that aggressive water lavage was the best method for human corrosive dermal exposures; however, this review did not compare water lavage to other decontamination methods [7]. Kashetsky et al. [8] summarized available in vivo human model data investigating decontamination with water-only and soap and water solutions, finding that water alone achieved complete decontamination in only 52.6% of decontamination outcomes, whereas soap and water provided partial decontamination in 92.9% of decontamination outcomes [8]. Kashetsky et al. [8] concluded that water-only and soap and water solutions provided incomplete decontamination. Similarly, reviews by Burli et al. [9] and Chiang et al. [10] investigated water-only and soap and water solutions for decontamination of chemicals in in vivo animal models and in vitro human models, respectively, all concluding that these solutions yield incomplete decontamination. These other reviews in the series did not focus on in vitro animal models which may provide great benefit for the future of dermal decontamination studies. In vitro animal models, if they provide similar results to other models, allow research to be performed in a more controlled chemical environment, provide less risk to both animals and humans, and may lower the cost of conducting research. Although in vivo animal models provide the greatest confidence levels, these benefits may allow greater advancement in dermal decontamination research. Thus, this systematic review summarizes water and/or soap and water decontamination when compared to other solutions using in vitro animal models.

Methods

The Preferred Reporting Items for Systematic Reviews and Meta-Analysis (PRISMA) guidelines were used to guide the methodology and reporting (Fig. 6.1) [11]. On December 11, 2020, a comprehensive database search was conducted using Embase, PubMed, MEDLINE, Web of Science, and Google Scholar. The search terms "cutaneous" or "skin" or "dermal" or "percutaneous" and "decontamination" or "decontaminant" or "skin decontamination" were used. There were no language, geographical, or date restrictions used to limit the articles. Articles were included if they met the following five criteria: chemical decontamination of the skin, decontamination with water and/or soap and water with quantitative data provided, experimental studies, data in English language, and in vitro animal models. The original pool of 363 articles pulled from database searches included reviews and experiments conducted across all models and were cut to the five articles included if they provided quantitative experimental data on in vitro animal models.

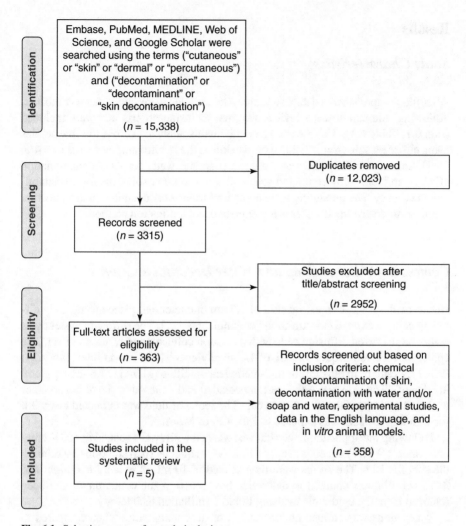

Fig. 6.1 Selection process for study inclusion

The data were pulled from the literature by one researcher (M.G.) and verified by two others (N.K., A.F.). Articles were screened using title and abstract reviews for inclusion. Conflicts surrounding data extraction were discussed and resolved by an additional independent researcher (H.M.). Data collected included the type of skin contaminant, concentration of contaminant, type of in vitro animal model used, number of models, decontamination solutions used, method of decontamination, and outcomes observed. Only descriptive analyses were conducted due to the heterogeneity between outcomes reported across studies.

Results

Study Characteristics

After the comprehensive database search, 363 articles were pulled from databases. Following title and abstract review, five met inclusion criteria and were included (Fig. 6.1, Table 6.1). There were 11 contaminants analyzed across the five studies using either rat skin ($n = 1/5$, 20%) or pig skin as the in vitro animal model ($n = 4/5$, 80%). One study compared water only to soap and water for its decontamination efficacy, and one study compared soap and water to other solutions for decontamination efficacy. The remaining three compared water-only decontamination to other solutions to determine if water is a complete decontamination method.

Comparing Water to Soap and Water Decontamination

Hewitt et al. (1995) clipped rat skin of 1.7 cm diameter and placed samples in diffusion cells to expose the skin to the contaminants [12]. The diffusion system was composed of seven diffusion cells with a fraction collector and water collector. The epidermis received aliquots of 5 µL of 4,4′-methylenebis[2-chloroaniline] (MbOCA) (9.7–17.7 µg/cm^2 in ethanol) or 4,4′-methylenedianiline (MDA) (17.6–21.6 µg/cm^2 in ethanol). The skin was either left unoccluded and exposed to the atmosphere or occluded and covered with a Teflon cap. The receptor fluid was collected every 2 h for 72 h that the skin was exposed to MbOCA or MDA.

Following the application, the skin was washed with swabs soaked in 100% ethanol, water, 1% (v/v) aqueous soap, or 10% (v/v) aqueous soap solutions by rubbing the skin for 10 s. The swabs were then soaked in 10 mL of ethanol overnight and 3×1 mL aliquots counted to determine how much of the contaminant had been removed from the epidermis by using liquid scintillation technology.

Water alone was an incomplete method of decontamination when compared to 10% soap solution and ethanol for both MbOCA and MDA contaminants. Water alone removed 10.4 ± 4.8% of applied dose of MbOCA in unoccluded rat skin samples and 13.0 ± 5.0% in occluded samples. Ten percent soap solution was the most effective decontamination solution and removed 33 ± 9.6% MbOCA from unoccluded rat skin and 31.0 ± 10.3% from occluded samples.

Water alone removed 17.9 ± 1.8% MDA contaminant from unoccluded rat skin samples and 10.2 ± 3.1% from occluded skin. Ten percent soap solution was again the most effective decontamination solution and removed 35.0 ± 10.0% MDA from unoccluded skin and 24.0 ± 7.7% from occluded skin. Therefore, the authors concluded that liquid hand soap facilitates the uptake of the contaminants into solution, but only when present at high concentrations such as 10%. These authors highlighted the importance of not only the method of decontamination but the timeliness of decontamination as well, stating that the skin must be washed almost immediately or at least within 30 min of exposure for maximum effect. It is important to

Table 6.1 Summary of efficacy using water and/or soap and water decontamination methods

Author (year)	Model (sample size)	Method of decontamination	Contaminant(s) (concentration/dose)	Result
Hewitt et al. (1995) [12]	Rat (n = 6)	1. 100% water	(a) 4,4'-Methylenebis[2-chloroanaline]	(1a) Unoccluded skin, 10.4 ± 4.8%; occluded skin, 13.0 ± 5%
			(b) 4,4'-methylenedianaline	(1b) Unoccluded skin, 17.9 ± 1.8%; occluded skin, 10.2 ± 3.1%
		2. 1% (v/v) aqueous solution	(5 µL of MbOCA (9.7–17.7 µg/cm² in ethanol))	(2a) Unoccluded skin, 15.4 ± 3.8%; occluded skin, 19.8 ± 5.1%
		3. 10% (v/v) aqueous solution		(2b) Unoccluded skin, 20.0 ± 1.2%; occluded skin, 15.3 ± 2.1%
		4. 100% Ethanol		(3a) Unoccluded skin, 33.0 ± 9.6%; occluded skin, 31.0 ± 10.3%
				(3b) Unoccluded skin, 35.0 ± 10.0%; occluded skin, 24.0 ± 7.7%
				(4a) Unoccluded skin, 29.5 ± 11.9%; occluded skin, 28.3 ± 13.7%
				(4b) Unoccluded skin, 27.7 ± 7.8%; occluded skin, 23.9 ± 5.6%
Campbell et al. (2000) [13]	Porcine (n = 9)	10% Ivory liquid and water	(a) Glyphosate	(a) Average recovery: 49 ± 14%
			(b) Alachlor	(b) Average recovery: 52 ± 12%
			(c) Methyl parathion	(c) Average recovery: 50 ± 19%
			(d) Trifluralin	(d) Average recovery: 56 ± 13%
			(0.5, 2.0, or 8.0 µg/cm²)	
Monteiro-Riviere et al. (2001) [14]	Porcine (n = 4)	100% water	Phenol	Peak concentration using water wash: at 23 min, 15.4 µg/mL
			(400 µL of 89% phenol)	Peak concentration using control: at 45 min, 19.9 µg/mL
Pavlikova et al. (2018) [15]	Porcine (not disclosed)	100% water	Paraoxon (5 µL of 97% pure POX)	34 ± 5.7% removed
Tazrart et al. (2018) [16]	Porcine (n = 6)	100% water	(a) Americium	(a) 80 ± 4% of contaminant removed
			(b) Plutonium	(b) 70 ± 15% of contaminant removed
			(c) Plutonium-TBP	(c) 82 ± 10% of contaminant removed
			(300 µL of aqueous solution)	

note that these same results were not observed using in vitro human models in the same study, thus highlighting the important point that in vitro animal results may not always represent effects seen in humans.

Comparing Soap and Water to Other Decontamination Solutions

Campbell et al. [13] chose four pesticides to contaminate porcine skin based on a wide range of water solubilities [13]. The four were glyphosate, alachlor, methyl parathion, and trifluralin. Decontaminants tested included 1-propanol, 10% soap and water, polyethylene glycol (PEG), and D-TAM (a commercial decontamination product).

Porcine skin was cut into 45 cm × 60 cm clippings and rinsed with soap and water. The skin was placed between two layers of plexiglass. Beneath the skin and plexiglass, a layer of gauze soaked in saline was placed to maintain moisture. The top of the plexiglass was cut to allow a loading zone for contaminants. Pesticide solutions were applied to the skin in two 40 µL drops and spread with a glass rod over the specimen. An initial experiment was conducted to determine how much of the pesticide remained on the rod by applying carbon-labeled pesticide to a skin sample with the glass rod. An alcohol wipe then wiped the remaining pesticide from the rod, and 0.03–0.5% of the pesticide did not make it onto the porcine skin sample. Three different quantities of pesticide were applied to skin samples, 0.5, 2.0, and 8.0 µg/cm^2, in order to test if the amount of pesticide removed by solvents differed by initial application. The pesticide was allowed to dry on the skin for 90 min.

Each skin sample was wiped with cotton gauze soaked in 0.5 mL of wipe solution of a particular solvent: 1-propanol, 10% soap and water, polyethylene glycol (PEG), and D-TAM. The gauze wiped each skin for 15 passes before being placed in a 20 mL scintillation vial. Following the wipe, skin samples were placed at −20 °C before pesticide remains were analyzed. Skin samples were placed in Soluene-350, an organic base used to create liquid scintillation solutions, and 1 mL of this was placed in 15 mL of Insta-Fluor. The amount of isotope of ^{14}C found in the 1 mL sample was then compared to the amount of skin tissue solubilized in Soluene-350 to determine the pesticide amount left on the skin.

Results for glyphosate recovery showed that at all three pesticide levels, 0.5, 2.0, and 8.0 µg/cm^2, 1-propanol, 10% soap and water, and PEG removed similar amounts of glyphosate from the skin. These three solvents removed a greater percentage of solvent at the 2.0 and 8.0 µg/cm^2 level compared to the 0.5 µg/cm^2 level. D-TAM solution only showed significant difference in pesticide removal between the 0.5 and 8.0 µg/cm^2 levels.

Alachlor recovery showed similar patterns for both 1-propanol and 10% soap and water with different pesticide removal observed for each level of pesticide treatment used. For both D-TAM and PEG, the amount of pesticide initially applied did not correspond with differential recovery.

All four solvents removed greater amounts of pesticide when 2.0 or 8.0 μg/cm^2 of methyl parathion was applied compared to 0.5 μg/cm^2, but there was no statistical difference in removal of pesticide for any solvent when either of the upper loading levels was used. This same pattern was observed with trifluralin.

Overall recovery patterns showed that 1-propanol showed significantly higher overall recovery of the four pesticides compared to the other three solvents. Soap and water showed significantly higher recovery of pesticide compared to PEG and D-TAM, but there was no significant difference in recovery between solvents when looking at the pesticides glyphosate, alachlor, and methyl parathion. With trifluralin, 1-propanol was the most effective method for decontamination, but this was not statistically different than using soap and water for decontamination of this pesticide. Campbell et al. [13] also conducted experiments in which the decontamination solvents applied were applied prior to contaminant application. In these experiments, 0.5 mL of wipe solution was spread over skin samples. Any extra solvent was removed with gauze, and the pesticide was added 30 min later. Interestingly, pretreatment with any of the decontaminants actually decreased the recovery of both alachlor and glyphosate. This is of relevance, as it suggests that decontamination solvents should not be applied prophylactically in high-risk scenarios.

Comparing Water to Other Decontamination Solutions

Monteiro-Riviere et al. [14] used an IPPSF in vitro porcine skin model to test the effectiveness of phenol decontamination using a 15-min water wash, PEG-400, or isopropyl alcohol (IPA) [14]. IPPSF model has typical anatomy and circulation patterns compared to live skin of a weanling pig. Two skin samples were created and collected 48 h later. They were then washed with saline solution and placed in perfusion chambers where they were perfused for 1 h before phenol was applied. A Stomahesive template of 1.0 × 2.8 cm area was placed on the flap in order to shield it during dosing. Four hundred microliter of 89% phenol was added to the template that was occluded with Scotch tape. The flap was exposed for 1 min and the phenol pad removed.

The skin was then washed with either a 15-min water wash, a 1-min water wash followed by a 1-min PEG-400 wash followed by seven consecutive 1-min water washes, or a 1-min water wash followed by a 1-min IPA wash followed by seven consecutive 1-min water washes. After each wash, the dose template was cut, and the flap was added back to the perfusion chamber. This chamber was used to gather samples of 1 mL arterial and 1 mL venous perfusate at 5, 15, 30, 60, 90, 105, and 120 min after exposure and wash. After 120 min, samples were collected every 30 min up to 6 h. Samples were stored at −20 °C for 8 h. The tissue was then stored in 10% neutral buffered formalin (NBF). Each sample from the perfusion chamber was then placed on a glass tube and deproteinized with 1 mL of acetonitrile. This sample was centrifuged and analyzed using Waters HPLC column at 270 nm.

Peak concentration of phenol was observed for no treatment models in the perfusate at 45 min at 19.9 µg/mL. Peak concentration of phenol for IPA-treated flaps was also observed at this time at 12.8 µg/mL. For both water- and PEG-400-treated flaps, the peak phenol was observed at 23 min and was 15.4 µg/mL and 10.2 µg/mL, respectively. There was a significant difference in phenol decontaminated observed between the unwashed control and the three treatments; however, there was no statistically significant difference between the three treatments in decontamination of phenol.

Pavlikova et al. [15] utilized an in vitro pig skin model to determine the effectiveness of water versus other detergents in decontamination of paraoxon (POX) [15]. Dorsal skin from white domestic pigs was cut and stored at −20 °C before use. Before exposure to POX, the skin was thawed for 24 h at 8 °C. After thawing, skin samples were placed in a Franz-type glass diffusion cell where they were exposed to the receptor fluid. Buffered saline containing 4% bovine serum albumin was used as the fluid. The total skin surface of 1.77 cm² was exposed to 5 µL of POX using a micropipette. The skin sample was washed after 1 min using the glass diffusion cell and a showering system with the supply tube and skin sample being placed 34 mm apart.

Differing flow rates of showering system, rinsing volume, and concentration of detergent were tested, but for the comparison of water to other detergents in effectiveness of decontamination of POX, a flow rate of 16 mL s⁻¹, a rising volume of 100 mL, and a detergent concentration of 5% were chosen. There were 30 detergents tested for decontamination of POX, and water only proved more effective than one of the 30 detergents in the decontamination of POX from skin samples. Water washed off 34.0 ± 5.7% of POX from skin samples, while Spolapon AES 253 washed 26.8 ± 10.9% of POX from the skin samples when flow rate of contaminant was set at 16 mL s⁻¹, rinsing volume of 100 mL was set, and 5% detergent solution was used. Spolapon AES 253 improved in its decontamination compared to water as flow rate increased to 25 mL s⁻¹ and rinsing volume increased to 200 mL. The remaining 29 detergent solutions were significantly more effective at decontaminating POX than water.

Tazrart et al. [16] used in vitro pig skin models to compare effectiveness in decontamination of three different actinide compounds using water versus cleansing gels or diethylenetriamine pentaacetic acid (DTPA) gels [16]. Skin samples were taken from pig ears following euthanasia and cut to 0.64 cm² surface area samples. They were placed in Franz diffusion cells between the donor and receptor compartments and washed with buffered saline. Samples were exposed to an equilibration time for 30 min at 35 °C and then deposited with 4 kBq of one of the three actinide solutions: ²⁴¹Am, ²³⁸/²³⁹Pu, and ²³⁸/²³⁹Pu complexed to TBP in dodecane. They were exposed to the actinides for 2 h, and then the actinide was removed.

The decontamination methods used were water, Trait Rouge 1:1 v/v with water, 7.2 mg of Fuller's earth, 500 mM DTPA, 500 mM LIHOPO, 500 mM HEDP, Osmogel, and two DTPA gel formulations. Five hundred microliter of solution was used for each wash, and 0.3 g of gel was added to test its decontamination ability. Each decontaminant was added to the skin sample following 2 h of exposure to actinide with a compress placed on top. A cotton bud spread the decontaminant over the skin for 30 s, and the compress was then removed. This was repeated three times using a different compress each time. Following the third collection, the skin was washed with a final drying swab to determine if any contaminant remained on the skin.

Radioactivity measurements were then taken from receptor compartments by drying them and wet washing the residues in HNO_3 and H_2O_2. Skin samples were dried in an oven at a maximum temperature of 500 °C for 52 h. They were then washed with the sample solutions as the receptor compartment. The donor compartment, skin, and decontamination solutions used liquid scintillation counting to determine the amount of radioactivity. Radioactivity was measured on the cotton buds, compresses, and drying swabs by measuring gamma and X-radiation with a germanium detector.

For the americium contamination, about 6% of contaminant remained on the skin for the control solution after the three washes. Trait Rouge, DTPA, and LIHOPO were more effective at removing americium from the skin samples compared to water only. Trait Rouge recovered 90 ± 3% of americium, and DTPA solution recovered 90 ± 6%. This is compared to the recovery using water of 80 ± 4%. However, there was not any difference in decontamination efficacy between DTPA, Trait Rouge, LIHOPO, and HEDP. This same result was shown for the contaminant, plutonium, with water alone proving an inferior decontamination method compared to DTPA, Trait Rouge, LIHOPO, and HEDP. Trait Rouge recovered 92 ± 4% of plutonium, and DTPA solution recovered 91 ± 5%. This is compared to the recovery using water of 70 ± 15%. This result was not shown, however, for plutonium-TBP, with water proving to be as effective as the other decontamination solutions. Trait Rouge recovered 84 ± 12% of plutonium-TBP, and DTPA solution recovered 90 ± 3%. This is compared to the recovery using water of 82 ± 10%.

Discussion

This overview combed the literature for water and/or soap and water skin decontamination of a variety of contaminants compared to different solutions using in vitro animal models. When comparing water to just soap and water using MbOCA and MDA contaminants, water proved less effective in decontamination. In the comparison of soap and water to other decontamination methods, all four contaminants, glyphosate, alachlor, methyl parathion, and trifluralin, were as effectively removed using soap and water, PEG, D-TAM, and 1-propanol. In comparing water to PEG-400 and IPA washes of a phenol decontaminant, water proved as effective at removing phenol from the skin samples. In an additional study, water was compared to 30 detergents for removing paraoxon from skin samples and was shown to be an inferior decontamination method when compared to 29/30 of the detergents used. Finally, water was compared to other decontamination methods in its ability to remove three types of actinides from skin samples. Water proved inferior to other methods for both the removal of americium and plutonium, but it proved as effective as DTPA, Trait Rouge, LIHOPO, and HEDP at removing plutonium-TBP from in vitro skin models. Overall, water proved ineffective compared to other decontamination methods for 5/7 of the contaminants tested. Soap and water proved to be as effective as other decontamination methods for 4/4 of the contaminants tested and more effective than water alone for 2/2 of the contaminants tested.

The field of dermal decontamination has traditionally found decontamination with water leads to better dermal clinical outcomes when compared to controls. Brent [7] found in his review that early water lavage led to fewer burns and shorter hospital stays in patients with hydrofluoric acid burns, and early decontamination with water worked more effectively than controls in patients [7]. However, this review does not have a group of decontamination strategies for comparison. Additionally, the review mentions that water should not be used in decontamination for alkali metals, as hydration causes bases to form.

Water decontaminates the skin by diluting the chemical agent, rinsing off the contaminant, decreasing chemical reaction rates on the skin, minimizing metabolism and inflammation, and restoring the normal skin pH [17]. Systematic reviews by Kashetsky et al. [8], Burli et al. [9], and Chiang et al. [10] which summarize available studies with in vivo human and animal data and in vitro human data, respectively, all concluded that these solutions achieve partial decontamination in the majority of decontamination outcomes [8–10]. However, available in vivo animal data shows mortality outcomes in approximately 6% of cases that used water-only and soap and water decontamination solution. Further, there are exceptions to using water as first-line decontamination including chemical exposures to metallic sodium, lithium, and potassium. These alkali metals should not be irrigated with water [9].

Water with soap has been theorized to work more effectively than water alone due to increased ability for chemical hydrolysis and ability to dissolve contaminants, but the results vary greatly by type of contaminant [18]. However, regardless of if water and/or soap and water is used, decontamination via these two methods may be inferior to other methods, as shown by the results of this review indicating that water alone proves inferior to other decontamination methods for five of the seven contaminants considered using in vitro animal models. This may lead to chemical contaminant on the skin that can lead to toxic clinical effects such as chemical burns, chemical poisoning, and systemic effects on the body. Thus, it is important to continue developing more decontamination solutions that have the essential qualities of effective decontaminants: effective, rapid action, do not increase absorption of the contaminant (lack of a wash-in effect), do not further damage the skin barrier, accessible, easy to remove, and affordable [19].

Different factors affect the initial amount of contaminant absorbed in the skin. Absorption of a chemical through the epidermis occurs more effectively for lipophilic contaminants compared to hydrophilic ones, thus leading to higher levels of cutaneous contaminant levels [20]. In addition, smaller molecules can penetrate the skin barrier more easily, and generally those with lower molecular weights can accumulate at higher rates within the skin [21]. In addition, the longer the contaminant is in contact with the skin surface before decontamination, the more difficult the removal of the contaminant may be [22]. All these factors may have contributed to how effective water and/or soap and water contamination was compared to other decontamination solutions across the studies.

There are also a wide variety of factors that contribute to the effectiveness of decontamination. First and most obviously, the greater the amount of initial contaminant used, the greater the levels of contamination that must be removed through decontamination. In addition, the length of time the contaminant is in contact with the skin may greatly affect how effective decontamination methods are, with less time of exposure resulting in better decontamination results, as shown by the results of the Campbell et al. [13] study looking at the removal of four pesticides from the dermis included in this study [23]. Finally, the length of decontamination efforts and amount of decontaminant used may greatly affect the amount of contaminant recovered, with greater lengths of time and greater levels of decontaminant used leading to better outcomes [19]. This is supported by the results of Pavlikova et al. [15] study in removing paraoxon from porcine skin samples where decontamination was improved by increasing rinsing volume and flow rate to a certain level. These components of study design for the literature reviewed likely also influenced the effectiveness of water and/or soap and water in removing the contaminants from the models.

There are important shortcomings of this systematic review. First, the small sample size of articles that met inclusion criteria made it difficult to compare water and/ or soap and water's decontamination efficacy to other decontamination methods across a wide range of contaminants. In addition, the results shared across studies were heterogenous and difficult to compare. The methods used for determining the effectiveness of decontamination across solutions also varied greatly.

Finally, this review solely looked at in vitro animal models, which do differ in their biochemical and physiological response to contaminants and decontamination methods when compared to in vivo human skin. In vitro models only look at cells in isolation and not as a part of a complex metabolic system, so it is difficult to apply findings from in vitro studies to how they would respond in an entire human model. In addition, the use of animal models limits the ability to extrapolate data to human models because humans have a different genetic profile and perform different biological processes compared to the pig and rat models used. Because of this, the conclusions drawn from this review cannot be generalized to practice within humans and may highlight the importance of in vivo human models in developing effective dermal decontamination methods. However, organizations such as the Food and Drug Administration (FDA) have recently pushed for the continued advancement of in vitro and in vivo animal models for clinical studies that would not be plausible using in vivo animal models. These studies could gain information on the effects of drugs or processes that would be unethical to perform on humans and with the use of additional models provide greater confidence in results [24].

Conclusion

Water and/or soap and water have traditionally been used as the primary method of decontamination for dermal contamination, but this study using in vitro animal models revealed that water alone often provides incomplete dermal decontamination when compared to other decontamination methods. However, the limited number of studies comparing water and/or soap and water decontamination strategies using in vitro animal model reveals a greater need for research to determine which contaminants may effectively be decontaminated from the skin using water and/or soap and water and which contaminants are more effectively removed using other decontamination solutions. There is limited ability to extrapolate the data from in vitro animal models to human models, so when it is safe and appropriate, it is best to determine the ideal decontamination method using in vivo human models.

Additional research must also be performed on the chemical and metabolic nature of skin contaminants, as we believe that standardized decontamination strategies can be created based on the chemical nature of contaminants and how they interact with the skin. Finally, additional research should be conducted on how the contaminants are absorbed and distributed throughout the layers of the skin, as this may indicate which types of contamination methods are most appropriate. Taken together, utilization of pharmacokinetic data, as utilized here, has added to our understanding of the complex issues involved in decontamination. Much remains to be accomplished in our knowledge of the complexities. The reader is referred to *Skin Decontamination: A Comprehensive Clinical Research Guide* [25] and other publications in this series for additional information.

Acknowledgments None.

Conflict of Interest None.

Funding Sources None.

References

1. Clarkson ED, Gordon RK. Rapid decontamination of chemical warfare agents from skin. In: Handbook of toxicology of chemical warfare agents. London: Academic Press; 2020. https://doi.org/10.1016/b978-0-12-819090-6.00073-8.
2. Kuca K, Pohanka M. Chemical warfare agents. EXS. 2010;100:543–58. https://pubmed-ncbi-nlm-nih-gov.qe2a-proxy.mun.ca/20358695/.
3. Chilcott R, et al. PRISM guidance for chemical incidents, Volume 1: Strategic guidance for mass casualty disrobe and decontamination. Washington, DC: Biomedical Advanced Research Development Authority; 2015.
4. Law RM, Ngo MA, Maibach HI. Twenty clinically pertinent factors/observations for percutaneous absorption in humans. Am J Clin Dermatol. 2020;21(1):85–95. https://doi.org/10.1007/s40257-019-00480-4.

5. Moody RP, Maibach HI. Skin decontamination: importance of the wash-in effect. Food Chem Toxicol. 2006;44(11):1783–8. https://doi.org/10.1016/j.fct.2006.05.020.
6. Magnano GC, Rui F, Larese Filon F. Skin decontamination procedures against potential hazards substances exposure. Chem Biol Interact. 2021;344:109481. https://doi.org/10.1016/j.cbi.2021.109481.
7. Brent J. Water-based solutions are the best decontaminating fluids for dermal corrosive exposures: a mini review. Clin Toxicol. 2013;51(8):731–6. https://doi.org/10.3109/1556365 0.2013.838628.
8. Kashetsky N, Law RM, Maibach HI. Efficacy of water skin decontamination in vivo in humans: a systematic review. J Appl Toxicol. 2022;42:346. https://doi.org/10.1002/jat.4230.
9. Burli A, Kashetsky N, Feschuk A, Law RM, Maibach HI. Efficacy of soap and water based skin decontamination using in vivo animal models: a systematic review. J Toxicol Environ Health B Crit Rev. 2021;24(7):325–36. https://doi.org/10.1080/10937404.2021.1943087.
10. Chiang C, Kashetsky N, Feschuk A, Burli A, Law R, Maibach H. Efficacy of water-based skin decontamination of occupational chemicals using in vitro human skin models: a systematic review. J Toxicol Environ Health B Crit Rev. 2021;24(7):337–53. https://doi.org/10.108 0/10937404.2021.1957048.
11. Page MJ, McKenzie JE, Bossuyt PM, Boutron I, Hoffmann TC, Mulrow CD, Shamseer L, Tetzlaff JM, Akl EA, Brennan SE, Chou R, Glanville J, Grimshaw JM, Hróbjartsson A, Lalu MM, Li T, Loder EW, Mayo-Wilson E, McDonald S, McGuinness LA, Stewart LA, Thomas J, Tricco AC, Welch VA, Whiting P, Moher D. The PRISMA 2020 statement: an updated guideline for reporting systematic reviews. BMJ. 2021;372:N71. https://doi.org/10.1136/BMJ.N71.
12. Hewitt P. Decontamination procedures after in vitro topical exposure of human and rat skin to 4,4′-methylenebis[2-chloroaniline] and 4,4′-methylenedianiline. Fundam Appl Toxicol. 1995;26(1):91–8. https://doi.org/10.1006/faat.1995.1078.
13. Campbell JL, Smith MA, Eiteman MA, Williams PL, Boeniger MF. Comparison of solvents for removing pesticides from skin using an in vitro porcine model. Am Ind Hyg Assoc J. 2000;61(1):82–8. https://doi.org/10.1202/0002-8894(2000)061<0082:COSFRP>2.0.CO;2.
14. Monteiro-Riviere NA, Inman AO, Jackson H, Dunn B, Dimond S. Efficacy of topical phenol decontamination strategies on severity of acute phenol chemical burns and dermal absorption: in vitro and in vivo studies in pig skin. Toxicol Ind Health. 2001;17(4):95–104. https://doi.org/10.1191/0748233701th095oa.
15. Pavlikova R, Misik J, Cabal J, Marek J, Kuca K. In vitro skin decontamination of paraoxon - wet-type cleansing effect of selected detergents. Cutan Ocul Toxicol. 2018;37(1):77–83. https://doi.org/10.1080/15569527.2017.1354216.
16. Tazrart A, Bolzinger MA, Lamart S, Coudert S, Angulo JF, Jandard V, Briançon S, Griffiths NM. Actinide-contaminated skin: comparing decontamination efficacy of water, cleansing gels, and DTPA gels. Health Phys. 2018;115(1):12–20. https://doi.org/10.1097/HP.0000000000000814.
17. Houston M, Hendrickson RG. Decontamination. Crit Care Clin. 2005;21(4):653. https://doi.org/10.1016/j.ccc.2005.06.001.
18. Hall AH, Maibach HI. Water decontamination of chemical skin/eye splashes: a critical review. Cutan Ocul Toxicol. 2006;25(2):67–83. https://doi.org/10.1080/15569520600695520.
19. Chan HP, Zhai H, Hui X, Maibach HI. Skin decontamination: principles and perspectives. Toxicol Ind Health. 2013;29(10):955–68. https://doi.org/10.1177/0748233712448112.
20. Potts RO, Guy RH. Predicting skin permeability. Pharm Res. 1992;9(5):663–9. https://doi.org/10.1023/A:1015810312465.
21. Buckley TJ, Sapkota A, Cardello N, Dellarco MJ, Klingner TD. A rational approach to skin decontamination; 2000
22. Wester R, Maibach H. Dermal decontamination and percutaneous absorption. In: Percutaneous absorption: drugs, cosmetics, mechanisms, methodology. Drugs and the pharmaceutical sciences. 4th ed. London: Routledge; 2005. p. 313–26. https://doi.org/10.1201/9780849359033-23.

23. Boeniger M. Skin decontamination of chemical exposures. Washington, DC: National Institute for Occupational Health and Safety; 2005.
24. Byrne J, et al. FDA public workshop summary: advancing animal models for antibacterial drug development. Antimicrob Agents Chemother. 2021;65(1):e01983–20. https://doi.org/10.1128/AAC.01983-20.
25. Zhu H, Maibach H. Skin decontamination: a comprehensive clinical research guide. Cham: Springer Nature; 2020.

Chapter 7
Dermal Decontamination with Readily Available Dry Products

Saisha Nandamuri, Aileen M. Feschuk, and Howard I. Maibach

Introduction

Dry decontamination is a general term for decontamination of compounds (e.g., chemicals, biological particles, or other liquids or solids) without the use of water or other liquids [1]. Decontamination is of interest, due to the threats of chemical warfare and accidents with toxic industrial chemicals [2]. In fact, more than 13 million workers in the United States are potentially exposed to chemicals that can be absorbed through the skin [3]. In addition, chemical warfare is arguably one of the most brutal methods of mass destruction, and they are relatively easy to produce and can cause mass casualties with small quantities [4]. However, universal decontamination guidelines are lacking due to limited research which mainly points to soap and water as a decontamination solution.

Soap and water are often considered the gold standard for dermal decontamination partly due to general accessibility, which in turn makes it time effective. Though soap and water is a widely accepted option, it is not a universal decontaminant. In fact, recent systematic reviews have generally concluded that soap and/or water methods often result in incomplete decontamination [5–8]. This may be partially attributable to the "wash-in" effect, which is when wet decontamination actually enhances the percutaneous penetration of the contaminant [9].

According to Chilcott et al. [10], wet decontamination should be used when the contaminant is a form of toxic, radioactive, or biological solid. Additionally, wet

S. Nandamuri
University of California San Francisco, San Francisco, CA, USA

A. M. Feschuk (✉)
Faculty of Medicine, Memorial University of Newfoundland, St. John's, NL, Canada
e-mail: amfeschuk@mun.ca

H. I. Maibach
Department of Dermatology, University of California San Francisco, San Francisco, CA, USA

© The Author(s), under exclusive license to Springer Nature Switzerland AG 2022
A. M. Feschuk et al. (eds.), *Dermal Absorption and Decontamination*,
https://doi.org/10.1007/978-3-031-09222-0_7

decontamination is preferred for the decontamination of corrosive liquids (e.g., strong acids or oxidizing agents) [10]. However, there are situations where dry decontamination holds benefits over wet decontamination. For example, Chilcott et al. [10] stated that dry decontamination is at least as effective and typically safer than wet decontamination and should be used for the decontamination of any non-corrosive liquid insult (e.g., sulfur mustard, nerve agents, liquid pesticides, etc.). In addition, wet decontamination should not be used following exposure to water-reactive chemicals (e.g., lithium, sodium, or potassium metals, phosphorus penta-chloride). In mass casualties occurring in extremely cold conditions, dry decontamination may be preferential to wet in order to prevent additional causalities due to hypothermia [1]. Additionally, people may not always have accessibility to clean water or water in copious amounts, and dry decontamination does not require an immediate source of water, so it may be preferred in these circumstances [10]. Additionally, the solid waste produced by dry decontamination is easier to contain than the effluent produced by wet decontamination [10].

There are dry decontamination methods which have proven quite efficacious, but are not readily available to the public in an emergency setting. For example, Fuller's earth is an absorbing powder that generally allows for rapid and reliable decontami-nation [11]. In addition, highly effective decontamination gel (DDGel) is a sub-stance with a continuous thick consistency and can be applied to the skin, allowed to dry for 5 min, and then peeled off [12]. However, a fundamental principle of responding mass causalities is to "do the best you can for the most people with the resources you have" [1]. Neither Fuller's earth nor DDGel are items that are gener-ally accessible to the public. However, dry decontamination can also be done by blotting and rubbing the body with commonly found, readily available dry absor-bent materials (e.g., tissues, paper towels, diapers) [10, 13, 14].

Thus, the objective of this manuscript is to summarize and draw conclusions from articles investigating the efficacy of dry decontaminants that would be com-monly found and easily accessible (i.e., in households, workplaces, or ambulances).

Materials and Methods

Methodology of this manuscript followed the Preferred Reporting Items for Systematic Reviews and Meta-Analysis (PRISMA) guidelines [15]. On August 28, 2021, a search for dry decontamination papers was conducted using PubMed. Search terms included "dry decontamination" OR "non-wet decontamination." Articles were considered eligible for inclusion in this manuscript if they were (1) experimental studies, (2) removing contaminants without water or other liquids, (3) using easily/publicly accessible dry decontamination methods, and (4) reporting data in English language. There were no restrictions based on study model (i.e., animal model versus human model or in vivo versus in vitro).

Title/abstract screening was conducted by two independent researchers (S.N. and H.M.). Full-text review was conducted independently by two researchers (H.M. and

A.F.). Data extraction was completed by two independent researchers (S.N., A.F.) and verified by one independent researcher (H.M.). Data on study characteristics, animal models, chemical contaminants, decontamination, decontamination analysis, and outcomes were extracted. Due to the large degree of heterogeneity between studies, descriptive analyses were conducted.

Results

Study Characteristics

After title/abstract screening of 427 studies, 11 studies moved on to full-text review, and seven studies met eligibility criteria and were therefore included in this review. The authors, study models, dry decontaminants used, methods of dry decontamination, methods of analyzing dry decontamination, contaminants tested, and main conclusions of each of these studies can be found in Table 7.1.

Study Findings

Kassouf et al. [16] studied four test materials including Ambulance Service decontamination sponge, blue roll, Maxiflex dressing, and green absorbent pad for dry decontamination efficacy in an ex vivo diffusion cell system containing pig skin. Radioactive ^{14}C-labelled contaminants methyl salicylate (MS), parathion (PT), diethyl malonate (DEM), phorate (PH), and potassium cyanide (KCN) were the test stimulants used. All contaminants were diluted to 0.25 μCi/μL. Experiments consisted of six test groups, with $n = 6$ replicants for each group. The test groups included (1) a control group (no decontamination), (2) a rinse-wash-rinse (R-W-R) decontamination group, (3) a green absorbent pad decontamination group, (4) a Maxiflex dressing decontamination group, (5) a blue roll decontamination group, and (6) an Ambulance Service decontamination sponge decontamination group. The R-W-R group served as a wet decontamination protocol to compare the four dry decontamination agents (groups 3, 4, 5, and 6) and involved the following protocol: rinsing with 10 mL detergent solution, dabbing with dry gauze, and rinsing again with 10 mL tap water.

Decontamination was performed 15 min after skin contamination. Each of the four dry decontamination products was cut into 5-cm-diameter swatches and applied directly to the skin surface for 5 s. Receptor fluid samples were taken at baseline and then every 10 min up to 1 h following contamination. Following the decontamination period, all skin samples were swabbed to collect residual contaminants. Then, all skin samples were imaged using digital autoradiography and finally dissolved in Soluene-350.

Table 7.1 Overview of data extracted from experimental studies including study model, dry decontaminant used, method in which the dry decontamination was used, method of analyzing decontamination, and main conclusions

Authors	Study model	Dry decontaminant	Method of dry decontamination	Time from exposure to decontamination	Method of analyzing decontamination	Contaminants tested	Main conclusions
Kassouf et al. [16]	Ex vivo pig skin	Blue roll	Decontaminant (5 cm diameter) swatches applied directly to skin surface for 5 s	15 min	Intensity and area of ^{14}C-labeled contaminants determined on autoradiography	Methyl salicylate	Dry decontamination generally effective, and more effective than wet protocols, against liquid contaminants
	$n = 36$ (six treatments, six repetitions each)	Sponge			Liquid scintillation counting performed on skin surface swabs, dissolved skin samples, and receptor fluid samples	Parathion	Wet decontamination should be used for non-liquid contaminants
		Green pad				Diethyl malonate	
		Maxiflex dressing				Phorate	
						Potassium cyanide	
Hall et al. [17]	In vivo pig skin	WoundStat	WoundStat (2 g) applied, left for 1 h, and removed with cotton swabs and surgical gauze	30 s	Biophysical measurements taken at baseline and hourly post exposure (cutaneous blood flow (laser Doppler imaging), skin barrier integrity (transepidermal water loss), skin color (skin reflectance spectroscopy), skin surface temperature (infrared thermography), and toxicokinetics)	Sulfur mustard	WoundStat is suitable for reducing the absorption and toxicity of chemical warfare agents
	$n = 12$ (six control group, six decontamination group)				Gross clinical observations made		
	Number of wounded skin test sites: (1) in control group = 2/3, (2) in decontamination group = 3/4				Microscopic skin structure changes investigated postmortem		

Reference	Model	Product	Procedure	Time	Analysis	Contaminant	Findings
Amlôt et al. [13]	In vivo human skin	Blue roll	Blue roll or incontinence pads used to rub, blot, or rub and blot contaminant application site for 5 s	15 min	Fluorescent images taken pre- and post-decontamination analyzed to determine level of contaminant spread	Methyl salicylate	The method of decontamination, i.e., blotting, rubbing, or blotting and rubbing, largely influences decontamination efficacy, with blotting and rubbing demonstrating the most consistently significant decontamination
	n = 60 (20 participants, three repetitions each)	Incontinence pads			Amount of contaminant recovered from swabs and tape-strips determined using headspace gas chromatography/mass spectrometry		
Chilcott et al. [18, 19]	In vivo human skin n = 86	Wound dressing	Wound dressing used to decontaminate from head to toe (10-s blotting followed by 10-s rubbing per main body area)	Not specified	Whole-body fluorescent imaging to visualize simulant distribution	Combination of methyl salicylate, curcumin, and baby oil	The "triple protocol" was the most consistently effective protocol significantly reducing methyl salicylate recoveries in all contamination sites
	(nine treatment groups each with between n = 7 and n = 11)				High-performance liquid chromatography to quantify recovery of methyl salicylate in swab samples		When used properly, dry decontamination of initially contaminated sites had an overall effectiveness of 99%
Matar et al. [20]	In vitro human hair and porcine skin n = 54 (four single study groups, five combination study groups each with six repeats)	Trauma dressing	Trauma dressing disk (38.5 cm^2) and weight placed on top of skin/hair left for 5 s. Dressing turned over, tinfoil disk placed over the dressing, and weight placed over that for another 5 s	4 min	Scintillation counting of contaminant radioactivity in samples (donor chamber air, flannel and towel swatches, dissolved skin tissue, shower effluent, trauma dressing)	Methyl salicylate	Dry decontamination significant in reducing the amount of bioavailable contaminant
						Phorate	Dry decontamination not significant in the decontamination of hair
						Sodium fluoroacetate	
						Potassium cyanide	

(continued)

Table 7.1 (continued)

Authors	Study model	Dry decontaminant	Method of dry decontamination	Time from exposure to decontamination	Method of analyzing decontamination	Contaminants tested	Main conclusions
Larner et al. [21]	In vivo human skin and hair n = 115 (48 volunteers attending varying number of sessions. Each of the 11 treatment groups contained n = 10, 11, or 12)	Wound dressing	Wipe face (10 s), wipe hands (10 s), wipe body (30 s), and wipe hair (10 s)	4 min	Particle analysis of the full-body fluorescent imaging followed by calculations of the total residual contaminated fluorescent area	Combination of methyl salicylate, fluorophore [curcumin], and mineral oil	Dry decontamination alone did not result in significant decreases in contamination when compared to controls
					Liquid chromatography and thermal desorption chromatography to measure residual contaminants in hair, skin, decontamination materials, and air samples		Dry decontamination prior to LPS or TD did significantly reduce contamination
					Liquid chromatography-mass spectrometry analysis of urine samples looking for salicyluric acid (primary metabolite of methyl salicylate)		The "triple protocol" (dry decontamination + LPS + TD) was the most effective method tested
Southworth et al. [14]	In vivo human skin n = 48 (12 volunteers each completing four decontamination conditions)	White roll	As many pieces of white roll folded in half twice as needed were used to blot and rub skin starting from shoulders and working to feet for 3 min (or as much time as needed)	15 min	Gas chromatography-tandem mass spectrometry used to measure simulant remaining on the skin following decontamination	Combination of methyl salicylate, vegetable oil, and a UV fluorescent compound	Wet, dry, and COMBINED protocols were all efficacious in significantly reducing the recovery of contaminant compared to controls
					UV imaging to detect fluorophores		Combined dry and wet decontamination protocols were significantly superior to wet or dry protocols alone
					24-h urine analysis of MeS		

Efficacy of decontamination was determined by analyzing the intensity and area of ^{14}C-labeled contaminants on autoradiography. Additionally, liquid scintillation counting was performed on the skin surface swabs, the dissolved skin samples, and the receptor fluid samples. Together, these values were used in the following equation to determine the amount of each contaminant not removed through decontamination, $\%R = ((Q_1 + Q_2 + Q_3)/Q_0) \times 100$, where $\%R$ equals the residual percentage of applied dose, Q_1 equals the amount of contaminant recovered from skin surface swabs, Q_2 equals the amount of contaminant recovered from solubilized skin samples, Q_3 equals the amount of contaminant recovered from the receptor fluid, and Q_0 equals the applied dose.

The green pad and blue roll were statistically significant in reducing the skin surface spreading of ^{14}C-MS. The green pad, Maxiflex dressing, and blue roll were statistically significant in reducing the residual amount of MS. The green pad was significantly more effective than the R-W-R method and the decontamination sponge at removing ^{14}C-MS.

Decontamination of phorate followed similar patterns to MS. However, reduction of skin surface spreading of ^{14}C-PH was also significant with Maxiflex dressing. Additionally, the R-W-R method was statistically not as effective at reducing skin surface spreading compared to the "green pads," Maxiflex dressing, or blue roll.

Only the blue roll was able to significantly reduce the spreading of ^{14}C-PT. However, the green pad, Maxiflex dressing, and blue roll were all able to significantly reduce PT skin contamination.

All of the dry test products were ineffective in decontamination of powder KCN. However, R-W-R was significant in reducing both the skin surface spreading and residual amounts of powder KCN.

Finally, other than the "sponge," all dry decontamination products significantly reduced ^{14}C-DEM skin surface spreading and residual.

In summary, Kassouf et al. [16] found that readily available dry contamination materials, Maxiflex dressing, blue roll, and green pad, are readily available dry decontamination options with results superior to wet decontamination for three out of five chemical stimulants tested. Dry decontamination using a sponge was less effective than wet decontamination. In the test conditions described, wet decontamination worked better than dry decontamination for KCN and DEM contamination. Authors concluded that, in general, dry decontamination materials were more effective in the dermal decontamination of liquid insults, while wet decontamination was more effective for the decontamination of non-liquid insults.

Hall et al. [17] studied the WoundStat, an FDA-approved clay-based substance, as a decontaminant for radiolabeled sulfur mustard (^{14}C-SM) using pigs as an in vivo model. Six pigs were assigned to each experimental group: (1) no decontamination (control) group and (2) decontamination group. All test skin sites were located on the dorsum of the pig. Test skin sites in the control group pigs included (1) a damaged skin site, (2) a damaged skin site exposed to SM, and (3) a non-damaged, non-SM-exposed site. Test skin sites in the decontamination group pigs included (1) a damaged skin site, (2) a damaged skin site exposed to WoundStat, (3) a damaged skin site exposed to WoundStat and SM, and (4) a non-damaged, non-SM-exposed, non-WoundStat-exposed site. "Damaged skin" was skin which had an ~3 cm^2 area of 100 μm depth of the skin removed via dermatome. Decontamination test sites receiving WoundStat were treated with 2 g at 30 s post exposure for 1 h. Test sites receiving SM were treated with 10 μL delivered as a discrete droplet. After 1 h, SM and/or WoundStat were removed using cotton swabs and surgical gauze.

To determine the efficacy of WoundStat decontamination, biophysical measurements were made pre-exposure and hourly post exposure (with the first post-exposure measurements taken ~1 min following the removal of SM and/or WoundStat). The biophysical measurements taken included cutaneous blood flow (laser Doppler imaging), skin barrier integrity (transepidermal water loss), skin color (skin reflectance spectroscopy), skin surface temperature (infrared thermography), and toxicokinetics. In addition, gross clinical observations were made, and microscopic skin structure changes were investigated postmortem.

Hall et al. [17] found that WoundStat was effective in preventing advanced signs of SM dermal toxicity including ulceration. In addition, WoundStat improved exposure site blood flow and significantly reduced the amount of contaminant recovery from the skin (solubilized skin samples post decontamination) (70% reduction) and skin surface swabs (99%), blood (45% reduction), and liver at 6 h post exposure. Hall et al. [17] concluded that applying WoundStat immediately after ^{14}C-SM exposure can decrease dermal absorption and delay the onset of systemic effects.

Amlôt et al. [13] investigated the efficacy of two readily available dry decontaminants. Human volunteers ($n = 20$) were exposed to 10 μL of contaminant (10 mg of curcumin per 1 mL of 99.9% methyl salicylate) on each forearm, with the dominant forearm serving as a control and non-dominant forearm receiving decontamination. A UV box was used to take fluorescent images at baseline, immediately after contamination, and 13 min after contamination in order to monitor the spread of simulant. Decontamination with either blue roll (squares of 10 × 10 cm) or incontinence pads (4-ply 25 cm^2) was employed 15 min after exposure, and participants were instructed to either rub, blot, or rub and blot the contaminant application site for 5 s. Another UV-illuminated photograph was taken post decontamination. Each participant returned on two more occasions, over the course of 3 weeks, and was told to use a different decontamination method each time.

After the final image was taken, application sites (both decontamination and control) were swabbed with a dry cotton wool bud, an ethanol-soaked cotton wool bud, and finally another dry cotton wool bud. Additionally, each application site (both decontamination and control) underwent tape-strip sampling. The images were analyzed for fluorescence, and the pre-decontamination area was subtracted from the post-decontamination area, indicating the level of spread of the contaminant due to decontamination (therefore, a negative value indicated a decrease in spread). The efficacy of decontamination was also determined by the amount of contaminant recovered by the swabs and tape-strips using headspace gas chromatography/mass spectrometry, with a lower amount indicating that decontamination was more successful.

In terms of spread of the simulant (analysis of the UV-illuminated images), no trends of significance were identified between decontaminants ("blue roll" or incontinence pads) or decontamination method (blotting, rubbing, or blotting and rubbing). The amount of methyl salicylate recovered from the cotton swabs following decontamination showed a significant difference when compared to controls for both the blot and the blot and rub methods of decontamination. Rubbing alone did not produce a significant difference when compared to the control. Tape-strip methyl salicylate recovery was used to indicate the amount of simulant permeated into the stratum corneum. There was a significant difference in the amount of methyl salicylate recovered from the tape-strips following decontamination using the blot and rub method when compared to controls. The difference was not significant for blotting or rubbing alone.

Amlôt et al. [13] concluded that there was no significant difference in the decontamination efficacy of the blue roll versus the incontinence pads. However, the method of decontamination, i.e., blotting, rubbing, or blotting and rubbing, was key to the efficacy of decontamination.

Chilcott et al. [18, 19] studied the effectiveness of the "triple protocol" of sequential dry decontamination, ladder pipe system (LPS), and technical decontamination (TD), in vivo. The experiment was conducted as a large-scale exercise or a "mock mass exposure." There were a total of nine treatment groups which tested the three methods of decontamination alone and in combinations. The contaminant was comprised of a 9:1 ratio of curcumin dissolved in methyl salicylate (10 mg/mL solution) and baby oil. This was applied to the back of the head, upper chest, and palm of the right hand of participants via a spray resulting in an 8-cm-diameter circular area of contamination. Dry decontamination involved following the PRISM guidelines [10]. Decontamination was performed as quickly as logistically possible, but there was no specific, predetermined time point at which decontamination occurred. Participants used wound dressing to decontaminate from head to toe (10-s blotting followed by 10-s rubbing per main body area). LPS involved parking two fire engines in parallel and creating a central corridor of 3.7 m wide into which the side nozzles released high-volume low-pressure water mist. Participants underwent a 15-s rinse in the middle of the corridor, during which they were told to rub themselves with their hands from head down. The participants were then given a towel to dry themselves with for 30 s. TD took place in specialized decontamination units containing six overhead hoses, in which participants were instructed to wipe themselves down with a 10 mL baby shampoo-penetrated washcloth for 90 s. Participants were then given a clean towel to dry themselves.

Three skin swabs were sampled from eight anatomical sites on each volunteer. The first and last cotton swabs were dry, while the second cotton swabs were immersed in propan-2-ol prior to use. The efficacy of decontamination was analyzed using whole-body fluorescent imaging to visualize simulant distribution. Additionally, the recovery of methyl salicylate in swab samples was quantified using high-performance liquid chromatography. Relative effectiveness of each decontamination protocol was calculated using the reduction in contamination (quantity of simulant recovered from the skin) as a percentage of the corresponding control value.

Chilcott et al. [18, 19] found that the "triple protocol" was the most consistently effective protocol and resulted in significantly reduced methyl salicylate recoveries in all contamination sites. Interestingly, dry decontamination was only statistically significant in one contamination site, until video evidence showed two outliers who did failed to engage in dry decontamination, even though they were instructed to do so. When these outliers were removed, dry decontamination was found to result in significant reduction in methyl salicylate recovery from the hair, right palm, and chest. In fact, they determined that when used properly, dry decontamination of the initially contaminated sites had an overall effectiveness of 99%. From the UV images, they found there were no significant differences in the spread of contaminant. In other words, decontamination did not cause significant transfer of contaminant from application sites to non-application sites.

Matar et al. [20] also studied the "triple protocol" of sequential dry decontamination, LPS, and TD, but in vitro. The three methods were tested on their own, and in different combinations to determine decontamination efficacy, and comprised a total of nine treatment groups. Human hair and porcine skin were exposed to either methyl salicylate (MS), phorate (PHR), sodium fluoroacetate (SFA), or potassium cyanide (KCN) using a hybrid in vitro diffusion cell described by Matar et al. [22] for the evaluation of hair and skin decontamination simultaneously. Twenty microliter of one of the four radiolabelled contaminants was added to the skin, while another 20 μL was added to the hair (total dose of 40 μL). At 4 min post exposure, sterile trauma dressings (cut into 38.5 cm² disks) with a weight placed on top were used for dry decontamination of the skin and hair. The dressing and weight were left for 5 s, before the dressing was turned over, and a tinfoil disk was placed over the dressing, and the weight was placed on top of that for another 5 s. The tinfoil disk and dressing then underwent digital autoradiography imaging. The dressing was applied for 5 s on each side for dry decontamination. In combination protocols where LPS was employed, it was performed for 15 s at 8 min post exposure. This involved shower with water at a temperature of 10 °C and flow rate of 10 mL/min. Shower effluent was collected post decontamination, in addition to an 11 × 11 cm towel which was used for hair and skin drying. In combination protocols where TD was employed, it occurred at 12 min post exposure. This involved a water temperature of 35 °C and a flow rate of 74 mL/min. The diffusion cells were open and tilted so that the skin and hair could be rubbed with a 3 × 3 cm flannel impregnated with 100 μL of shampoo. Shower effluent was collected. The skin and hair were then dried with a towel swatch, which was subsequently collected along with the flannel for digital autoradiography imaging. Throughout the experiments, 75 mL of air was sampled from the donor chamber every minute. All samples underwent liquid scintillation counting to detect radioactivity, which was then used to determine the quantities of radiolabelled contaminant in each.

Within the same manuscript, Matar et al. [20] also described the investigation of residual hair contamination after decontamination with "triple protocol" at different intervals post exposure, and the off gassing of hair after exposure to sulfur mustard or phorate (PHR) and subsequent decontamination, in order to assess the risk of secondary contamination. However, neither of these studies investigated dry decontamination on its own, and therefore, it is difficult to draw comparative conclusions about dry decontamination efficacy based on these aspects of the article.

Matar et al. [20] found that the amount of recovered bioavailable fraction ("the total amount of receptor fluid, remaining within the skin and on the skin surface") or on the hair was significantly smaller than controls for all nine treatment groups. There were no statistically significant differences between decontamination protocols for the skin with the exception of dry decontamination compared to the "triple protocol," for all four contaminants tested. Additionally, there were significant differences between dry decontamination versus the dry decontamination plus TD combination and the dry decontamination versus the LPS plus TD combination for contaminants SFA and KCN. Additionally, dry decontamination was effective in reducing the amount of all four of the contaminants in the hair compared to controls. However, the reduction was not statistically significant after dry decontamination, but was for all other decontamination protocols. A statistical difference was present between dry decontamination versus the "triple protocol" and dry decontamination versus the dry contamination plus LPS combination for contaminants SFA and KCN, respectively. Matar et al. [20] also noted that the majority of contaminant was removed by the decontamination method first performed and that in general dry decontamination was not as effective as wet decontamination for hair use.

Larner et al. [21] studied the effectiveness of dry decontamination, LPS, and TD (individually and in combination) for the decontamination of human hair and skin, in vivo. Although the latter two decontamination protocols are wet, dry decontamination was tested in isolation. Additionally, the influence of dry decontamination on later success of wet decontamination protocols was also assessed and is therefore relevant to this manuscript. The toxin of interest used was a mixture of methyl salicylate, fluorophore [curcumin], and mineral oil and was delivered as an aerosol in a dosing chamber (total dose 2 ± 0.1 g) for 5 s. After 4 min, dry decontamination with a wound dressing (25×75 cm) was completed via the following procedure: wipe face (10 s), wipe hands (10 s), wipe body (30 s), and wipe hair (10 s). Wound dressings were photographed on both sides in a fluorescent imaging booth and then placed in a jar and weighed. In combination protocols where the LPS was employed, it occurred at 8 min post exposure and involved walking the distance of the LPS hallway for 15 s and then completing a full 360-degree turn. In combination protocols where TD was employed, it occurred at 12 min post exposure and involved washing with a cotton washcloth containing 10 mL of shampoo for 90 s. The washcloth was then rung out and placed in a jar, which was then weighed. In both the LPS and TD protocols, participants were given disposable cotton towels to dry with for 30 s. Fluorescence photographs of both sides of the cotton towels were taken and placed in jars. Baseline air samples were taken from the decontamination booth at baseline and then at 6.5 and 11.5 min post exposure.

Three skin swab samples were taken from 28 different anatomical sites (15 ventral, 11 dorsal, 1 scalp, and 1 hair) on each volunteer at 18 min post exposure. The first and third swabs were performed with dry cotton pads, while the second was performed with a propan-2-ol-soaked cotton pad. Four swabs (1 and 4 with dry pads and 2 and 3 with propan-2-ol-soaked pads) were performed on the hair.

Fluorescent photographs were taken before (at baseline) and after each step of decontamination and again after hair and skin swabs were taken. Baseline urine samples were taken, followed by a 24-h urine collection post experiment.

The effectiveness of the decontamination methods were assessed by (1) particle analysis of the full-body fluorescent imaging followed by calculations of the total residual contaminated fluorescent area; (2) liquid chromatography and thermal desorption chromatography to measure residual contaminants in hair, skin, decontamination materials, and air samples; and (3) LC-MS analysis of urine samples looking for salicyluric acid (primary metabolite of methyl salicylate).

Larner et al. [21] found that while all of the individual decontamination protocols, including dry decontamination alone, resulted in qualitative reductions, none were significant in reducing the median amount of methyl salicylate from the back, hair, and scalp when compared to controls. However, authors found that dry decontamination prior to LPS or TD significantly reduced the amount of methyl salicylate skin contamination. The use of dry decontamination also decreased the secondary sources of contamination (off gassing of vapor and residual contaminant on washcloths and towels). Larner et al. [21] found that the "triple protocol" (dry decontamination, LPS, and TD) was the most efficacious protocol of those tested and resulted in an up to 16-fold decrease in contamination when compared to controls. Therefore, these authors concluded that dry decontamination, when executed promptly post exposure, and later followed by wet decontamination protocols result in an improvement in clinical outcomes. This could be of significance in situations where there is a delay in the deployment and arrival of wet decontamination resources.

Southworth [14] conducted a controlled crossover human volunteer study with randomized assignments. Decontamination protocols tested included no decontamination (control), wet decontamination, dry decontamination, and combined wet and dry decontamination. Two microliters of 1:1 (v/v) ratio of methyl salicylate in vegetable oil with 4 mg/mL of Invisible Red S (a UV fluorophore) was applied to analytic sites as the contaminant. Areas of contamination and subsequent decontamination included the shoulder, forearm, and calf.

Decontamination took place at 15 min post exposure, and although exposure sites were distinct anatomical areas, volunteers were instructed to decontamination as though their entire body had been contaminated. Dry decontamination utilized 25×25 cm pieces of white roll folded in half twice. The volunteers were instructed to use as many pieces of white roll as they required to blot and rub their skin beginning at the shoulders and working down, over a 3-min time period. Wet decontamination involved the following subsequent steps which each took place for 1 min (total 3 min): (1) rinse the body with clean water using 1 L jug provided, (2) wipe body in a downward motion from shoulders using a sponge and 0.5% detergent solution, and (3) rinse the body again using clean water and 1 L jug. In the combined dry and wet decontamination test group, the second protocol was started at 21 min post exposure.

UV images were collected at baseline and at 13, 19, 25, 28, and 40 min post exposure. Urine samples were collected at baseline and over 24 h post exposure. Tape-strip sampling was done 30 min post exposure.

The efficacy of decontamination was evaluated by determining the spread and intensity of contaminant on the skin using UV photo image analysis. Additionally, the amount of contaminant remaining on the skin (tape-strips) after decontamination was determined using gas chromatography-tandem mass spectrometry. Finally, urine samples were examined for methyl salicylate.

Southworth [14] found that there was a significant reduction in simulant recovered from the skin following all three decontamination protocols when compared to controls. In addition, combined wet and dry decontamination protocols were superior to either wet or dry protocols alone. In fact, 67% less contaminant was recovered from the skin that underwent the combined decontamination protocol rather than either the wet or dry decontamination protocol alone. These conclusions were supported both by UV imaging and skin sample analyses. However, there was no significant main effect of decontamination on the amount of contaminant present in urine when compared to controls, and authors concluded these samples were problematic and inconclusive. The authors hypothesized that participant compliance with 24-h urine collection and the urinary half-life of MeS contributed to the lack of difference in urine MeS levels among controls and participants. Authors proposed limiting urine sample collection at 8 h rather than 24 h post contamination to "improve protocol adherence by participants in future studies."

Discussion

Several important conclusions can be drawn from these studies. Firstly, of the seven studies investigated, all found that dry decontamination resulted in reductions in contamination. However, not all experiments within these articles showed that these reductions in contamination were significant.

Two out of four dry decontaminants resulted in the reduction of skin surface spreading, and three out of four dry decontaminants resulted in the reduction in the residual amount of contaminant in the Kassouf et al. [16] study. Hall et al. [17] showed that WoundStat was statistically significant in reducing the amount of contaminant recovered from the skin and on skin surface swabs. It should be noted that this was the only study that tested decontamination of wounded skin. Amlôt et al. [13] found that decontamination was significant in reduction of cotton swab contaminant recovery when compared to controls for both the blot and the blot and rub methods of decontamination. There was also a significant difference in the amount of methyl salicylate recovered from the tape-strips following decontamination using the blot and rub method when compared to controls. Chilcott et al. [18, 19] found that when performed properly, dry decontamination was statistically significant for all initially contaminated sites. Matar et al. [20] found that dry decontamination resulted in a significantly smaller bioavailable fraction of contaminant compared to controls. Larner et al. [21] found while dry decontamination alone was not statistically significant, dry decontamination prior to LPS or TD did result in significant contaminant reduction. Finally, Southworth et al. [14] found that significantly lower levels of contamination were recovered from samples that underwent each decontamination method compared to controls.

The fact that all dry decontamination methods tested resulted in reductions in contamination (whether at statistically significant levels or not) is of relevance considering some wet decontamination methods, such as soap and water, can result in an increase in contaminant absorption due to the "wash-in" effect [9]. As quoted from Lake et al. [1], one should "use the fastest approach that will cause the least harm and do the most good for the majority of the people." Dry decontamination with the readily available materials described in this review will likely be the fastest and most widely accessible method of decontamination available, and these results show that where dry decontamination may be inferior to specific decontaminants for specific insults, it appears that performing dry decontamination does not run the same risk of actually causing harm, like some wet decontaminants.

Prior to 2015, US Federal Guidelines (Primary Response Incident Scene Management [PRISM]) recommended first responders wait for specialist response teams to arrive on the scene for chemical decontamination. However, the UK Initial Operational Response Programme guidelines [23] recommend that dry decontamination should take place immediately after a contamination with a non-caustic chemical is suspected and then possibly be followed by wet decontamination. Additionally, the second edition of PRISM [10] recommends the "triple protocol" of decontamination: dry, ladder pipe, and technical.

This is of relevance given that all studies that tested combination decontamination methods (wet and dry) compared to individual methods showed that the combination methods were the most efficacious. These studies include Chilcott et al. [18, 19], who found that the "triple protocol" (dry decontamination plus LPS and TD) was the most effective. Similarly, Larner et al. [21] found that the "triple protocol" was significantly superior to other methods. Southworth et al. [14] found that the dry and wet decontamination protocol was superior to either dry or wet decontamination alone. Matar et al. [20] found while the "triple protocol" was the most effective, this difference was only statistically significant when compared to dry decontamination alone (not compared to LPS or TD alone). These studies also highlighted that dry decontamination can often serve as the first step in these combination decontamination protocols, and they can be improvised, using common household/workplace/ambulance items while waiting for the deployment and arrival of specialist/formal decontamination supplies.

Kassouf et al. [16] noted that the blue roll, sponge, green pad, and Maxiflex dressing were all chosen as they are materials commonly found in domestic and clinical environments. Similarly, Amlôt et al. [13] stated that they chose their decontaminants based on the fact that they are "readily available, absorbent materials" (incontinence pads and paper towel). Chilcott et al. [18, 19] used wound dressing as a dry decontaminant as it can be rapidly implemented and does not rely on specialist resources. Additionally, Larner et al. [21] highlighted the importance of having dry decontamination options that are readily available to employ while waiting for the deployment and organization of "more formal decontamination measures." Matar et al. [20] highlighted the importance of dry decontamination as an "improvised decontamination method" while waiting for "specialist" methods of decontamination like the technical decontamination they described. Finally, Southworth et al. [14] also highlighted the intentional testing for "readily available materials" that can be used in "improvised decontamination procedures."

Hall et al. [17] stated that the investigation of WoundStat is of relevance due to the fact that current decontamination practices are contraindicated for intrawound use and may even hinder wound healing. Given that, in many chemical exposure events (occupational accidents, chemical warfare), wounds are likely, it is helpful to have a decontaminating agent that is not only safe to use on wounded skin but actually also acts to stop bleeding [17]. Similar hemostatic agents may be present in ambulances and other emergency vehicles/locations, and therefore, WoundStat was considered a relatively accessible type of dry decontaminant.

As mentioned, Chilcott et al. [18, 19], Larner et al. [21], Matar et al. [20], and Southworth et al. [14] showed that combination protocols tend to be the most efficacious. This review also highlights another reason that future chemical exposure response guidelines should include not only decontaminant recommendations but also recommendations on the manner in which decontaminants are used. This was clear in the article by Amlôt et al. [13], who noted that blotting versus rubbing versus blotting and rubbing yielded different decontamination effectiveness. They concluded that the blotting and rubbing combination method was superior to either rubbing or blotting alone.

The importance of the manner in which the decontaminants are used was also highlighted by Southworth et al. [14]. This was the only study protocol which allowed subjects to use "as much decontaminant as they needed," whereas other protocols predefined the amount that was to be used. Southworth et al. [14] found that a higher number of white roll sheets used was associated with better decontamination (lower post-decontamination contaminant recovery). This is a point that should be interpreted with situational judgment in determining whether decontaminant supplies need to be rationed or not (i.e., single-person exposure versus mass exposures, respectively). If supplies are not limited, perhaps a large amount is more effective in decontamination; however, more studies should be conducted on this.

The Kassouf et al. [16] study also highlighted the importance of guidelines not only including information on decontaminants but also on the manner in which they are used. Their manuscript included a second study, in which they gave a group of ten volunteers detailed instructions on how to use the dry decontaminants, whereas a different group of 11 volunteers was told to use the product to remove contaminants from the skin and received no further guidance. The study measured whether the participants completed decontamination successfully (video observational analysis) and how the participants experienced the process (questionnaire). The measures observed on the video were whole-body decontamination, top-down decontamination to avoid cross contamination, and use of adequate blue roll. The instructed guided group was more successful at performing dry decontamination from top down than those in the no guidance group.

Guidance promoted volunteer adherence to safe and systematic decontamination steps which would likely lead to less cross contamination and more effective dry decontamination. The no guidance group perceived inadequate communication and had lower confidence in cleanliness after decontamination based on questionnaire responses.

This study exemplifies the importance of public education on the matter of decontamination protocols in case of dermal exposures to toxic compounds. Training of first responders and military personnel may not be adequate as there is a time lag between exposure and arrival of first responders. Additionally, Chilcott et al. [18, 19] followed up with EMS responders after their experimental simulations. The EMS responders noted that it was difficult to communicate with the volunteers and that giving instructions was challenging to coordinate. Therefore, public awareness and emergency readiness campaigns are important to keep communities safe.

Some limitations of this study included the heterogeneity in study protocols, which made interstudy comparisons difficult. Additionally, factors important to consider include the benefits and drawbacks of in vivo versus ex vivo versus in vitro findings and animal versus human models. While this study investigated a wide variety of study models, human in vivo methods tend to be considered the gold standard for dermal decontamination, but their use in experimentation is hindered due to ethical considerations.

Conclusion

There are specific situations in which dry decontamination holds benefits over wet decontamination, and these methods are available to most, as demonstrated in this study which investigated only dry decontamination methods commonly found in households/workplaces/ambulances. Important takeaways include that all studies investigated demonstrated that dry decontamination resulted in decreases in contamination. This is in contrast to some wet decontamination scenarios, where the amount of contamination is increased due to the "wash-in" effect. Additionally, these studies generally showed that not only the decontaminant but also the manner in which it is used (blotting versus rubbing, amount of decontamination used, and whether decontamination instructions are provided) is of importance. In all four studies in which combination protocols (dry and wet) were employed, they resulted in the most effective decontamination. These conclusions should be kept in mind in the event that a universal decontamination protocol is developed, though more studies are needed in order to provide greater insight into this important topic.

Acknowledgments None.

Conflicts of Interest None.

Funding Sources None.

References

1. Lake W, Schulze P, Gougelet R, Divarco S. Updated guidelines for mass casualty decontamination during a HAZMAT/weapon of mass destruction incident, Volumes I and II. 2013. https://apps.dtic.mil/sti/pdfs/ADA590069.pdf.
2. Schwartz MD, Hurst CG, Kirk AM, Reedy JDS, Braue HE. Reactive skin decontamination lotion (RSDL) for the decontamination of chemical warfare agent (CWA) dermal exposure. Curr Pharm Biotechnol. 2012;13(10):1971–9. https://doi.org/10.2174/138920112802273191.
3. National Institute for Occupational Safety and Health. Skin exposures and effects. Atlanta, GA: CDC; 2013. https://www.cdc.gov/niosh/topics/skin/default.html. Accessed 5 Dec 2021.
4. Ganesan K, Raza S, Vijayaraghavan R. Chemical warfare agents. J Pharm Bioalil Sci. 2010;2(3):166. https://doi.org/10.4103/0975-7406.68498.
5. Burli A, Kashetsky N, Feschuk A, Law RM, Maibach HI. Efficacy of soap and water based skin decontamination using in vivo animal models: a systematic review. J Toxicol Environ Health B. 2021;24(7):325–36. https://doi.org/10.1080/10937404.2021.1943087.
6. Chiang C, Kashetsky N, Feschuk A, Burli A, Law RM, Maibach HI. Efficacy of water-only or soap and water skin decontamination of chemical warfare agents or simulants using in vitro human models: a systematic review. J Appl Toxicol. 2021a;42:930. https://doi.org/10.1002/jat.4251.
7. Chiang C, Kashetsky N, Feschuk A, Burli A, Law R, Maibach H. Efficacy of water-based skin decontamination of occupational chemicals using in vitro human skin models: a systematic review. J Toxicol Environ Health B. 2021b;24(7):337–53. https://doi.org/10.1080/1093740 4.2021.1957048.
8. Green M, Kashetsky N, Feschuk AM, Maibach HI. Efficacy of soap and water-based skin decontamination using in vitro animal models: a systematic review. J Appl Toxicol. 2021;24:325. https://doi.org/10.1002/jat.4274.
9. Moody RP, Maibach HI. Skin decontamination: importance of the wash-in effect. Food Chem Toxicol. 2006;44(11):1783–8. https://doi.org/10.1016/j.fct.2006.05.020.
10. Chilcott RP, Larner J, Matar H. Primary Response Incident Scene Management (PRISM): guidance for the operational response to chemical incidents. Volume 1: Strategic guidance for mass casualty disrobe and decontaminate. 2nd ed. Washington, DC: Biomedical Advanced Research Development Authority; 2018. https://www.medicalcountermeasures.gov/BARDA/Documents/PRISM%20Volume%201_Strategic%20Guidance%20Second%20Edition.pdf.
11. Roul A, Le CAK, Gustin MP, Clavaud E, Verrier B, Pirot F, Falson F. Comparison of four different fuller's earth formulations in skin decontamination. J Appl Toxicol. 2017;37(12):1527–36. https://doi.org/10.1002/jat.3506.
12. Cao Y, Hui X, Zhu H, Elmahdy A, Maibach H. In vitro human skin permeation and decontamination of 2-chloroethyl ethyl sulfide (CEES) using Dermal Decontamination Gel (DDGel) and Reactive Skin Decontamination Lotion (RSDL). Toxicol Lett. 2018;291:86–91. https://doi.org/10.1016/j.toxlet.2018.04.015.
13. Amlôt R, Carter H, Riddle L, Larner J, Chilcott RP. Volunteer trials of a novel improvised dry decontamination protocol for use during mass casualty incidents as part of the UK'S Initial Operational Response (IOR). PLoS One. 2017;12(6):e0179309. https://doi.org/10.1371/journal.pone.0179309.
14. Southworth F, James T, Davidson L, Williams N, Finnie T, Marczylo T, Collins S, Amlôt R. A controlled cross-over study to evaluate the efficacy of improvised dry and wet emergency decontamination protocols for chemical incidents. PLoS One. 2020;15(11):e0239845. https://doi.org/10.1371/journal.pone.0239845.
15. Page MJ, McKenzie JE, Bossuyt PM, Boutron I, Hoffmann TC, Mulrow CD, Shamseer L, Tetzlaff, JM, Akl EA, Brennan SE, Chou R, Glanville J, Grimshaw JM, Hróbjartsson A, Lalu MM, Li T, Loder EW, Mayo-Wilson E, McDonald S, McGuinness LA, Stewart LA, Thomas J, Tricco AC, Welch VA, Whiting P, and Moher D. The PRISMA 2020 statement: An updated guideline for reporting systematic reviews. 2021;BMJ 372:n71. https://doi.org/10.1136/bmj.n71.

16. Kassouf N, Syed S, Larner J, Amlôt R, Chilcott RP. Evaluation of absorbent materials for use as ad hoc dry decontaminants during mass casualty incidents as part of the UK's Initial Operational Response (IOR). PLoS One. 2017;12(2):e0170966. https://doi.org/10.1371/journal.pone.0170966.

17. Hall CA, Lydon HL, Dalton CH, Chipman JK, Graham JS, Chilcott RP. The percutaneous toxicokinetics of Sulphur mustard in a damaged skin porcine model and the evaluation of WoundStat™ as a topical decontaminant. J Appl Toxicol. 2017;37(9):1036–45. https://doi.org/10.1002/jat.3453.

18. Chilcott RP, Larner J, Durrant A, Hughes P, Mahalingam D, Rivers S, Thomas E, Amer N, Barrett M, Matar H, Pinhal A, Jackson T, McCarthy-Barnett K, Reppucci J. Evaluation of US Federal Guidelines (Primary Response Incident Scene Management [PRISM]) for mass decontamination of casualties during the initial operational response to a chemical incident. Ann Emerg Med. 2019a;73(6):671–84. https://doi.org/10.1016/j.annemergmed.2018.06.042.

19. Chilcott RP, Larner J, Matar H. UK's initial operational response and specialist operational response to CBRN and HazMat incidents: a primer on decontamination protocols for healthcare professionals. Emerg Med J. 2019b;36:117. https://doi.org/10.1136/emermed-2018-207562.

20. Matar H, Pinhal A, Amer N, Barrett M, Thomas E, Hughes P, Larner J, Chilcott RP. Decontamination and management of contaminated hair following a CBRN or HazMat incident. Toxicol Sci. 2019;171(1):269–79. https://doi.org/10.1093/toxsci/kfz145.

21. Larner J, Durrant A, Hughes P, Mahalingam D, Rivers S, Matar H, Thomas E, Barrett M, Pinhal A, Amer N, Hall C, Jackson T, Catalani V, Chilcott RP. Efficacy of different hair and skin decontamination strategies with identification of associated hazards to first responders. Prehosp Emerg Care. 2019;24(3):355–68. https://doi.org/10.1080/10903127.2019.1636912.

22. Matar H, Amer N, Kansagra S, Pinhal A, Thomas E, Townend S, Larner J, Chilcott RP. Hybrid in vitro diffusion cell for simultaneous evaluation of hair and skin decontamination: temporal distribution of chemical contaminants. Sci Rep. 2018;8(1):16906. https://doi.org/10.1038/s41598-018-35105-z.

23. Home Office. Initial operational response to a CBRN incident. 2015. https://www.jesip.org.uk/uploads/media/pdf/CBRN%20JOPs/IOR_Guidance_V2_July_2015.pdf.

Chapter 8
A Review of Reactive Skin Decontamination Lotion Efficacy

Aileen M. Feschuk, Rebecca M. Law, and Howard I. Maibach

Abbreviations

CEES	2-Chloroethyl ethyl sulfide
CWA	Chemical warfare agent
DAM	2,3-Butanedione monoxime
DDGel	Dermal Decontamination Gel
DIMP	Diisopropyl methylphosphonate
FE	Fuller's earth
GM	Soman
M291 SDK	M291 Skin Decontamination Kit
POX	Paraoxon
PR	Protective ratio
PS104	Swedish decontamination powder 104
SM	Sulfur mustard
TIC	Toxic industrial chemical
VX	Venomous Agent 10

A. M. Feschuk (✉)
Faculty of Medicine, Memorial University of Newfoundland, St. John's, NL, Canada
e-mail: amfeschuk@mun.ca

R. M. Law
School of Pharmacy, Memorial University of Newfoundland, St. John's, NL, Canada

H. I. Maibach
Department of Dermatology, University of California San Francisco, San Francisco, CA, USA

Introduction

Chemical warfare agents (CWAs) caused 1.2 million casualties in the First World War [1]. Today, the threat of chemical warfare remains, in addition to the substantial risks posed by accidents with toxic industrial chemicals (TICs) [2]. Despite these threats, contemporary knowledge surrounding comparative efficacy of human skin decontaminating agents remains limited.

The skin is the first line of defense against CWAs and can provide a temporary barrier to agents which affect other tissues within the body [3]. However, some chemicals are toxic to the skin itself. Schwartz et al. [2] stated that dermal decontamination is the "single most important action" in preventing dermal absorption of CWAs and TICs. Therefore, rapid and effective decontamination following exposure to CWAs and TICs remains of utmost importance.

Classically, skin decontamination relies heavily on "wet" decontamination practices, which include washing the body with water or soap and water [4]. Alternatively, "dry" decontamination is based on adsorptive properties of powders, flours, or clay, including Fuller's earth (FE) [4]. FE is an absorbing powder that, when spread onto contaminated skin, absorbs toxic agents, due to its large surface area and selectivity for lipophilic molecules [5]. Another skin decontamination agent that has shown its effectiveness against multiple different CWAs and TICs is Reactive Skin Decontamination Lotion (RSDL) and hence has been endorsed by several governments. Both FE and the newer RSDL have been extensively used as skin decontamination agents, with research comparing their efficacy versus various toxins still being done today [6].

RSDL, developed by the Canadian Department of National Defense, was distributed as a lotion-impregnated sponge to Canadian troops in the First Gulf War in 1991 [7]. Subsequently, RSDL has been approved by the US Food and Drug Administration, Health Canada, Australian Therapeutic Goods Administration, and Israel Ministry of Health [7].

RSDL is composed of Dekon 139 and 2,3-butanedione monoxime (DAM) dissolved in a polyethylene glycol monomethyl ether and water solvent (US Department of Health and Human Services 2017), and when applied to contaminated skin, a nucleophilic substitution reaction occurs between DAM and the susceptible sites of the toxic substances [8], resulting in non-toxic products [9]. Therefore, the action of RSDL is at least threefold: (1) physical removal of the contaminant with the sponge, (2) dilution of the contaminant by RSDL solution, and (3) degradation of the contaminant by the active ingredients of RSDL. RSDL removes or neutralizes compounds such as tabun, soman (GD), sarin, cyclohexyl, Venomous Agent 10 (VX), VR, mustard gas, and T-2 toxin, from the skin [7].

VX is a toxin that is commonly used for skin decontamination studies [6, 10, 11]. VX is a man-made nerve agent developed in the United Kingdom in the 1950s as a chemical warfare agent, and it is a tasteless, odorless, oily liquid that is slow to evaporate [12].

Due to the vital importance, yet insufficiency, of conclusive data regarding skin decontamination of numerous CWAs and TICs, this systematic review compares efficacy of the widely used RSDL to other skin decontaminating agents.

Methods

A library scientist, Alison Farrell, was consulted to identify the online search engines most appropriate for this overview. The search engines used were PubMed, Web of Science, and Embase. The librarian also generated a search code used to do a general background search on skin decontaminating agents: (("Decontamination"[Mesh] OR decontamination[tiab] OR decontaminate[tiab] OR decontaminating[tiab]) AND ("Skin"[Mesh] OR skin[tiab]) AND (effective[tiab] OR efficacy[tiab] OR effectiveness[tiab] OR comparing[tiab] OR comparison[tiab] OR comparative[tiab])). This code was designed specifically for PubMed and was then altered for searching in Embase and Web of Science. Hits that were deemed relevant, based on their title and abstract, were uploaded to Covidence for further approval by two additional reviewers. Covidence is an online tool designed for the conduction of systematic reviews which is available at http://app.covidence.org through an institutional subscription at Memorial University Health Sciences Library.

The initial decontamination search generated 2662 studies. To focus on the scope, the decontamination method, RSDL, was chosen based on the fact that it is relatively new, appears highly effective, is in current use, and has been massively distributed worldwide. Emergent Biosolutions Inc. [7] states over 15 million packets of RSDL have been sold in over 35 countries. A comparison of RSDL to other decontamination agents would provide relative efficacies, i.e., put into perspective the effectiveness of other agents.

RSDL studies were retrieved in October 2020 from PubMed, Embase, and Web of Science, and all relevant articles were uploaded to Covidence. Duplicates between the search engines were automatically discarded in Covidence. Relevance of each article was judged based on title and abstract. Each abstract was then reviewed by two additional reviewers to determine whether the article would be included or not. The articles that passed the title and abstract review by all three reviewers were then examined in full. Publications that involved quantitative comparisons of RSDL to other decontaminating agents were retained and their results compiled and summarized. Multiple studies compared the efficacy of RSDL to other decontaminating agents in their ability to decontaminate hair. Only articles that involved quantitative comparisons of skin decontamination using RSDL to another decontaminating agent(s) were included.

Results

Searching RSDL in PubMed resulted in 35 hits; Web of Science, 31 hits; and Embase, 52 hits. Based on title and abstract, 32 articles from PubMed, 29 articles from Web of Science, and 38 articles from Embase were uploaded into a Covidence systematic review file. Covidence removed duplicates found between the three search engines, leaving 46 articles for review. Articles not in English were excluded. Of the remaining, 14 involved quantitative comparisons of skin decontamination using RSDL to another decontaminating agent(s). The 14 articles that involved quantitative comparisons of RSDL to other decontaminating agents were then sub-categorized by year of publication, type of study (in vitro versus in vivo), and model used (human versus animal) (Table 8.1). The toxin used and results of each study were documented (Table 8.2). An additional study (from a PubMed alert) e-published ahead of print in January 2021 was subsequently included.

Taysse et al. [13] compared the performance of RSDL and FE in vitro using domestic swine. These two decontaminating agents were tested against sulfur mustard (SM) and VX. Three days post exposure, RSDL was better than FE in preventing skin injury induced by SM based on reduced formation of perinuclear vacuoles and inflammation in the epidermis and dermis. Both RSDL and FE completely prevented cholinesterase inhibition usually caused by VX, indirectly indicating that both were successful in inhibiting toxin percutaneous absorption.

Then, Taysse et al. [14] compared the effectiveness of FE and RSDL against two CWAs: liquid SM and VX. One mouse group was exposed to 2 µL of neat SM and another exposed to 50 µg/kg of diluted VX and then decontaminated with either FE

Table 8.1 Authors, publication year, study type, and research model used for each paper involving quantitative comparisons of RSDL versus other agents for skin decontamination (found in PubMed, Web of Science, and Embase)

Authors	Year of publication	Type of study	Model
Taysse et al.	2007	In vitro	Domestic swine
Bjarnason et al.	2008	In vivo	Domestic swine
Bazire et al.	2010	In vivo	Human skin grafted onto hairless mice
Braue et al.	2011	In vivo	Guinea pigs
Braue et al.	2011	In vivo	Guinea pigs
Josse et al.	2011	In vitro	Domestic swine
Taysse et al.	2011	In vivo	Hairless mice
Rolland et al.	2012	In vitro	Domestic swine
Salerno et al.	2017	In vitro	Domestic swine
Thors et al.	2017	In vitro	Human skin
Cao et al.	2018	In vitro	Human skin
Cao et al.	2018	In vitro	Human skin
Thors et al.	2020	In vitro	Human skin
Thors et al.	2020	In vitro	Human skin
Dachir et al.	2021	In vivo	Domestic swine

Table 8.2 The toxin used and result of each paper involving quantitative comparisons of RSDL versus other agents for skin decontamination (found in PubMed, Web of Science, and Embase)

Study	Toxin	Result
Taysse et al. [13]	SM	Superior
Taysse et al. [13]	VX	Equal
Taysse et al. [14]	SM	Superior
Taysse et al. [14]	VX	Inferior
Bjarnason et al. [11]	VX	Superior
Bjarnason et al. [11]	VX/decontaminating agent mixture	Equal
Bazire et al. [10]	VX	Superior
Braue Jr. et al. [15]	GD	Superior
Braue Jr. et al. [16]	VX	Superior
Josse et al. [17]	VX	Equal
Rolland et al. [5]	VX	Superior
Salerno et al. [18]	POX	Equal
Cao et al. [19]	DIMP	Inferior
Cao et al. [20]	CEES	Inferior
Thors et al. [21]	VX	Superior
Thors et al. [22]	VX	Superior
Thors et al. [23]	Fentanyl	Inferior
Dachir et al. [6]	VX	Equal

Toxin legend: *SM* sulfur mustard, *VX* Venomous Agent 10, *GD* soman, *POX* paraoxon, *DIMP* diisopropyl methylphosphonate, *CEES* 2-chloroethyl ethyl sulfide, *VX-decontaminating agent* VX that was vigorously mixed for 5 min with the trial decontaminant prior to exposure. Result legend: *Superior* RSDL was the most effective decontaminant tested against the toxin of interest, *Equal* RSDL was equal in efficacy to at least one of the other decontaminating agents tested, against the toxin of interest, *Inferior* RSDL was not the most effective decontaminant tested against the toxin of interest

or RSDL, 5 min post exposure. Although both FE and RSDL reduced blisters 3 days following SM exposure, RSDL was more efficient than FE in reducing SM epidermal necrosis and erosion. However, RSDL failed to sufficiently prevent VX cholinesterase inhibition. This was true regardless of the ratio of decontaminant to toxicant used (RSDL 10, 20, 50). They used plasma cholinesterases as a surrogate marker of exposure and toxicity. Taysse et al. [14] concluded that only FE significantly reduced inhibition of cholinesterase in mice.

Bjarnason et al. [11] compared the efficacy of RSDL, FE, 0.5% hypochlorite, and soapy water in decontaminating anesthetized domestic swine 45 min after exposure to 5 × LD(50) VX. All domestic swine decontaminated with either RSDL or FE survived. However, half of the swine decontaminated with FE showed serious signs of VX poisoning. Decontamination of swine with 0.5% hypochlorite was less effective than RSDL and FE but still increased survival. Decontamination with soapy water was ineffective and resulted in death of all animals in that test group.

Effect of decontaminating the VX prior to its exposure to open wounds was also investigated. Decontaminating agents used included RSDL, FE, 0.5% hypochlorite, and soapy water. In order to test this, 5 × LD(50) VX was vigorously mixed for

5 min with the trial decontaminant and the mixture then placed onto a full-thickness skin wound. All swine in the dry FE-VX mixture test group survived and displayed no signs of organophosphate poisoning. However, a significant portion of the swine treated with an aqueous suspension of FE-VX mixture displayed signs of serious organophosphate poisoning. The animals in both the RSDL and 0.5% hypochlorite-VX mixture test groups survived and showed no symptoms of organophosphate poisoning. All soapy water-VX mixture animals died.

Bazire et al. [10] studied human skin decontamination in vivo by grafting human skin onto athymic nude mice ("HuSki model") and then exposing the grafted skin to a droplet of 40 μg VX diluted in distilled water 2 months later. This study compared a control group (no decontamination) to decontamination 20 min post exposure with FE, RSDL, or an aqueous detergent (Argos® group). At 2 h post exposure, all control animals died, 1/7 of the FE test group animals died, and 2/7 of the Argos® test group animals had died. None of the animals in the RSDL test group died 2 h post exposure. At 6 h post exposure, 5/7 of the animals in the FE test group died, and 6/7 of the animals in the Argos® test group died. In comparison, at 6 h post exposure, 3/7 of the animals in the RSDL group died. Bazire et al. [10] concluded that RSDL applied to the "HuSki model" 20 min post exposure was a more efficient decontaminant than either FE or Argos®.

Braue et al. in 2011 published companion articles, both comparing efficacy of four decontaminating agents, and Skin Exposure Reduction Paste Against Chemical Warfare Agents (SERPACWA), against toxic nerve agents. The four decontaminating agents used were RSDL, 0.5% bleach, 1% soapy water, and the M291 Skin Decontamination Kit (M291 SDK). In the first study, the toxic nerve agent used was VX and in the second study GD.

Hairless guinea pigs in the treatment group received VX (either neat or 5% VX in isopropyl alcohol solution) and then received a decontaminating agent 2 min later. The protective ratio (PR) was then determined for each treatment group. The PR is defined as "the median lethal dose [LD(50)] of the treatment group divided by the LD(50) of the untreated positive control animals" [15]. Then, a delayed decontamination time, LT(50), was determined for each decontaminating agent. The LT(50) is the "time at which 50% of the animals died in the test population following a 5-LD(50) challenge" [15]. The same procedure was repeated in the second study [16], utilizing GD instead of VX. Additionally, in the second study, only RSDL was used for delayed decontamination trials.

The first study found that RSDL provided the best protection, and 0.5% bleach and 1% soapy water provided less effective but good protection, against VX. M291 SDK did not provide significant protection against VX. The LT(50) values for RSDL, 0.5% bleach, and 1% soapy water were 31, 48, and 26 min, respectively. The second study found that RSDL provided significantly better protection against GD than the other decontaminants. The other decontaminants, bleach, soapy water, and M291 SDK, all provided significantly less protection against GD. Given that only RSDL provided significant protection against GD, it was the only decontaminating agent used in the delayed-decontamination portion of the study. The LT(50) time for RSDL against GD was only 4 min.

Josse et al. [17] used skin samples from domestic swine to determine the effectiveness of showering before decontamination. Decontaminating agents tested included FE, RSDL, Dakin (solution of 0.5% of sodium hypochlorite [24]), or baby wipes. Skin samples were decontaminated with one of the test agents either 30 min or 1 h post exposure, followed by 1 min of showering 1 h post exposure. Effectiveness of each skin decontamination procedure was determined by VX amount absorbed into, and permeated through, the skin 6 h post exposure.

Treatment with either RSDL or 0.5% hypochlorite 30 min post exposure, followed by 1 min of showering 1 h post exposure, was the most effective decontamination protocol; and the effectiveness of skin decontamination by FE was improved when followed with a shower, although this procedure was still not as effective as protocols using RSDL or 0.5% hypochlorite. There was no evidence that showering created a wash-in effect.

Rolland et al. [5] investigated efficacy of RSDL compared to FE in vitro using pig skin exposed to VX. Exposed hairy skin samples were decontaminated 45 min post exposure. Hair clipping and comparison of clipped vs. unclipped skin showed less viable skin when hair shafts were present. While FE was somewhat effective in the decontamination of the skin exposed to VX, RSDL was more efficient in reducing VX amount in both the skin and hair.

Salerno et al. [18] investigated decontamination of pig skin exposed to paraoxon (POX), in vitro. POX is a cholinesterase inhibitor, is the active metabolite of parathion (an insecticide), and is used as a pesticide, thereby making it a TIC [25]. The four methods of decontamination include powder nanometric cerium oxide [CeO(2)], aqueous nanometric cerium oxide solution [(CeO(2)-W)], FE, and RSDL. Decontaminating agents were applied to skin samples 1 h post exposure.

CeO(2)-W and RSDL were the most effective in the POX removal and that they decreased skin absorption by a factor of 6.4 when compared to control. Although FE was not as efficient as RSDL and CeO(2)-W at reducing the absorption of POX, it was still twice as efficient as CeO(2) powder.

Cao et al. [19] published companion articles comparing the efficacy of using RSDL and Dermal Decontamination Gel (DDGel) for in vitro human skin decontamination. These decontaminating agents were applied at two time points, 5 min and 90 min, and compared. In one paper [19], skin decontamination of diisopropyl methylphosphonate (DIMP) was investigated, and in the companion paper [20], decontamination of 2-chloroethyl ethyl sulfide (CEES) was investigated.

In the first study, radioactivity was measured with a liquid scintillation spectrometer in order to quantify the mass of (14)-C DIMP removed from the skin surface after decontamination. Compared to the control group, both RSDL and DDGel recovered over 90% of applied DIMP from the human skin. DDGel was slightly superior to RSDL in decontaminating human skin of DIMP.

The same method was used in the second study, this time to determine the mass of 14-C CEES removed from the skin surface after decontamination. Both RSDL and DDGel removed over 82% of CEES from human skin in vitro. However, DDGel had twice the decontamination efficacy factor of RSDL. DDGel also efficiently removed chemicals from the skin surface and significantly reduced CEES skin penetration and systemic absorption.

Thors et al. published three applicable papers, in 2017 and 2020; the first investigated decontamination efficacy of RSDL, Swedish decontamination powder 104 (PS104), FE, and the aqueous solution AlldecontMED. The four decontaminating agents were compared 5 or 30 min following dermal exposure to the nerve agent VX (neat or diluted with water to 20%). This efficacy was evaluated in vitro utilizing human skin. Different decontaminating procedures were also investigated (e.g., physical removal by sponge swabbing). Thors et al. [21] found that RSDL was superior in reducing penetration of VX (both neat and at 20% concentration) through the human skin samples, although FE and AlldecontMED both significantly reduced the penetration of VX (neat). Both RSDL and FE were more effective when applied 5 min post exposure, as opposed to 30 min post exposure. AlldecontMED showed similar decontamination efficacy at both time points. PS104 was insufficient in decontaminating the skin from VX at both time points. Using water, without any additional decontaminating agent, resulted in a significant reduction of VX skin penetration when performed 5 min post exposure, but not when performed at 30 min. They concluded that early initiation of decontamination using RSDL, left for 30 min, was the most effective treatment/protocol for preventing VX human skin penetration.

Subsequently, Thors et al. [21] evaluated several RSDL protocols for the efficacy to remove VX (neat) from human skin in vitro. Decontamination efficacy with the RSDL protocols was compared to the efficacy of washing skin with soapy water. Of the RSDL protocols evaluated, the one that demonstrated the greatest efficacy involved repeated swabbing with RSDL sponge and a skin-RSDL contact time of 10 min. They then repeated the protocol that was found to be favorable, 2 h after initial decontamination, which resulted in a transient increase in penetration of the remaining VX on the skin, but was followed by a rapidly declined rate of agent penetration. When soapy water was used for decontamination, significantly increased amounts of VX penetrated the skin. The authors hypothesized that this was caused by dilution of VX and skin hydration. However, this may relate to the washing-in phenomenon seen with percutaneous absorption [26]. The authors concluded that a slightly extended RSDL decontamination procedure improved efficacy and that skin decontamination of nerve agents should involve procedures consisting of low water content.

Then, Thors et al. [22] evaluated the use of different decontaminating agents for skin removal and/or degradation of synthetic opioids. Decontaminating agents included water, soapy water, AlldecontMED, and RSDL. Efficacy of each was evaluated following exposure to fentanyl in solution. Excluding the sponge-only procedure, all procedures decreased the amount of fentanyl hydrochloride and free base solutions penetrating the skin over a 24-h time period. They concluded that if the skin is exposed to small amounts of fentanyl in solution and in the form of solid powder, RSDL is sufficient to remove it but that soapy water is the best decontamination method for fentanyl.

Dachir et al. [6] compared the efficacy of RSDL and FE in the decontamination of domestic swine exposed to VX and SM. The efficacy of decontamination against VX was measured in terms of cholinesterase inhibition and clinical symptoms. The efficacy of decontamination against SM was measured in terms of lesion area and erythema. Both RSDL and FE were found to be highly effective in the decontamination of both agents. FE was more effective than RSDL when the exposure time was just 1 min and assessed 24 h later. However, there was no significant difference between RSDL and FE when assessed 7 days post exposure. Additionally, there was no significant difference between FE and RSDL for exposure times between 5 and 60 min. Although the authors concluded with recommending the use of FE over RSDL, this recommendation was based on other considerations such as shelf life and price.

Discussion

Of the 15 articles that involved quantitative comparisons of RSDL to other decontaminating agents, 2 by Taysse et al. [13] and 1 by Bjarnason et al. [11] each consisted of 2 parts, and each reached different conclusions. For this reason, each of these articles will be considered two articles, for a total of six.

Of the 18 articles reviewed, 9 concluded that RSDL was the most effective decontaminant against the toxin of interest. Taysse [13] concluded that RSDL was more effective than FE against SM. Taysse et al. came to the same conclusion in their 2011 study. Rolland et al. [5] found that RSDL was more efficient in VX decontamination than FE. Thors et al. [21] determined that RSDL was superior to PS104, FE, and AlldecontMED in decontamination of VX. Thors et al. [23] determined that RSDL was more effective than soapy water against VX. Bazire et al. [10] concluded that RSDL was more effective than both FE and Argos® against VX. In companion articles, Braue Jr. et al. [15, 16] concluded that RSDL was more effective than 0.5% bleach, 1% soapy water, and the M291 Swedish Decontamination Kit against VX and against GD. Bjarnason et al. [11] determined that RSDL was more effective than 0.5% hypochlorite, soapy water, and FE in decontaminating VX.

Four studies found that RSDL was not the most effective decontaminant tested against a certain toxin. Of these four, two, both by Cao et al. [19, 20], concluded that DDGel was more effective than RSDL in decontaminating the toxin of interest. In one study, the toxin was DIMP, and in the other, the toxin was CEES. Thors et al. [22] concluded that soapy water was more effective than RSDL in decontaminating fentanyl. Interestingly, de Bruin-Hoegée et al. [27] found that fentanyl is removed by RSDL kits but is not chemically inactivated by the lotion, which could account for why soapy water was found to be more effective than RSDL. Taysse et al. [14] determined that RSDL was not sufficient in decontaminating VX in mice, while FE was. Also of interest is that, in 2007, Taysse et al. had concluded that both FE and RSDL were effective in preventing cholinesterase inhibition due to VX, in guinea pigs. The authors attributed the differences in findings to differences in the decontamination procedures, rather than the agents themselves.

The most recent study by Dachir et al. [6] found similar efficacy between FE and RSDL in decontaminating sulfur mustard and VX. The only significant difference occurred when the exposure time was just 1 min, with FE being more effective than RSDL when assessed at 24 h after exposure, but there was no difference between FE and RSDL at 7 days. Furthermore, there was no difference between FE and RSDL for exposure times from 5 to 60 min.

The remaining four studies concluded RSDL displayed similar efficacy to at least one of the other decontaminating agents tested, against the toxin of interest. Bjarnason et al. [11] showed that when a RSDL-VX mixture or 0.5% hypochlorite-VX mixture was each separately applied to a wound, each mixture prevented symptoms of VX organophosphate poisoning. Josse et al. [17] showed that if applied 30 min post exposure, followed by a 1-min shower 1 h post exposure, both RSDL and 0.5% of sodium hypochlorite were equally as effective against VX. Taysse [13] showed that both RSDL and FE were completely effective in preventing cholinesterase inhibition usually associated with VX. Salerno et al. [18] showed that both RSDL and an aqueous solution of nanometric cerium oxide (CeO(2)-W) were effective in POX decontamination. Dachir et al. [6] found similar efficacy between FE and RSDL in decontaminating sulfur mustard and VX.

Considering that only 4 of 18 concluded that a decontaminating agent other than RSDL was the most effective tested against the toxin of interest, RSDL appears generally useful in protecting people from chemical warfare agents and accidents with TICs. However, there are limitations to the existing studies.

One limitation of the existing literature on skin decontamination is the lack of human in vivo studies to mimic toxic compounds. Structural changes to the skin and the absence of blood flow can affect penetration rates in in vitro studies [28]. However, it is generally accepted that if properly handled, frozen skin is a reasonable surrogate for non-frozen human skin [29]. In vivo studies using animal models provide supporting evidence, but not conclusive results, in terms of applicability to humans. Many articles reviewed used domestic swine or guinea pigs as an animal model for in vivo studies. Domestic swine and guinea pigs are generally considered suitable animal models for dermal studies, due to their similarities with humans in terms of skin composition [28]. The study by Bazire et al. [10] used human skin grafted onto mice as their test model and called it the "HuSki" model. Due to ethical constraints, the HuSki model may be the closest model to in vivo human skin that is possible for studies testing toxic compounds. It is of interest then that this study found that RSDL was more effective in decontaminating VX from the skin, than FE or, the aqueous detergent, Argos®. However, even though RSDL was the most efficient of those three decontaminants, 3/7 of the animals in the RSDL group still died by 6 h post exposure to VX.

Due to the shortage of human in vivo model data available, this systematic review explored all human and animal in vitro and in vivo decontamination data that fit our inclusion criteria. However, we acknowledge the heterogeneity of methods used by each study makes it difficult to conclusively advise for or against the use of RSDL against any and all contaminants. In the future, standardized testing protocols should be developed in order to allow for streamlined interstudy comparisons.

Another limitation includes the lack of data for multiple different CWAs and TICs. Of the 15 publications and 18 study models investigated, 10 used VX as the toxin of interest. One study used both SM and VX as toxins of interest. Two studies used SM, one used GD, one used POX, one used DIMP, one used CEES, and one used fentanyl. VX may be tested the most because it is the most potent of all nerve agents [12]. Despite this, conclusions made about decontamination of VX do not directly reflect decontamination of other toxins. Thus, for some of these toxins, there is only one evaluable comparative study of RSDL with other decontaminating agents.

Additionally, the decontaminating agent itself is not the only important factor in determining the success of decontamination. The protocol of decontamination (e.g., amount, concentration, use of sponge, etc.) influences the study outcome. This was evidenced by Taysse et al. studies, where different results were obtained in 2007 and 2011, when the same decontaminating agents but different decontaminating regimens were employed. Both the delay in application of the decontaminant and the time that the decontaminant is in contact with the skin are important considerations. Taysse et al. [14] stated that decontamination evaluation needs to be based on precisely determined protocols, which standardize the timing of decontamination. Additionally, Thors et al. [21] concluded that performing decontamination early is crucial for efficiently preventing penetration of VX into the epidermis.

Another important consideration of using RSDL for skin decontamination includes wound healing. In a study by Connolly et al. [30], skin exposed to RSDL displayed a decreased skin elasticity, a significant trans-epidermal water loss, an altered coloration, and an altered thickness and a decreased rate of wound healing when compared to non-RSDL-treated wounds. This is of significance because physical injuries are probable in the event of a CWA exposure.

Finally, consideration must be given as to whether using RSDL is safe in pregnancy. The active ingredient in RSDL, DAM, crosses the placental barrier, but the possibility of RSDL teratogenicity has not been well explored (US Department of Health and Human Services 2017).

Conclusion

There is much evidence supporting the use of RSDL as a decontaminating agent against CWAs and TICs. However, there are limitations and gaps in the data surrounding the use of RSDL, which highlight the need for continued research in this important field. Taken together, we intuit in vivo studies are often the most informative and human skin is preferred, followed (in order) by rhesus monkey, miniature (young) pig, and guinea pig. Dermatopharmacokinetic data often provides more robust data than lethal dose data. Due to the wide variety of industrial chemical spills, data providing for widely varying physical/chemical properties (molecular weight, lipid and water solubility, partition coefficients, melting points, hydrogen bonds, etc.) should help clarify the most efficient decontamination systems for the varied chemical world.

Author Contributions A. Feschuk performed the literature search—with additional sources from H. Maibach; A. Feschuk, R. Law, and H. Maibach systematically reviewed abstracts and full papers (on Covidence); A. Feschuk drafted the work; R. Law and H. Maibach critically revised the work at several time points.

Funding This research did not receive any specific grant from funding agencies in the public, commercial, or not-for-profit sectors.

References

1. Ganesan K, Raza SK, Vijayaraghavan R. Chemical warfare agents. J Pharm Bioallied Sci. 2010;2(3):166–78.
2. Schwartz MD, Hurst CG, Kirk MA, Reedy SJ, Braue EH Jr. Reactive skin decontamination lotion (RSDL) for the decontamination of chemical warfare agent (CWA) dermal exposure. Curr Pharm Biotechnol. 2012;13(10):1971–9.
3. U.S. Department of Health & Human Services. Reactive Skin Decontamination Lotion (RSDL)- Medical Countermeasures Database. Accessed 14 December 2020. https://chemm. hhs.gov/countermeasure_RSDL.htm.
4. Roul A, Le C, Gustin MP, Clavaud E, Verrier B, Pirot F, Falson F. Comparison of four different Fuller's earth formulations in skin decontamination. J Appl Toxicol. 2017;37(1):527–1536.
5. Rolland P, Bolzinger MA, Cruz C, Josse D, Briançon S. Hairy skin exposure to VX in vitro: effectiveness of delayed decontamination. Toxicol In Vitro. 2012;27(1):358–66.
6. Dachir S, Cohen M, Buch H, Kadar T. Skin decontamination efficacy of sulfur mustard and VX in the pig model: a comparison between Fuller's Earth and RSDL. Chem Biol Interact. 2021;25:109393. https://doi.org/10.1016/j.cbi.2021.109393.
7. Emergent Biosolutions Inc. RSDL. 2017. https://www.rsdl.com/about-rsdl/#history. Accessed 1 Dec 2020.
8. Fentabil M, Gebremedhin M, Barry J, Mikler J, Cochrane L. In vivo efficacy of the reactive skin decontamination lotion (RSDL®) kit against organophosphate and carbamate pesticides. Chem Biol Interact. 2020;318(1):108980.
9. Elsinghorst PW, Worek F, Koller M. Detoxification of organophosphorus pesticides and nerve agents through RSDL: efficacy evaluation by 31(P) NMR spectroscopy. Toxicol Lett. 2015;233(1):207–13.
10. Bazire A, Baubichon D, Cruz C, Bifarella R, Josse D. In vivo evaluation of skin decontaminants against chemical warfare agent VX. Clin Toxicol. 2010;50(9):807–8011.
11. Bjarnason S, Mikler J, Hill I, Tenn C, Garrett M, Caddy N, Sawyer TW. Comparison of selected skin decontaminant products and regimens against VX in domestic swine. Hum Exp Toxicol. 2008;27(3):253–61.
12. Centers for Disease Control and Prevention. Facts about VX. 2018. https://emergency.cdc. gov/agent/vx/basics/facts.asp#:~:text=VX%20is%20the%20most%20potentsomewhat%20 more%20toxic%20by%20inhalation. Accessed 4 Dec 2020.
13. Taysse L, Daulon S, Delamanche S, Bellier B, Breton P. Skin decontamination of mustards and organophosphates: comparative efficiency of RSDL and Fuller's earth in domestic swine. Hum Exp Toxicol. 2007;26(2):135–41.

14. Taysse L, Dorandeu F, Daulon S, Foquin A, Perrier N, Lallement G, Breton P. Cutaneous challenge with chemical warfare agents in the SKH-1 hairless mouse (II): effects of some currently used skin decontaminants (RSDL and Fuller's earth) against liquid sulphur mustard and VX exposure. Hum Exp Toxicol. 2011;30(6):491–8.
15. Braue EH Jr, Smith KH, Doxzon BF, Lumpkin HL, Clarkson ED. Efficacy studies of reactive skin decontamination lotion, M291 skin decontamination kit, 0.5% bleach, 1% soapy water, and skin exposure reduction paste against chemical warfare agents, part 1: guinea pigs challenged with VX. Cutan Ocul Toxicol. 2011a;30(1):15–28.
16. Braue EH Jr, Smith KH, Doxzon BF, Lumpkin HL, Clarkson ED. Efficacy studies of reactive skin decontamination lotion, M291 skin decontamination kit, 0.5% bleach, 1% soapy water, and skin exposure reduction paste against chemical warfare agents, part 2: guinea pigs challenged with soman. Cutan Ocul Toxicol. 2011b;30(1):29–37.
17. Josse D, Barrier G, Cruz C, Ferrante MC, Berthelot N. P1336: Delayed decontamination effectiveness following skin exposure to the chemical warfare agent VX. Toxicol Lett. 2011;205(1):163.
18. Salerno A, Devers T, Bolzinger MA, Pelletier J, Josse D, Briançon S. In vitro skin decontamination of the organophosphorus pesticide paraoxon with nanometric cerium oxide CeO(2). Chem Biol Interact. 2017;267(1):57–66.
19. Cao Y, Hui X, Elmahdy A, Maibach H. In vitro human skin permeation and decontamination of diisopropyl methylphosphonate (DIMP) using dermal decontamination gel (DDGel) and reactive skin decontamination lotion (RSDL) at different timepoints. Toxicol Lett. 2018a;299(1):118–23.
20. Cao Y, Hui X, Zhu H, Elmahdy A, Maibach H. In vitro human skin permeation and decontamination of 2-chloroethyl ethyl sulfide (CEES) using dermal decontamination gel (DDGel) and reactive skin decontamination lotion (RSDL). Toxicol Lett. 2018b;291(1):86–91.
21. Thors L, Koch M, Wigenstam E, Koch B, Hägglund L, Bucht A. Comparison of skin decontamination efficacy of commercial decontamination products following exposure to VX on human skin. Chem Biol Interact. 2017;273(1):82–9.
22. Thors L, Oberg L, Forsberg E, Wigenstam E, Larsson A, Bucht A. Skin penetration and decontamination efficacy following human skin exposure to fentanyl. Toxicol In Vitro. 2020a;67(1):104914.
23. Thors L, Wigenstam E, Qvarnström J, Hägglund L, Bucht A. Improved skin decontamination efficacy for the nerve agent VX. Chem Biol Interact. 2020b;325(1):109135.
24. Ueno C, Mullens C, Luh J, Wooden W. Historical review of Dakin's solution application. J Plast Reconstr Aesthet Surg. 2018;71(1):49–55.
25. National Centre for Biotechnology Information. PubChem compound summary for CID 9395, paraoxon. 2021. https://pubchem.ncbi.nlm.nih.gov/compound/Paraoxon. Accessed 19 May 2021.
26. Law RM, Ngo MA, Maibach HI. Clinically pertinent factors/observations for percutaneous absorption in humans. Am J Clin Dermatol. 2020;21(1):85–95.
27. de Bruin-Hoegée M, de Koning MC, Cochrane L, Joosen MJA. Contact transfer risk from fentanyl-contaminated RSDL kits. Toxicol Lett. 2020;319(1):237–41.
28. Joosen MJ, van den Berg RM, de Jong AL, van der Schans MJ, Noort D, Langenberg JP. The impact of skin decontamination on the time window for effective treatment of percutaneous VX exposure. Chem Biol Interact. 2016;267(1):48–56.
29. Bronaugh RL, Maibach HI. In vitro percutaneous absorption: principles, fundamentals and applications. Boca Raton: CRC; 1991.
30. Connolly JM, Stevenson RS, Railer RF, Clark OE, Whitten KA, Lee-Stubbs RB, Anderson DR. Impairment of wound healing by reactive skin decontamination lotion (RSDL(®)) in a Göttingen minipig(®) model. Cutan Ocul Toxicol. 2020;39(2):143–57.

Chapter 9
Aqueous Suspensions of Fuller's Earth Potentiate the Adsorption Capacities of Paraoxon and Improve Skin Decontamination Properties

Alix Danoy, Kardelen Durmaz, Margaux Paoletti, Laetitia Vachez, Annick Roul, Jérôme Sohier, and Bernard Verrier

Introduction

Fuller's earth (FE) is a clay that has been used for hundreds of years for woolen fulling in order to clean wool to eliminate oils, dirt, and impurities [1]. Due to its adsorptive capacities, modern uses of FE have been extensively developed, ranging from absorbent for cat litter to carrier for fertilizers or active ingredient in cosmetic products [2]. Interestingly, one of its most intriguing uses concerns dry skin decontamination in the military field. Indeed, chemical warfare agent (CWA) still represents a threat, both for civilian [3–5] and military populations. Organophosphorus compounds (OPCs) are among the most detected chemical compounds in the environment due to their use as pesticides [such as paraoxon (POX)] and nerve agents (tabun, sarin, soman, VX) [6]. Because most OPCs have a low volatility, their absorption through the dermal route remains predominant in comparison with the

Supplementary Information The online version contains supplementary material available at [https://doi.org/10.1007/978-3-031-09222-0_9].

A. Danoy · K. Durmaz (✉) · M. Paoletti · L. Vachez · J. Sohier · B. Verrier
UMR 5305: Laboratoire de Biologie Tissulaire et d'Ingénierie Thérapeutique, Institut de Biologie et Chimie des Protéines, CNRS/Université Claude Bernard Lyon 1, Lyon Cedex 07, France
e-mail: kardelen.durmaz@ibcp.fr

A. Roul
UMR 5305: Laboratoire de Biologie Tissulaire et d'Ingénierie Thérapeutique, Institut de Biologie et Chimie des Protéines, CNRS/Université Claude Bernard Lyon 1, Lyon Cedex 07, France

Pôle Santé, Direction Générale de la Sécurité Civile et de la Gestion des Crises, Ministère de l'Intérieur, Paris, France

A. M. Feschuk et al. (eds.), *Dermal Absorption and Decontamination*, https://doi.org/10.1007/978-3-031-09222-0_9

respiratory one [7, 8], meaning that any system acting by adsorption and displacement of the toxic agent from the skin surface could be an efficient decontaminant product. Thus, FE, which is unexpansive, easy to obtain, and composed of layers with high ion exchange capacities [9] favoring interaction with OPCs, has largely been used for OPC decontamination. As illustrated by previous ex vivo and in vivo studies, this phyllosilicate has been shown to be the reference agent applied for skin decontamination following CWA exposure [10–12].

FE is a dusty agent that easily induces aerosols, favoring the propagation of contaminated dust and particles which could be inhaled by surrounding people and thus represents a new threat by cross-contamination [13]. One way to bypass this problem could be the use of water suspension of FE as recently described [14]. Even if most of the OPC materials have low water solubility (e.g., POX is soluble at 2.4 g/L), an aqueous suspension of FE could offer a strong added value for decontamination. In their paper, Roul and collaborators [14] have shown that aqueous suspension of FE (10 g into 100 mL) limits skin penetration of 4-cyanophenol. Thus, suspension's decontamination efficacy of this compound was proved to be better than FE powder or water alone, meaning that the contaminant is better entrapped.

In order to further investigate these observations, we decided to analyze the decontaminant properties of different concentrations of FE suspension to highlight a potential dose effect decontamination efficacy. As skin is the first barrier to protect the body from external assaults, especially with OPC, we have explored the penetration of an OPC through this semipermeable barrier to analyze if FE suspensions could diminish it. Ex vivo diffusion assays were done with specific derived Franz cells [15] (see Fig. S1 in Supplementary Data) allowing multiple runs at the same time and ensuring strong reproducibility. These devices consist of donor and receiver compartments separated by a membrane, making it possible to mimic passive cutaneous diffusion [16]. Pig skin is commonly used as a predictive model for human skin permeability because of the histological and pathophysiological similarities between the two species [17, 18]. Although expensive and difficult to obtain, human skin remains the best model for ex vivo penetration study seeing as no interspecies extrapolation is needed [19, 20].

The primary aim of this study was to investigate the toxicity of different FE aqueous suspensions. This analysis is essential because the water in the suspension could favor the release of toxic compounds, such as heavy metals entrapped into Fuller's earth aggregates, jeopardizing the use of such a decontamination system. The evaluation has been done in vitro on skin cells and in vivo on *Danio rerio* embryos. After toxicological validation of the suspensions, their effectiveness as a decontamination tool has been evaluated ex vivo with skin diffusion assays. POX was used as a simulant agent for VX [21, 22] and chose for its lower toxicity and its intrinsic properties (see Table S1 in Supplementary Data). Furthermore, both pig ear and human abdominal skins have been used as a model in order to determine if pig ear skin can be considered as a good predictive model of human skin for this contaminant.

Materials and Methods

Material

Fuller's earth (FE) was purchased as a free powder with adsorptive properties available for the firefighter decontamination process (NBC-Sys, France).

Toxicity

In Vitro Cell Toxicity

Normal human dermal fibroblasts (NHDF), passages 9–12, were cultured in Dulbecco's Modified Eagle Medium (DMEM) supplemented with 10% fetal bovine serum and 1% penicillin-streptomycin (5000 U/mL). Human primary keratinocytes (HPK) extracted from foreskin, passages 1–4, were cultured in keratinocytes-SFM medium supplemented with bovine pituitary extract, 1% penicillin-streptomycin (5000 U/mL), epidermal growth factor, and $CaCl_2$. Both cell lineages were maintained in a 37 °C incubator (Heracell 150i, Thermo Fisher Scientific, USA), under 5% CO_2 and 95% humidity. All the compounds for the cell media were purchased from Gibco (Thermo Fisher Scientific, USA). Three FE suspensions were prepared, respectively, 5%, 9.1%, and 15% w/w, in PBS 1× (Gibco, USA) and then filtered on 0.22 μm single-use polycarbonate filters (Merck Millipore, USA). The filtered supernatants were left at room temperature until they were added into cells for 30 min of incubation before washing with cell media and cell viability evaluation by the MTT technique. Cytotoxicity assays were done 40 h after the coating of a 96-well plate with a density of 10,000 or 15,000 cells per well for, respectively, NHDF and HPK, with MTT cytotoxicity assay reagent from Sigma-Aldrich (USA) as described by the protocol.

The values for the culture media and tested ones (i.e., PBS 1×, SD 5%, and the three supernatants from the three FE suspensions) were compared and statistically analyzed using a two-way ANOVA coupled with Dunnett's multiple comparison post hoc analysis.

In Vivo *Danio rerio* Toxicity

Fish embryo toxicity test (FET) on zebrafish (*Danio rerio*) was made in agreement with the OECD 236 guideline (see Fig. S2 in Supplementary Data). Briefly, zebrafish were obtained from Institut de Génomique Fonctionnelle de Lyon (IGFL) where they were maintained in a closed flow-through system with a temperature of 26 °C ± 1 °C and a 16 h light/8 h dark cycle. After fertilization, newly fertilized eggs were collected and selected under a binocular microscope: embryos with normal development staging from the zygote stage to the gastrula stage were distributed on a 24-well plate (Thermo Fisher Scientific, USA), one embryo per well. One condition per plate was tested: 3,4-dichloroaniline (Sigma-Aldrich, France) at 8 µg/mL used as negative control, aquarium water (E3) used as positive control, and FE suspensions in water aquarium at 5%, 9.1%, and 15% w/w. Every well was filled with 2 mL of solution, and embryo viability was assessed every 24 h using microscope and toxicological endpoints as criterions (coagulated embryo, absence of heartbeat, non-detachment of the tail, absence of somite formation) for 4 days. Alive fishes were analyzed to determine if they had any morphological abnormalities before observing their mobility with a Zebrabox equipped with Zebralab software (Viewpoint Behavior Technology, France) by 5 min light cycle exposition before 3 min dark cycle.

The values for the aquarium media (E3) and tested ones (i.e., 3.4-dichloroaniline and the three FE aqueous suspensions) were compared and statistically analyzed using a two-way ANOVA coupled with Dunnett's multiple comparison post hoc analysis.

Ex Vivo Cell Diffusion Assays

VitroPharma® (patent no. WO2013057401) was used as a cell diffusion system (see Fig. S1 in Supplementary Data). Dermatomed skin at 500 µm, either from pig ear or human abdomen, with a diffusion-available area of 0.71 cm² was mounted in the system with the dermis facing the receptor compartment filled with 5 mL of PBS 1× as receptor media. Heated magnetic stirrer was used to heat receptor fluid to 37 °C ± 1 °C, which allowed the skin to be at 32 °C (i.e., the physiological average temperature of human skin surface), and to homogenize it with a magnetic rod according to the OECD 428 guideline.

Skin Explants

Frozen pig ears (Proviskin, France) obtained from a slaughterhouse were thawed, shaved, and dermatomed (Aesculap GA 630 model) at 500 µm. Individual disks of 2 cm² were cut off to fit into a VitroPharma system. Abdominal human skin (Proviskin, France) was obtained after approval from women who have had abdominal plastic surgery and stored as frozen 2 cm² disks dermatomed at 500 µm. Before the experiment, each skin explant was controlled with a caliper in order to have a homogeneous thickness of 500 µm ± 50 µm, and skin integrity was visually assessed by microscopy.

Decontamination Protocols

Contaminated skins were obtained after the deposit of 10 $\mu L/cm^2$ of paraoxon-diethyl (Sigma-Aldrich, France) (paraoxon or POX) as a simulant of VX nerve agent. In accordance with the standard NF X52–122, decontamination was realized after 30 min to evaluate decontamination efficiency for delayed decontamination. For dry decontamination, 0.16 g/cm^2 of Fuller's earth (NBC-Sys, France) was applied. Wet decontamination occurs through the use of water (Otec®, Aguettant, France) or FE aqueous suspensions prepared at 5%, 9.1%, and 15% w/w using Otec® water (Aguettant, France). In each case, 102 $\mu L/cm^2$ of liquid was deposited. For both decontamination protocols, the decontaminant was left on the skin for 2 min before being removed, and then the skin was dry by patting with a pad.

Collection and Treatment of Samples

To determine POX penetration kinetics, 500 μL of fluid receptor was collected over time (1, 2, 4, 6, 8, 10, and 24 h of diffusion) and replaced by 500 μL of fresh media. After the set exposure period of 24 h, VitroPharma® diffusion cells were dismantled, and the surface of skin sample was wiped with an absorbent paper in order to recover the fraction of POX remaining on the skin. Skin layers were separated using the cyanoacrylate glue method [23] for *stratum corneum* (SC), and immersion into PBS 1× heated at 60 °C for epidermis and dermis. For each sample, POX was extracted for 24 h into HPLC-grade ethanol before HPLC-UV quantification.

Quantification by HPLC-UV

The concentration of POX was determined by liquid chromatography using a quaternary pump (Agilent Technologies 1260 Infinity), vial autosampler (Agilent Technologies 1260 Infinity II), and photodiode array detector (Agilent Technologies 1200 Series). The mobile phase was composed by 52.25% of methanol (HPLC grade, Carlo Erba, Italy), 42.75% of Milli-Q water (ultrapure analytical water with $r = 18$ $m\Omega/cm$, Millipore, USA), and 5% of glacial acetic acid (HPLC grade, Carlo Erba, Italy), the whole at a flow rate of 0.7 mL/min. 10 μL of sample were brought to the C18 Clipeus column (5 μm, 100×40 mm) heated at 40 °C. POX was identified at 269 nm UV wavelength with a retention time of 5.9 min [23]. The linearity of the method was assessed for POX concentration in the range of 1.95–2000 ng/mL ($R^2 = 0.999$) with a limit of detection (LOD) of 0.31 ng/mL and a limit of quantification (LOQ) of 1.95 ng/mL.

The value for the kinetic profiles and for the quantification into cell diffusion compartments and skin layers was compared between them and statistically analyzed using a one-way ANOVA coupled with either Dunnett's or Tukey's multiple comparison post hoc analysis.

Ex Vivo Evaluation of a Skin Decontaminant

Skin decontamination methods need to be evaluated and compared to each other in order to determine the most effective one, based on skin penetration data. Ex vivo decontamination efficiency has been calculated as follows to compare skin decontamination methods:

$$DE(\%) = \frac{(Q3T+Q4T)-(Q3+Q4)}{Q3T+Q4T} \times 100$$

where $Q3$ is the amount of POX present into skin layers (SC + epidermis + dermis) at the end of the experiment, $Q4$ is the amount of POX in the receptor (meaning that it passed through the skin) at the end of the experiment, and T is for control samples.

According to the standard NF X52–122, skin decontamination has an impact on functional prognosis because of its ability to capture the contaminant on the skin's surface. The improvement of the functional prognosis for each decontamination method has been calculated as follows:

$$FP = \frac{Q2T+Q3T+Q4T}{Q2+Q3+Q4}$$

where $Q2$ is the amount of POX present on the skin after decontamination, $Q3$ is the amount of POX present into skin layers (SC + epidermis + dermis) at the end of the experiment, $Q4$ is the amount of POX in the receptor (meaning that it passed through the skin) at the end of the experiment, and T is for control samples.

Statistical Analysis

Data was statistically analyzed using GraphPad Prism Version 7.0 software (San Diego, CA, USA). All of the data are presented as the mean ± SD, where $n = 4$ for in vitro cell toxicity experiments, $n = 3$ for in vivo *Danio rerio* toxicity experiments, and $n = 6$ for ex vivo skin decontamination assays. The statistical difference between groups was analyzed using either unpaired t test, one-way ANOVA, or two-way ANOVA tests, followed by specific multiple comparison post hoc tests as mentioned with each observed parameter individually.

Results

Toxicity of Fuller's Earth Suspensions

Fuller's earth is a heterogeneous smectite composed of particles sizing from nanometers to millimeters, corresponding to heavy metal particles and elementary clay aggregates. In order to assess its toxicity, it is necessary to take into account the presence of these different populations and to identify appropriate toxicity tests. First, in vitro experiments were performed using 0.22 μm filtered FE suspensions, on two different skin cells to identify ultrafiltrable toxicity, such as heavy metal or nanoparticles. In parallel, the toxicity of the whole suspensions was assessed in vivo on a zebrafish embryo model to determine the potential side effects of clay aggregates.

FE Suspensions' Supernatant Cytotoxicity

The toxicity of particles with a size <0.22 μm was evaluated in vitro on two types of skin cells: human primary keratinocytes (HPK) and normal human dermal fibroblasts (NHDF) after 30 min of contact (see "Materials and Methods," section "In Vitro Cell Toxicity"). As keratinocytes compose the top skin layer, which is epidermis, they are the first ones in contact with the product. Regardless of the concentration of the suspensions, no toxic effect on cell viability of FE supernatant was observed, in comparison with the two negative controls: cell media and PBS 1× (Fig. 9.1). NHDF, on the other hand, are found in the dermis under the epidermis: they are in contact with an external element only in the case of a skin lesion. Interestingly, PBS 1× in which the suspensions were made also exhibits a significant toxic effect on NHDF, which indicates that the suspensions are not more toxic than PBS (Fig. 9.1).

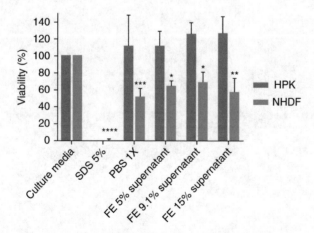

Fig. 9.1 In vitro cell toxicity of FE supernatants filtered (size <0.22 μm) from FE PBS 1× suspensions at different concentrations, on human primary keratinocytes (HPK) and normal human dermal fibroblasts (NHDF) ($n = 4$ for each). Results were statistically analyzed using a two-way ANOVA, followed by Dunnett's multiple comparison tests using culture media as control treatment. Values are presented as mean ± SD. *$p < 0.05$; **$p < 0.01$; ***$p < 0.005$; ****$p < 0.0001$

In Vivo Toxicity of FE Suspensions

To address a potential toxicity due to the FE suspension concentration, *Danio rerio* fish embryos have been immerged for 4 days into different amounts of FE suspensions, respectively, 5, 9.1, and 15% w/w. Their viability was assessed as described in section "In Vivo *Danio rerio* Toxicity" using optical microscopy. Observations have been done to differentiate embryos without and with morphological abnormalities such as development default, curved tail, or cardiac edema (Fig. 9.2). The presented figure is a picture of the viability after 4 days of immersion, meaning that fish embryos that have died on previous days are also counted.

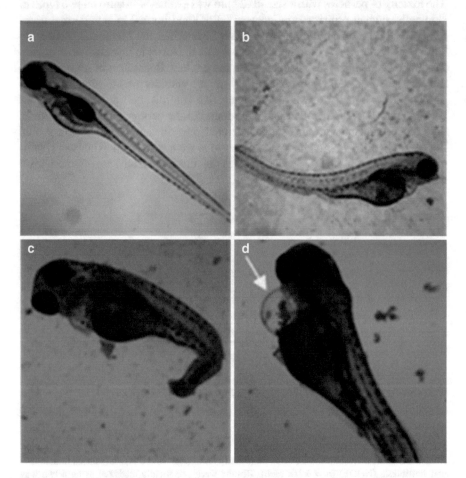

Fig. 9.2 Morphological observation of 4-day-old *Danio rerio*. (**a**) Normal development; (**b**) global development default; (**c**) curved tail; (**d**) cardiac edema

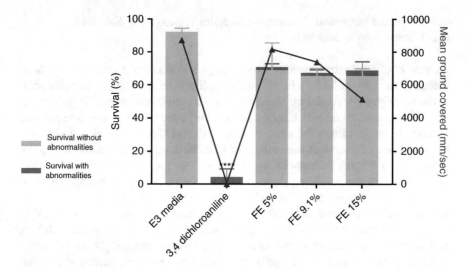

Fig. 9.3 Survival rate of *Danio rerio* with and without morphological abnormalities and mean ground covered after 4 days on immersion in aquarium media (E3), negative control (3,4-dichloroaniline), and three different concentrations of FE aqueous suspensions into E3 media (n = 3 for each). Results were statistically analyzed using a two-way ANOVA, followed by Dunnett's multiple comparison tests using E3 medium as control treatment. Values are presented as mean ± SD. ****$p < 0.0001$

No significant difference was observed on global survival and the occurrence of anomalies depending on the suspensions' concentration (Fig. 9.3). When analyzing the mean ground covered for 3 min of light after 4 days of immersion, the 15% suspension impacts fish mobility but not significantly. However, as 15% of FE implies a strong increase in water viscosity, we could not exclude that these observations are due to physical impairment of fish mobility.

Ex Vivo Decontamination Assays

Most of the ex vivo skin diffusion experiments are done on pig skin [17], which is also true for skin decontamination studies [18, 24]. This model is widely used as a human skin penetration model due to the respect of the physiopathology in relation to human skin [25]. Nevertheless, it is still necessary to compare penetration profile for a given molecule on both skin origins as they differ slightly, leading to misleading extrapolations on human decontamination efficiency [26, 27].

Differences in Paraoxon Penetration Kinetics Through Pig Ear Skin and Human Abdominal Skin

Ex vivo POX penetration kinetics through pig ear skin is linear over time for 24 h, reaching the value of 13.59 ± 0.78% of the applied dose found in the receptor compartment (Fig. 9.4). At the opposite, ex vivo skin diffusion on human abdominal skin follows a more complex kinetics. Indeed, the penetration seems to take place in several stages: it follows the same pattern as the one for pig ear skin during 4 h before a strong increase in the amount of POX in the receptor. From 8 h of POX diffusion, significant differences are observed between pig ear skin and human abdominal skin profiles. These observations are supported by the quantification of POX into each compartment that makes up the diffusion cell, i.e., the skin surface, the skin, and the receptor, and each skin layer, i.e., the *stratum corneum* (SC), epidermis, and dermis (Table 9.1). Stronger significant differences between both skin origins are found in the receptor and in the skin surface, whereas pig ear epidermis contains significantly lower quantity of contaminant than the human abdominal epidermis.

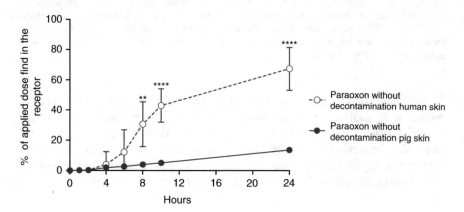

Fig. 9.4 Ex vivo POX penetration assessment through pig ear skin and human abdominal skin without decontamination: kinetic of diffusion of applied POX dose through the skin for 24 h ($n = 6$ for each time). Results were statistically analyzed using unpaired t test. Values are presented as mean ± SD. $**p < 0.01$; $****p < 0.0001$

Table 9.1 Percentage of the applied dose of POX found at the skin surface, trapped into skin layers, and passed through the skin after 24 h of diffusion without decontamination method into pig ear skin and human abdominal skin ($n = 6$ for each)

Skin model	Skin surface (%)	*Stratum corneum* (%)	Epidermis (%)	Dermis (%)	Receptor (%)
Pig ear skin	69.84****	5.55	0.64*	2.21	13.59****
Human abdominal skin	3.82	3.13	1.57	3.99	67.46

Results were statistically analyzed using unpaired t test. Values are presented as mean. $*p < 0.05$. $****p < 0.0001$

Efficacy of FE Suspension Compared to FE Powder and Water

After assessing the POX penetration profiles on both skin origin explants, decontamination efficiencies of FE powder, water, and FE 9.1% suspension were evaluated into both pig and human skins. This suspension concentration was chosen as it was the one developed by Roul et al. [14] that has proven to have a better decontamination efficiency than FE powder or water alone for 4-cyanophenol skin decontamination.

The same decontamination protocol was applied for each decontamination method, and the kinetics of POX penetration through the skin were evaluated for 24 h (Fig. 9.5). The profiles of the contaminant penetration curves differ according to the type of decontaminant used but not according to the nature of the skin. After 8–10 h of diffusion, a plateau is observable when the decontamination was done with the 9.1% suspension, whereas for FE powder and water decontamination, there is only an inflection point in the curve. Despite these observations, there is not significant difference in the quantity of POX found in the receptor after 24 h of diffusion, depending on the decontamination methods or skin origins.

At the end of the experiment, POX quantification in each skin layer highlighted differences between decontaminants and skin origins (Table 9.2). Indeed, after FE powder decontamination, POX significantly accumulates in the SC regardless of the skin nature. Furthermore, for this condition, when contaminant content in human abdominal skin is compared with the one in pig ear skin, a significant difference showing an accumulation in favor of the first one is observed for the skin surface, epidermis, and dermis. Tested decontamination formulations are effective on both pig ear and human abdominal skins, with an increased efficiency between FE powder, water, and FE 9.1% suspension.

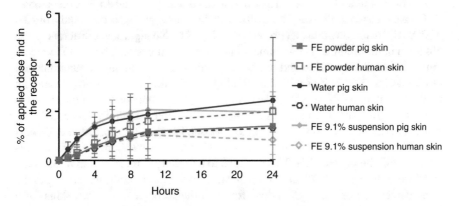

Fig. 9.5 Ex vivo POX penetration assessment through pig ear skin and human abdominal skin with three decontamination methods following the same protocol (FE powder, water, and FE 9.1% aqueous suspension): kinetic of diffusion of applied POX dose through the skin for 24 h ($n = 6$ for each time). Results were statistically analyzed using a two-way ANOVA, followed by Tukey's multiple comparison tests. Values are presented as mean ± SD

Table 9.2 Percentage of the applied dose of POX found at the skin surface, trapped into skin layers, and passed through the skin after 24 h of diffusion with three different decontamination methods (FE powder, water, FE 9.1% suspension) into pig ear skin and human abdominal skin ($n = 6$ for each)

Decontamination method	Skin model	Skin surface (%)	Stratum corneum (%)	Epidermis (%)	Dermis (%)	Receptor (%)
FE powder	Pig ear skin	0.89	3.18*	0.30	0.36	1.43
	Human abdominal skin	5.28***	3.98**	1.71**	3.48**	2.01
Water	Pig ear skin	0.78	0.21	0.05	0.09	2.45
	Human abdominal skin	0.56	0.59	0.24	0.46	1.33
FE 9.1% suspension	Pig ear skin	0.06	0	0.01	0.02	1.99
	Human abdominal skin	0.48	0.87	0.29	0.29	0.85

Results were statistically analyzed using a one-way ANOVA, followed by Tukey's multiple comparison tests between each skin origin and decontamination methods. Values are presented as mean. *$p < 0.05$; **$p < 0.01$; ***$p < 0.0001$

Relationship Between FE Suspensions' Concentration and Decontamination Efficiency

The added value of the FE 9.1% suspension compared to FE powder in terms of POX accumulation in the SC has been illustrated by Table 9.2. Then, a dose effect of FE concentration has been further investigated using 5% and 15% suspensions.

For each concentration, a plateau effect in the kinetic profile is observed from 8 h of POX diffusion onwards, as presented in Fig. 9.6. No significant differences are observed in the amount of contaminant in the receptor depending on the FE concentration for each suspension and on the skin origin. The contaminant quantification in skin layers after 24 h of diffusion highlights some differences mostly depending on the skin nature (Table 9.3). Indeed, higher POX accumulation into the skin surface, epidermis, and dermis for the human skin decontamination with FE 5% suspensions is mainly due to an outlier in the dataset. For the SC compartment, there is a significant accumulation of the contaminant in the human abdominal skin in comparison with the pig ear skin. This can lead to a prolonged release even if the penetration kinetics of the POX shows a plateau from 8 h in human skin, leading to the same percentage of the applied dose found in the receptor in the two skins for a given decontamination method.

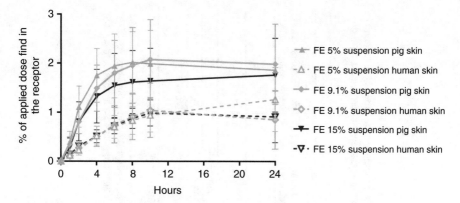

Fig. 9.6 Ex vivo POX penetration assessment through pig ear skin and human abdominal skin with FE aqueous suspensions as decontaminant at three different concentrations (5%, 9.1%, and 15%): kinetic of diffusion through the skin for 24 h ($n = 6$ for each time). Results were statistically analyzed using a two-way ANOVA, followed by Tukey's multiple comparison tests. Values are presented as mean ± SD

Table 9.3 Percentage of the applied dose of POX found at the skin surface, trapped into skin layers, and passed through the skin after 24 h of diffusion with FE aqueous suspensions as decontaminant at three different concentrations (5%, 9.1%, 15%) into pig ear skin and human abdominal skin ($n = 6$ for each)

Decontamination method	Skin model	Skin surface (%)	*Stratum corneum* (%)	Epidermis (%)	Dermis (%)	Receptor (%)
FE 5% suspension	Pig ear skin	0.06*[(a)]	0.02**[(b)]	0*[(e)]	0.07*[(f)]	1.86
	Human abdominal skin	0.83[(a)]	0.81[(b)]	0.28	0.40[(f)]	1.26
FE 9.1% suspension	Pig ear skin	0.06*[(a)]	0***[(c)]	0.01*[(e)]	0.02*[(f)]	1.99
	Human abdominal skin	0.48	0.87[(c)]	0.29[(e)]	0.29	0.85
FE 15% suspension	Pig ear skin	0.12*[(a)]	0.16*[(d)]	0*[(e)]	0.04*[(f)]	1.76
	Human abdominal skin	0.53	0.78[(d)]	0.18	0.13	0.91

Results were statistically analyzed using a one-way ANOVA, followed by Tukey's multiple comparison tests: comparison was made between all the values for given compartment and significance is by comparison with the letter (i.e., for skin surface, values are only significantly different to the one for human abdominal skin decontaminated with FE 5% suspension). Values are presented as mean. $*p < 0.05$; $**p < 0.01$; $***p < 0.005$

Comparison of Skin Origins and of Decontamination Methods

Decontamination methods were evaluated in comparison with POX skin contamination alone for both pig and human skins (Table 9.4). The quantity of contaminant absorbed by the skin, meaning found in the *stratum corneum*, the epidermis, the

Table 9.4 Evaluation of skin decontamination methods following the quantity of POX absorbed by the skin (i.e., the percentage of the applied dose found in the *stratum corneum*, the epidermis, the dermis, and the receptor), the in vitro decontamination efficiency, and the functional prognosis improvement depending on skin origin ($n = 6$ for each)

Decontamination method	Pig ear skin			Human abdominal skin		
	Quantity of POX absorbed by the skin (%)	In vitro decontamination efficiency	Functional prognosis improvement factor	Quantity of POX absorbed by the skin (%)	In vitro decontamination efficiency	Functional prognosis improvement factor
No decontamination	21.77****[a]; ****	–	–	76.15[b]	–	–
Fuller's earth powder	5.27****[a]	75.81%	23.18	11.18[c]; ****[b]	85.32%[d]	14.53
Water	2.81****[a]	87.11%	48.71	2.62****[b][c]	96.55%****[d]	31.81
FE 5% suspension	1.95****[a]	91.04%**	53.19*	2.75****[b][c]	96.39%****[d]	23.51
FE 9.1% suspension	2.01****[a]	90.75%**	53.10	2.30****[b][c]	96.98%****[d]	36.14
FE 15% suspension	1.96****[a]	91.01%**	71.5	2.00****[b][c]	97.38%****[d]	34.21

Results were statistically analyzed using unpaired t test for the comparison of each value of pig ear skin and human abdominal skin; and a one-way ANOVA, followed by Tukey's multiple comparison test, was used to compare values between them for a given skin origin. Values are presented as mean. *$p < 0.05$; **$p < 0.01$; ****$p < 0.0001$

dermis, and the receptor compartment, is significantly lower when decontamination methods are applied, no matter which type. Furthermore, for the same applied dose, the quantity of POX absorbed by human abdominal skin is significantly higher than the one for pig ear skin.

For both skin models, in vitro decontamination efficiency of FE powder is the lowest. Whereas there are no significant differences for the in vitro decontamination efficiencies depending on the decontamination method applied on pig ear skin, wet decontamination is significantly more effective than dry decontamination into human abdominal skin. The use of FE suspensions into pig ear skin leads to significant lower decontamination efficiency values than the ones on human abdominal skin with the same aqueous decontaminants. Thus, it appears that pig ear skin is a good predictive model for the assessment of the decontamination efficiency because there is no risk of overestimation when extrapolated to human skin.

The functional prognosis improvement factor defined as the ability of each decontaminant to capture the contaminant on the skin surface (see "Materials and Methods," section "Ex Vivo Evaluation of a Skin Decontaminant") is not impacted by the type of decontamination method used for a given skin origin. Although FE powder decontamination presents the lowest value in both skins, there are no significant differences with wet decontamination. However, the use of FE 5% suspension induces an increase of the functional prognosis improvement factor significantly higher in the pig ear skin than in the human abdominal skin: these results can be explained by an exceptional value in the human skin dataset, increasing the global percentage of contaminant found on the skin surface. This factor cannot be used to significantly classify decontamination methods according to their efficiency.

The more pronounced effect of the suspensions on pig ear skin is explained by histological differences with human skin, which will be discussed in the next session.

Discussion

The toxicity of clays in general is not very well documented, and even more surprising when Fuller's earth (FE) is concerned, in particular its potential unsafe use regarding skin contact. First of all, when analyzing the toxicity of ultrafiltrable compounds released by water suspension of FE, our in vitro skin cell toxicity tests on filtered supernatant illustrated two information. Keratinocytes, which are cells from the epidermis, are not impacted in their viability by the application of neither PBS 1× or various concentrated supernatants of filtered FE suspensions. Although the measured toxicity of PBS 1× on NHDF can be attributed to their structural differences with HPKs (due to a stronger resilience and tolerance to external aggressions), it allows to determine that FE supernatants do not induce a higher cytotoxicity than PBS 1×. Han et al. [28] previously demonstrated that clay suspensions at 1000 µg/mL are not toxic on human skin fibroblasts (CCD986sk), whereas Sandri et al. [29] shaded this purpose by the observation of a tendency of a decrease in cell viability of NHDF incubated with montmorillonite nanocomposites from 150 to 300 µg/mL. However, in vitro toxicity assessment is highly dependent on the clay mineral and its structure in addition of the nature of the cell line [30]. Based on suspensions' effect of raw FE, the results on keratinocytes are in accordance with the ones of Janer et al. [31] that recorded low toxicity of FE supernatants. To our knowledge, it is the first study that characterizes FE's intrinsic toxicity using a *Danio rerio* model. Most of the time, this type of experiment allows to determine the adsorption properties of clays in order to diminish environmental water contamination [32, 33]. Here, the classical fish embryo toxicity test was coupled with a mobility test: no suspension has an effect of fish viability, while the more concentrated one has an impact on mobility. These results are in accordance with the ones of Abdel-Wahhab et al. [34] and Dwyer et al. [35] who gave ingested clays to rats and chickens in order to detoxify them after toxin ingestion. Neither models showed toxicity, leading to the conclusion that clays are safe to use. Taken together, in vitro and in vivo toxicity tests suggest that FE suspensions are safe to use on undamaged and healthy skin in a concentration range from 5 to 9.1% w/w.

Furthermore, pig ear skin was studied as a predictive model for ex vivo human skin decontamination studies of paraoxon as a model for VX organophosphorus compound. Indeed, although human excised skin is considered as the gold standard for in vitro skin penetration experiments [36], its use is complicated due to ethical and supply difficulties. The presence of the papillary body and the large content in elastic tissue of its dermis in addition to the highly differentiated epidermis make pig skin a good substitute for human skin to assess ex vivo skin penetration. Just like for human skin, pig skin presents differences in terms of permeability as a function of the age, sex, or anatomical region. In et al. [25] compared the histological and functional anatomical regions of porcine skin, including the ear, with human abdominal skin. Several significant differences have been identified, in particular for the SC, the dermo-epidermal interface, and the dermis thickness that are larger in the human model. These variations in layer thickness lead to a significant difference in the epidermal–dermal thickness ratio: 1:19 for human abdominal skin versus 1:14 for pig ear skin. It means that even if both explants are dermatomed at 500 µm, the pig one has a larger dermal hydrophilic component. Despite these differences, skin from the pig ear is the more appropriate anatomical site in order to predict human skin penetration [37–39]. Penetration abilities of various compounds are impacted by the skin nature which is mainly greater for animal skin than for human skin, leading to a possible overestimation of the human percutaneous absorption [40, 41].

The receptor medium could also influence POX penetration behavior between human and pig skins. However, various studies have shown that the receptor medium does not modify the differences of contaminant penetration between pig and human skins. For instance, a study by Boudry et al. [37] showed a higher parathion penetration in pig skin compared to human skin (7.5% against 20.7%) while using Eagle medium supplemented with BSA and gentamycin as receptor medium. Similarly, Chilcott et al. [11] showed that the absorption of sulfur mustard through pig ear skin was 2.6 times higher than that of human skin using 50% aqueous ethanol in the receptor medium. Finally, other studies showed that using another receptor medium, such as ethanol and water (1:1) [8, 42] or HBSS [43], does not impact the penetration of compounds through the skin. The use of different membrane origins at the interface of the diffusion device can lead to differences in the evaluation in skin decontaminants [11]. Despite this, pig ear skin can be used as a cheap predictive model for human skin POX diffusion and its decontamination studies, whereas reconstructed skin could not be because of its weak barrier function [39].

The improvement of decontamination efficiency for FE aqueous suspensions in comparison to FE powder or water alone can be explained by the molecular structure of the particles. Clays, more particularly smectites, are compounds of negatively charged organized units called lamellas, spaced by cations and water molecules, that are then organized as particles and further as aggregates [44]. Generally speaking, the adsorption model for this type of material is based on pore diffusion through and inside aggregates before sorption by intern particles [45]. This sorption mechanism was validated for pesticides: diffusion occurs through migration inside aggregates and their pores leading to the adsorption on the solid phase inside the aggregate before reaching a local equilibrium between the concentration in the pore solution and the locally absorbed concentration [46]. Although the interlamellar space is filled with cations, it remains the privileged area for chemical sorption with aggregates' surface [47]. The nature of exchangeable cations and their degree of isomorphic substitution as well as the clay chemical composition are going to be key factors to understand clays' wettability properties with water [48]. Indeed, when clays are added in aqueous media, aggregates become oriented and ordered [44]: lamellas are separated by water molecule layers, and an increase in micropore size is observed as the result of the increase of basal space, leading to a bigger BET surface area (the Brunauer, Emmett, and Teller method permits to measure the surface areas) [49]. Hydration sequence is well described for smectite clay: first, an external hydration occurs on mesopore with single layers of water before filling of interlamellar spaces and osmotic swelling.

With the use of FE suspensions, new hidden and non-accessible adsorption territories are released [45], which explains the decontamination efficiency improvement of water suspensions in comparison with dry FE. Nevertheless, this phenomenon is limited because the intercalation of molecules into interlamellar spaces is controlled by two parameters: attractive forces and cation exchange capacity [50]. This restriction explains the absence of a relationship between the concentration of suspensions and decontamination efficiency or functional prognosis improvement factor. All decontamination methods tested are significantly effective, but depending on the decontaminant, different mechanisms are involved: for dry decontamination with FE as a powder, there is contaminant adsorption and fixation site saturation leading to free contaminant available to pass through skin layers. The excess contaminant will accumulate in the SC because of its lipophilic properties and create a tank reservoir that allows a delayed release and a later contamination which is represented by a low functional prognosis, in accordance with the one found by Salerno et al. [23] for FE powder applied on pig ear skin. To the opposite, wet decontamination with water alone allows only physical displacement, and no adsorption with FE is involved. Thus, aqueous suspensions of FE used as innovative wet decontamination potentiate FE powder decontamination ability with the emergence of new adsorption sites as a result of interlamellar swelling induced by water molecules. As it was already detailed for pesticide sorption by wet soils, contaminant will migrate by a diffusion phenomenon into aggregates' internal pores filled with water [46].

Conclusion

Fuller's earth (FE) is a smectite clay well known for its adsorbent properties used for household or skin decontamination. This compound is very heterogeneous in terms of nature and particle size as it is mostly composed of elementary clay aggregates and few amounts of minerals such as heavy metals. Our results clearly indicate that the aqueous suspension of FE, regardless of its concentration, does not promote the release of toxic compounds from the clay. We have identified a minimal dose of 5% FE suspension in water as an optimal concentration for ex vivo dermal decontamination of paraoxon when loaded on porcine or human skin explants. Indeed, water suspension increases the decontaminant properties of FE, as noticed by the disappearance of a *stratum corneum* reservoir of paraoxon. All together, these results are in favor of the use of water suspension of FE as a new tool to organophosphate decontamination.

Acknowledgments We would like to thank Julien Rouleau for his advices during all the project, the PRECI (IGFL Lyon, SFR Biosciences) for animal housing and facilities, Damien Salmon for the supply of VitroPharma® device, and Damien Ficheux and Maxime Dzikowski for the help for HPLC-UV method development. We would like to thank Fanny Charriaud for English language and style corrections.

CRediT Authorship Contribution Statement Alix Danoy: conceptualization; methodology; formal analysis; investigation; writing—original draft; writing—review and editing. Kardelen Durmaz: investigation. Margaux Paoletti: investigation. Laetitia Vachez: methodology; investigation. Annick Roul: conceptualization. Jérôme Sohier: review and editing. Bernard Verrier: conceptualization; resources; writing—review and editing; supervision; funding acquisition.

Funding This research was funded by the Direction Générale de l'Armement DGA who paid Alix Danoy as PhD student, Laetitia Vachez is a recipient from ANR-16-CE20–0002-01 (FishRNAVax), and most part of this work has been funded by CNRS grant to Bernard Verrier.

References

1. Kherdekar G, Adivarekar RV. Effect of different wool scouring techniques on physical properties of wool fiber. Int J Mod Trends Eng Res. 2017;4(5):163–7. https://doi.org/10.23883/ijrter.2017.3527.ndvmi.
2. Rehan I, Khan MZ, Rehan K, Sultana S, Rehman MU, Muhammad R, Ikram M, Anwar H. Quantitative analysis of Fuller's earth using laser-induced breakdown spectroscopy and

inductively coupled plasma/optical emission spectroscopy. Appl Optics. 2019;58(16):4227–33. https://doi.org/10.1364/AO.58.004227.

3. Ciottone GR. Toxidrome recognition in chemical-weapons attacks. N Engl J Med. 2018;378(17):1611–20. https://doi.org/10.1056/NEJMra1705224.

4. Haines DD, Fox SC. Acute and long-term impact of chemical weapons: lessons from the Iran–Iraq war. Forensic Sci Rev. 2014;26(2):97–114.

5. Pitschmann V. Overall view of chemical and biochemical weapons. Toxins. 2014;6(6):1761–84. https://doi.org/10.3390/toxins6061761.

6. Naughton SX, Terry AV. Neurotoxicity in acute and repeated organophosphate exposure. Toxicology. 2018;408:101–12. https://doi.org/10.1016/j.tox.2018.08.011.

7. John H, Balszuweit F, Kehe K, Worek F, Thiermann H. Chapter 56—Toxicokinetic aspects of nerve agents and vesicants. In: Gupta RC, editor. Handbook of toxicology of chemical warfare agents. 2nd ed. New York: Academic Press; 2015. p. 817–56. https://doi.org/10.1016/B978-0-12-800159-2.00056-7.

8. Thors L, Koch B, Koch M, Hägglund L, Bucht A. In vitro human skin penetration model for organophosphorus compounds with different physicochemical properties. Toxicol In Vitro. 2016;32:198–204. https://doi.org/10.1016/j.tiv.2016.01.003.

9. Taylor L, Brown T, Benham A, Lusty P, Minchin D. World mineral production 2000–2004. Nottingham: British Geological Survey; 2006. http://www.bgs.ac.uk/mineralsuk/.

10. Bjarnason S, Mikler J, Hill I, Tenn C, Garrett M, Caddy N, Sawyer TW. Comparison of selected skin decontaminant products and regimens against VX in domestic swine. Hum Exp Toxicol. 2008;27(3):253–61. https://doi.org/10.1177/0960327108090269.

11. Chilcott RP, Jenner J, Hotchkiss SA, Rice P. In vitro skin absorption and decontamination of sulphur mustard: comparison of human and pig-ear skin. J Appl Toxicol. 2001;21(4):279–83. https://doi.org/10.1002/jat.755.

12. Taysse L, Dorandeu F, Daulon S, Foquin A, Perrier N, Lallement G, Breton P. Cutaneous challenge with chemical warfare agents in the SKH-1 hairless mouse (II): effects of some currently used skin decontaminants (RSDL and Fuller's earth) against liquid sulphur mustard and VX exposure. Hum Exp Toxicol. 2011;30(6):491–8. https://doi.org/10.1177/0960327110373616.

13. Denet E, Espina-Benitez MB, Pitault I, Pollet T, Blaha D, Bolzinger M-A, Rodriguez-Nava V, Briançon S. Metal oxide nanoparticles for the decontamination of toxic chemical and biological compounds. Int J Pharm. 2020;583:119373. https://doi.org/10.1016/j.ijpharm.2020.119373.

14. Roul A, Le C-A-K, Gustin M-P, Clavaud E, Verrier B, Pirot F, Falson F. Comparison of four different fuller's earth formulations in skin decontamination. J Appl Toxicol. 2017;37(12):1527–36. https://doi.org/10.1002/jat.3506.

15. Salmon D, Gilbert E, Gioia B, Haftek M, Pivot C, Verrier B, Pirot F. New easy handling and sampling device for bioavailability screening of topical formulations. Eur J Dermatol. 2015;25(Suppl 1):23–9. https://doi.org/10.1684/ejd.2015.2551.

16. Misik J, Pavlikova R, Cabal J, Kuca K. Method of static diffusion cells for assessment of pesticides skin permeation. Mil Med Sci Lett. 2011;80:46–51. https://doi.org/10.31482/mmsl.2011.007.

17. Godin B, Touitou E. Transdermal skin delivery: predictions for humans from in vivo, ex vivo and animal models. Adv Drug Deliv Rev. 2007;59(11):1152–61. https://doi.org/10.1016/j.addr.2007.07.004.

18. Matar H, Larner J, Kansagra S, Atkinson KL, Skamarauskas JT, Amlot R, Chilcott RP. Design and characterisation of a novel in vitro skin diffusion cell system for assessing mass casualty decontamination systems. Toxicol In Vitro. 2014;28(4):492–501. https://doi.org/10.1016/j.tiv.2014.01.001.

19. Hui X, Domoradzki JY, Maibach HC. In vitro study to determine decontamination of 3,5-dichloro-2,4,6-trifluoropyridine (DCTFP) from human skin. Food Chem Toxicol. 2012;50(7):2496–502. https://doi.org/10.1016/j.fct.2012.03.069.

20. Moore CA, Wilkinson SC, Blain PG, Dunn M, Aust GA, Williams FM. Percutaneous absorption and distribution of organophosphates (chlorpyrifos and dichlorvos) following dermal

exposure and decontamination scenarios using in vitro human skin model. Toxicol Lett. 2014;229(1):66–72. https://doi.org/10.1016/j.toxlet.2014.06.008.

21. Bartelt-Hunt SL, Knappe DRU, Barlaz MA. A review of chemical warfare agent simulants for the study of environmental behavior. Crit Rev Environ Sci Technol. 2008;38(2):112–36. https://doi.org/10.1080/10643380701643650.

22. Sellik A, Pollet T, Ouvry L, Briançon S, Fessi H, Hartmann DJ, Renaud FNR. Degradation of paraoxon (VX chemical agent simulant) and bacteria by magnesium oxide depends on the crystalline structure of magnesium oxide. Chem Biol Interact. 2017;267:67–73. https://doi.org/10.1016/j.cbi.2016.11.023.

23. Salerno A, Devers T, Bolzinger M-A, Pelletier J, Josse D, Briançon S. In vitro skin decontamination of the organophosphorus pesticide paraoxon with nanometric cerium oxide CeO_2. Chem Biol Interact. 2017;267:57–66. https://doi.org/10.1016/j.cbi.2016.04.035.

24. Taysse L, Daulon S, Delamanche S, Bellier B, Breton P. Skin decontamination of mustards and organophosphates: comparative efficiency of RSDL and Fuller's earth in domestic swine. Hum Exp Toxicol. 2007;26(2):135–41. https://doi.org/10.1177/0960327107071866.

25. In MK, Richardson KC, Loewa A, Hedtrich S, Kaessmeyer S, Plendl J. Histological and functional comparisons of four anatomical regions of porcine skin with human abdominal skin. Anat Histol Embryol. 2019;48(3):207–17. https://doi.org/10.1111/ahe.12425.

26. Jung EC, Maibach HI. Animal models for percutaneous absorption. J Appl Toxicol. 2015;35(1):1–10. https://doi.org/10.1002/jat.3004.

27. Netzlaff F, Lehr C-M, Wertz PW, Schaefer UF. The human epidermis models EpiSkin®, SkinEthic® and EpiDerm®: an evaluation of morphology and their suitability for testing phototoxicity, irritancy, corrosivity, and substance transport. Eur J Pharm Biopharm. 2005;60(2):167–78. https://doi.org/10.1016/j.ejpb.2005.03.004.

28. Han H-K, Lee Y-C, Lee M-Y, Patil AJ, Shin H-J. Magnesium and calcium organophyllosilicates: synthesis and in vitro cytotoxicity study. ACS Appl Mater Interfaces. 2011;3(7):2564–72. https://doi.org/10.1021/am200406k.

29. Sandri G, Bonferoni MC, Ferrari F, Rossi S, Aguzzi C, Mori M, Grisoli P, Cerezo P, Tenci M, Viseras C, Caramella C. Montmorillonite–chitosan–silver sulfadiazine nanocomposites for topical treatment of chronic skin lesions: in vitro biocompatibility, antibacterial efficacy and gap closure cell motility properties. Carbohydr Polym. 2014;102:970–7. https://doi.org/10.1016/j.carbpol.2013.10.029.

30. Maisanaba S, Pichardo S, Puerto M, Gutiérrez-Praena D, Cameán AM, Jos A. Toxicological evaluation of clay minerals and derived nanocomposites: a review. Environ Res. 2015;138:233–54. https://doi.org/10.1016/j.envres.2014.12.024.

31. Janer G, Fernández-Rosas E, del Molino EM, González-Gálvez D, Vilar G, López-Iglesias C, Ermini V, Vázquez-Campos S. In vitro toxicity of functionalised nanoclays is mainly driven by the presence of organic modifiers. Nanotoxicology. 2014;8(3):279–94. https://doi.org/10.3109/17435390.2013.776123.

32. Gupta GS, Dhawan A, Shanker R. Montmorillonite clay alters toxicity of silver nanoparticles in zebrafish (*Danio rerio*) eleutheroembryo. Chemosphere. 2016;163:242–51. https://doi.org/10.1016/j.chemosphere.2016.08.032.

33. Kansara K, Paruthi A, Misra SK, Karakoti AS, Kumar A. Montmorillonite clay and humic acid modulate the behavior of copper oxide nanoparticles in aqueous environment and induces developmental defects in zebrafish embryo. Environ Pollut. 2019;255(Pt 2):113313. https://doi.org/10.1016/j.envpol.2019.113313.

34. Abdel-Wahhab MA, Nada SA, Amra HA. Effect of aluminosilicates and bentonite on aflatoxin-induced developmental toxicity in rat. J Appl Toxicol. 1999;19(3):199–204. https://doi.org/10.1002/(sici)1099-1263(199905/06)19:3<199::aid-jat558>3.0.co;2-d.

35. Dwyer M, Kubena L, Harvey R, Mayura K, Sarr A, Buckley S, Bailey R, Phillips T. Effects of inorganic adsorbents and cyclopiazonic acid in broiler chickens. Poult Sci. 1997;76(8):1141–9. https://doi.org/10.1093/ps/76.8.1141.

36. Barbero AM, Frasch HF. Pig and guinea pig skin as surrogates for human in vitro penetration studies: a quantitative review. Toxicol In Vitro. 2009;23(1):1–13. https://doi.org/10.1016/j.tiv.2008.10.008.

37. Boudry I, Blanck O, Cruz C, Blanck M, Vallet V, Bazire A, Capt A, Josse D, Lallement G. Percutaneous penetration and absorption of parathion using human and pig skin models in vitro and human skin grafted onto nude mouse skin model in vivo. J Appl Toxicol. 2008;28(5):645–57. https://doi.org/10.1002/jat.1317.

38. Gerstel D, Jacques-Jamin C, Schepky A, Cubberley R, Eilstein J, Grégoire S, Hewitt N, Klaric M, Rothe H, Duplan H. Comparison of protocols for measuring cosmetic ingredient distribution in human and pig skin. Toxicol In Vitro. 2016;34:153–60. https://doi.org/10.1016/j.tiv.2016.03.012.

39. Schmook FP, Meingassner JG, Billich A. Comparison of human skin or epidermis models with human and animal skin in in-vitro percutaneous absorption. Int J Pharm. 2001;215(1–2):51–6. https://doi.org/10.1016/s0378-5173(00)00665-7.

40. Kraeling MEK, Topping VD, Keltner ZM, Belgrave KR, Bailey KD, Gao X, Yourick JJ. In vitro percutaneous penetration of silver nanoparticles in pig and human skin. Regul Toxicol Pharmacol. 2018;95:314–22. https://doi.org/10.1016/j.yrtph.2018.04.006.

41. Vallet V, Cruz C, Josse D, Bazire A, Lallement G, Boudry I. In vitro percutaneous penetration of organophosphorus compounds using full-thickness and split-thickness pig and human skin. Toxicol In Vitro. 2007;21(6):1182–90. https://doi.org/10.1016/j.tiv.2007.03.007.

42. Dalton C, Hall C, Lydon H, Jenner J, Chipman JK, Graham JS, Chilcott RP. The percutaneous absorption of soman in a damaged skin porcine model and the evaluation of WoundStat™ as a topical decontaminant. Cutan Ocul Toxicol. 2018;37(2):172–9. https://doi.org/10.1080/15569527.2017.1365883.

43. Bignon C, Amigoni S, Devers T, Guittard F. Barrier cream based on CeO₂ nanoparticles grafted polymer as an active compound against the penetration of organophosphates. Chem Biol Interact. 2017;267:17–24. https://doi.org/10.1016/j.cbi.2016.03.002.

44. Salles F, Bildstein O, Douillard JM, Jullien M, Raynal J, Van Damme H. On the cation dependence of interlamellar and interparticular water and swelling in smectite clays. Langmuir. 2010;26(7):5028–37. https://doi.org/10.1021/la1002868.

45. van Beinum W, Beulke S, Brown CD. Pesticide sorption and diffusion in natural clay loam aggregates. J Agric Food Chem. 2005;53(23):9146–54. https://doi.org/10.1021/jf050928g.

46. Villaverde J, van Beinum W, Beulke S, Brown CD. The kinetics of sorption by retarded diffusion into soil aggregate pores. Environ Sci Technol. 2009;43(21):8227–32. https://doi.org/10.1021/es9015052.

47. Shah KJ, Pan S-Y, Shukla AD, Shah DO, Chiang P-C. Mechanism of organic pollutants sorption from aqueous solution by cationic tunable organoclays. J Colloid Interface Sci. 2018;529:90–9. https://doi.org/10.1016/j.jcis.2018.05.094.

48. Iannuccelli V, Maretti E, Sacchetti F, Romagnoli M, Bellini A, Truzzi E, Miselli P, Leo E. Characterization of natural clays from ITALIAN deposits with focus on elemental composition and exchange estimated by EDX analysis: potential pharmaceutical and cosmetic uses. Clays Clay Miner. 2016;64(6):719–31. https://doi.org/10.1346/CCMN.2016.064038.

49. Bertella F, Pergher SBC. Scale up pillaring: a study of the parameters that influence the process. Materials. 2017;10(7):712. https://doi.org/10.3390/ma10070712.

50. Moraes JDD, Bertolino SRA, Cuffini SL, Ducart DF, Bretzke PE, Leonardi GR. Clay minerals: properties and applications to dermocosmetic products and perspectives of natural raw materials for therapeutic purposes—a review. Int J Pharm. 2017;534(1–2):213–9. https://doi.org/10.1016/j.ijpharm.2017.10.031.

Chapter 10
Development of a Next Generation Military Skin Decontaminant: Initial Efficacy Studies of Zirconium Hydroxide

Hazem Matar, Shawn Stevenson, Robert P. Chilcott, and Kevin Morrissey

Introduction

Chemicals in war have been used to debilitate armies and gain a tactical advantage on the battlefield since at least 256 AD [1]. One of the earliest documented uses of chemical warfare agents was during the First World War when chlorine, phosgene and sulphur mustard (HD), along with other blister agents, were used at the battle of Flanders near Ypres, Belgium, in July 1917 [2]. Despite legal treaties prohibiting their use, chemical warfare agents have been deployed on several occasions in recent history, such as the Iran–Iraq War (1980), the sarin attack on the Tokyo underground system (1995), assassination of Kim Jong-nam (2017) using VX and the attempted execution of the Russian ex-spy Sergei Skripal (2018) using a nerve agent.

Chemical warfare agents are generally classified based upon their mode of action. Nerve agents achieve their toxicity by overstimulating the body's nervous system, ultimately resulting in respiratory paralysis and death. Blister agents (vesicants) primarily affect the skin, lungs, eyes and mucosal membranes. Blood agents interfere with the body's metabolic processes, impeding the function of vital biochemical pathways. Incapacitating agents can vary in their mode of action but are designed to temporarily render individuals incapable of performing their tasks by

H. Matar (✉) · R. P. Chilcott
Research Centre for Topical Drug Delivery and Toxicology, University of Hertfordshire, Hatfield, UK
e-mail: h.matar@herts.ac.uk; r.chilcott@herts.ac.uk

S. Stevenson · K. Morrissey
Combat Capabilities Development Command Chemical Biological Center, Aberdeen Proving Ground, MD, USA
e-mail: shawn.m.stevenson7.civ@army.mil; kevin.m.morrissey.civ@army.mil

© The Author(s), under exclusive license to Springer Nature Switzerland AG 2022
A. M. Feschuk et al. (eds.), *Dermal Absorption and Decontamination*,
https://doi.org/10.1007/978-3-031-09222-0_10

exerting either physiological or mental effects. Choking agents target and damage the lungs, causing pulmonary oedema and in sufficient dose death due to asphyxiation.

Generally, the routes of exposure depend upon the physicochemical properties of chemical warfare agents – an obvious example being volatility. Typically, non-volatile chemicals of a molecular weight less than 500 Da are generally regarded as dermal hazards, given their ability to persist and be absorbed into the body via direct skin contact. In contrast, volatile chemicals can evaporate and disperse, therefore posing a greater hazard via inhalation. It should also be noted that chemical vapours also pose a dermal hazard, as vesicant vapours can still elicit an adverse dermal response [3]. The onset of symptoms is usually dependent upon route of exposure, not taking into account injection; the rate of absorption is fastest via inhalation and generally slowest via percutaneous exposure.

Reacting to and dealing with nefarious releases of chemical warfare agents differ in the context of military and civilian scenarios. The obvious advantage for military personnel over civilians is that they are generally prepared for reacting to chemical, biological, radiological or nuclear (CBRN) incidents and have access to personal protective equipment (PPE) such as respirators and suits. Additionally, antidotes are more readily available (where possible); for instance, oxime auto-injectors may be carried by soldiers. Moreover, chemical agents may be detected and identified much more rapidly by military personnel using readily deployed detection equipment. Further countermeasures that are more suitable for military applications involve the use of prophylactics and topical skin protectants (barrier creams). However, these measures still do not fully mitigate against the likelihood of direct skin exposure.

One common strategy (process) that applies to both military and civilian situations is the implementation of decontamination. Decontamination can be defined as "the process of removing hazardous material(s) both on or available to the external surfaces of the body in order to reduce local or systemic exposure to a contaminant and thus minimise the risk of subsequent adverse health effects" [4]. Typically, decontamination is conducted by physical removal or by chemical neutralisation. Physical removal methodologies aim to absorb/sequester contaminants, whereas chemical neutralisation aims to modify the structure of the contaminant in order to reduce or eliminate toxicity by hydrolysis, oxidation or other chemical means [5]. The lack of clean water on the battlefield has ultimately led to the development of personal products to decontaminate skin following exposure to chemical warfare agents [6]. A decontaminant should possess certain desirable qualities: effective, rapid mode of action, minimal skin irritation or disruption to the barrier function of the skin, ease of disposal, minimal residual contamination and easily obtained/affordable [5–7]. Products that decontaminate by physical removal include (but are not limited to) Fuller's earth, Dutch powder, Ambergard and M291; their mode of action is fundamentally based upon physical absorption, while they may exhibit some elements of chemical neutralisation [8]. The relative importance of physical removal versus chemical neutralisation is often debated with regard to skin decontamination. Some researchers advocate the primary objective should be physical removal, as in some cases, neutralising properties of some decontaminants are not as rapid as physical removal [7]. In contrast, the rationale of rapid neutralisation is that it should prevent the absorption of intact toxic agent, which is regarded as the primary objective [9]. At present, the main disadvantage of neutralising agents is the lack of a single substance capable of neutralising a wide range of agents.

There are a range of "neutralising" decontamination products designed against chemical warfare agents [10]. Historically, 0.5% hypochlorite solution has been used as the universal reactive decontaminant of choice, because of its alleged ability to denature chemical and biological warfare agents [6]. However, it has been contraindicated against wounds affected by sulphur mustard, as they may exacerbate sulphur mustard-induced lesions [11]. Further developments of neutralising products included a polyurethane sponge impregnated with a specific enzyme (recombinant acetylcholinesterase) which could hydrolyse organophosphate nerve agents [12], although it was prone to rapid saturation due to stoichiometric reactions [9]. However, the most commercially successful is Reactive Skin Decontamination Lotion (RSDL), which is currently in service in a number of countries. RSDL was designed to absorb/solubilise and neutralise chemical warfare agents and can be administered as a lotion or via a sponge soaked with the lotion. The first generation of RSDL comprised two main components: a solvent and an oxime. The solvent was designed to solubilise chemical warfare agents away from the skin, while the oxime reacted with chemical warfare agents to produce less toxic breakdown products [13]. RSDL has been shown to be more efficacious than Fuller's earth against sulphur mustard and VX in domestic swine when decontamination is commenced within 5 min of exposure [14].

An ideal decontaminant would both sequester (absorb) and neutralise chemical warfare agents, thus mitigating cross contamination and reducing the amount of agent available. One such marketed product which incorporates these traits is FAST-ACT®. It is a white nano-powder comprising titanium and magnesium oxides and claims to neutralise chemical warfare agents by hydrolysis and dehydrohalogenation (fast-act.com). However, there is limited dermal toxicity data available for its use on skin. This, coupled with slow reaction rates for specific agents with magnesium oxide ($t_{1/2}$ 68 h) question its suitability as skin decontaminant [15, 16]. Metal oxides have demonstrated their suitability as catalysts for the degradation of chemical warfare agents [17].

Zirconium hydroxide ($Zr(OH)_4$) is a white powder metal oxide and is generally used as precursor for zirconium compounds for use in a wide range of applications such as antiperspirants, paint driers and inks. Zirconium hydroxide encompasses its absorption properties due to its high porosity and surface area. Its neutralising properties are attributed to the basic terminal hydroxyl groups and the acidic bridging groups [18, 19], yielding both Brønsted and Lewis acid and base sites of varying strengths [20–24]. Reactivity rates determined by nuclear magnetic resonance (NMR) have demonstrated rapid neutralisation for VX ($t_{1/2}$ 1 min) to ethyl methylphosphonic acid (EMPA) and 2-(diisopropylamino)ethanethiol [18], soman (GD; $t_{1/2}$ 8.7 min) to pinacolyl methylphosphonic acid (PMPA) and sulphur mustard (HD; $t_{1/2}$ 138 min) to several vinyls and thiodiglycol [18].

There have been no studies assessing the potential for $Zr(OH)_4$ to be used a skin decontaminant. Therefore, prior to embarking on a large multi-year research programme, initial studies were performed to assess various simple formulations of $Zr(OH)_4$ using a synthetic skin membrane against chemical warfare agents prior to evaluating the skin surface decontamination of "optimal" formulations with porcine skin.

Materials and Methods

Chemicals

The synthesis, use and destruction of sulphur mustard (HD), soman (GD) and VX were conducted in accordance with the Chemical Weapons Convention. The chemical agents were synthesised by DEVCOM CBC (Maryland, USA) and were reported to be >85% pure (as determined by NMR or GC-MS). Personnel handling the chemical contaminants were fully trained and certified for such activities.

Isopropanol, 1-nonanol, acetonitrile and chloroform all reported to be >98% were purchased from Sigma-Aldrich, USA. Deionised water was produced from the municipal supply and purified using an in-house GE Osmonics, Model E4-11000-DLX reverse osmosis water purification system (Silver Lake, WI). Zirconium hydroxide type B was purchased from Guild Associates Inc. (Dublin, OH). Zirconium hydroxide type C was supplied by Luxfer MEL Technologies (Flemington, NJ), and Reactive Skin Decontamination Lotion (RSDL) was purchased from First Line Technologies (Chantilly, VA).

Experimental Approach

An initial screening study was performed using Strat-M™ (Millipore, MA, USA). Strat-M™ is a synthetic two-layer system designed to mimic the interaction of a wide range of chemical compounds with human skin. The products with the best efficacy were those that resulted in the lowest remaining agent and were taken forward to be evaluated using porcine skin.

Screening Experiment

Discs of Strat-M™ (4.9 cm²) were placed into individual polystyrene petri dishes, and each disc received a nominal 4 g m⁻² challenge applied as a 2 µL droplet of either GD, HD or VX. The contaminated panels were covered for a period of 5 min prior to decontamination. Decontamination treatments comprised a rinse-only control group where 120 mL of water was applied as 6×20 mL aliquots at a flow rate of 1 L min^{-1} to the surface in a vertical orientation. Two types of $Zr(OH)_4$ powder in a range of solvents were evaluated (Table 10.1). Decontaminant powders were applied over the entire surface area of the panel and liquid formulations (250 µL) dispensed via a positive displacement pipette, ensuring the entire surface area of the disc was covered.

Differences between the two types of $Zr(OH)_4$ are detailed in Table 10.2. Type B consists of very small crystallites that form larger agglomerates, whereas type C consists of much larger, spherical particles (Fig. 10.1). Decontaminants remained in situ on the surface of the panel for 10 min before being removed by rinsing with

Table 10.1 Formulations of zirconium hydroxide used for Strat-M™ evaluations

$Zr(OH)_4$ type	$Zr(OH)_4$ mass used	Solvent	Comments
B	3.7	None	Powder alone
		1-Nonanol	Weight % = 100
		DI water	
		Isopropyl alcohol (IPA)	
C	3.7	None	Powder alone
		1-Nonanol	Weight % = 53
		DI water	
		Isopropyl alcohol (IPA)	
	1.25	30/70 v/v, IPA/DI water	Weight % = 25
		50/50 v/v, IPA/DI water	
		70/30 v/v, IPA/DI water	

Table 10.2 Characteristics of zirconium hydroxide as a function of type

Parameter	Type B	Type C
Micropore volume (cc/g)	0.17	0.20
Total pore volume (cc/g)	0.38	0.48
Hydroxyl ratios, O/Zr	3.4	3.6
Hydroxyl ratios, % terminal	21	35

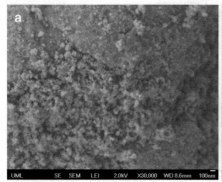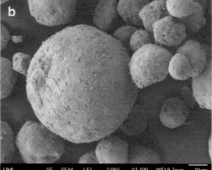

Fig. 10.1 Scanning electron micrograph images of zirconium type B (**a**) and type C (**b**)

120 mL of deionised water (applied as 6×20 mL aliquots at a flow rate of 1 L min^{-1}). The Strat-M™ discs were then placed in glass vials containing 20 mL of chloroform, acetonitrile or isopropanol to extract HD, GD and VX, respectively. The amount of agent remaining within the discs of Strat-M™ was determined via gas chromatography coupled with mass spectrometry (GC-MS) or liquid chromatography coupled with mass spectrometry (LC-MS).

Decontamination of Porcine Skin

Experiments using excised porcine skin were performed in a similar manner as the Strat-M studies. Yorkshire mix (white) female pig skin from the dorsal aspect (5 months old) was supplied by Lampire Biological Laboratories, PA, USA. The skin was prepared by removing the hair with an electric clipper and the skin washed to remove debris, blood and faecal matter. Excess subcutaneous fat was removed and the skin cut into 1 in. × 1 in. square sections and wrapped in aluminium foil. The skin was stored at −20 °C for a maximum of 6 months prior to use.

Prior to commencement of each study, the skin was removed from cold storage and allowed to equilibrate to room temperature prior to being contaminated. Each section of porcine skin received a 3.1 g m^{-2} challenge applied as one 2 μL droplet of HD, GD or VX. Decontamination was initiated 5 min postexposure and comprised five different treatments (Table 10.3). The decontaminants remained in situ for 10 min before rinsing the products off the skin. The skin was then placed in glass vials containing 40 mL of chloroform, acetonitrile or isopropanol to extract HD, GD and VX, respectively. The amount of agent remaining within the sections of porcine skin was determined via GC-MS or LC-MS.

Table 10.3 Decontaminants used for porcine skin evaluations

Formulation	Decontaminant state	Mass or volume used	Description
Rinse only	Liquid	120 mL	Skin sections were rinsed with 120 mL of deionised water (applied as 6 × 20 mL aliquots, at a flow rate of 1 L min^{-1}) in a vertical orientation
Zr(OH)$_4$ type C powder	Solid	0.25 g	Powder alone
Zr(OH)$_4$ type C powder (rubbed)	Solid	0.25 g	Powder applied and rubbed into the skin clockwise (three full rotations)
RSDL liquid	Liquid	0.25 mL	Applied using a positive displacement pipette
RSDL kit	Liquid and sponge	0.25 mL	Lotion applied as 250 μL and immediately rubbed using sponge

Results

Screening Experiment Using Strat-M™

Generally, the absorption of sulphur mustard (HD) was greater than that of soman (GD) or VX into the Strat-M™ discs (Fig. 10.2). The administration of zirconium hydroxide powders alone outperformed the formulations containing carrier solvents (except for VX; Fig. 10.2). Interestingly, the top performer for VX was $Zr(OH)_4$ type B in DI water as indicated by the lowest average mass of VX remaining within Strat-M™ (Fig. 10.2). Mostly, the presence of either $Zr(OH)_4$ type B or C in each carrier solvent tended to decrease the amount absorbed into Strat-M™ when compared to solvent alone (1-nonanol was not evaluated against VX; Fig. 10.2). Furthermore, rinse only tended to elicit the greatest amount of agent recovered from Strat-M™.

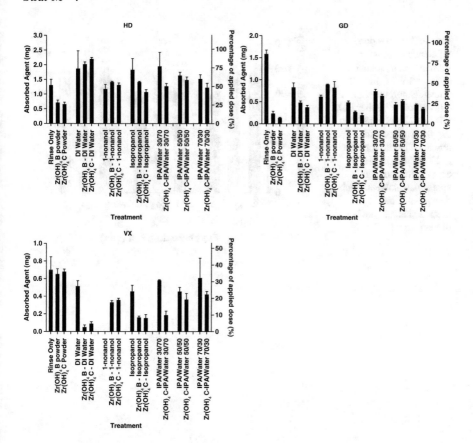

Fig. 10.2 Amount of sulphur mustard (HD), soman (GD) and VX remaining on Strat-M™ discs (4.9 cm²) following decontamination. A 2 µL droplet of HD, GD or VX was applied to the surface and decontamination performed 5 min postexposure. All data points are mean ± standard deviation of between 3 and 10 replicates

Decontamination Efficacy with Porcine Skin

An initial pre-test was performed to confirm the extraction efficiency of HD, GD and VX from porcine skin over varying exposure durations (Fig. 10.3). Overall, the extraction efficiency from pig skin was >94% of the applied dose except for GD exposed for 60 min (Fig. 10.3). The results indicate that the agent can be successfully recovered from pig skin using current extraction solvents.

Generally, the removal of HD, GD and VX from pig skin was least effective when rinse only was performed (Fig. 10.4). The application of RSDL was not as effective as the application of RSDL with rubbing across all agents. The efficacy results for $Zr(OH)_4$ type C resulted in similar or greater performance than the RSDL treatments. The application of $Zr(OH)_4$ type C by rubbing increased efficacy for GD and VX when compared to not rubbing, except for skin contaminated with HD (Fig. 10.4).

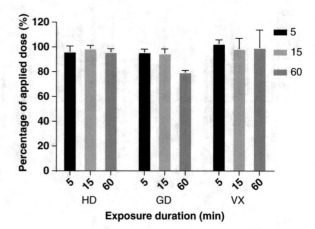

Fig. 10.3 Extraction efficiency of sulphur mustard (HD), soman (GD) and VX from full thickness porcine skin. A 2 µL droplet of either HD, GD or VX was applied to the skin surface and remained in situ for either 5, 15 or 60 min prior to being extracted in an appropriate solvent. Each data point is the mean ± standard deviation of 3 replicates

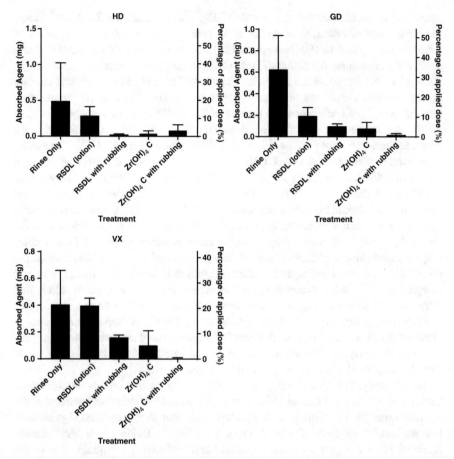

Fig. 10.4 Amount of sulphur mustard (HD), soman (GD) and VX remaining within full thickness porcine skin following decontamination. A 2 μL droplet of either HD, GD or VX was applied to the skin surface and decontamination initiated 5 min postexposure. Where applicable, decontaminants remained in situ for 10 min prior to being removed and the skin extracted to determine the amount of agent absorbed within the skin. All data points are mean ± standard deviations of 3 replicates

Discussion

This study identified and assessed the suitability of zirconium hydroxide ($Zr(OH)_4$) as a potential skin decontaminant. The initial study demonstrated that the application of the dry powder alone was more effective than formulations containing solvents and that decontamination of pig skin was as effective as the currently fielded product RSDL. However, it should be noted that these studies were proof-of-concept studies and further tests will be performed.

The use of Strat-M™ as a surrogate for skin was justified because previous work has demonstrated that chemicals exhibit similar diffusion and partition parameters compared to excised human and rat skin [25]. Furthermore, the Strat-M™ model has demonstrated potential as an initial screening tool for the down-selection of formulations related to skin absorption [26]. However, it should be noted that this study did not evaluate the extent of penetration through the membrane but what was retained within the substrate following exposure. The amount of chemical warfare agents retained within the Strat-M™ within this study tended to be greater than porcine skin. This further justifies the use of Strat-M™ as a conservative model to potentially screen decontamination products. However, there was a difference between Strat-M™ and porcine skin with $Zr(OH)_4$ decontaminated VX. The results with porcine skin showed that $Zr(OH)_4$ C powder was more effective on pig skin than Strat-M™ (0.1 mg as opposed to 0.6 mg, respectively), which is likely due to the increased absorption into Strat-M compared to pig skin. However, future studies using Strat-M should contain a non-decontaminated control. A limitation of using synthetic membranes is lack of anatomical skin surface features such as hair follicles, ridges and sulci which may, in some circumstances, provide a further challenge for assessing decontamination efficacy. Traditionally, porcine skin is often the model of choice as a surrogate for human skin due to similarities in structure and morphology [27, 28]. Furthermore, another advantage of using porcine skin is that if the product is assessed using porcine in vivo models, it will serve as a direct comparison for determining toxicokinetic parameters. This is of importance as decontamination efficacy against chemical warfare agents cannot be performed on human subjects. However, in vivo animal studies can be negated if appropriate safe simulants are identified and evaluated in human volunteer trials.

Interestingly, $Zr(OH)_4$ powders in the absence of carrier liquids demonstrated the highest efficacy for GD and HD, while each powder in deionised water was the top performer for VX. This was unexpected result, due to the reported high absorptive and neutralising capacity of $Zr(OH)_4$ for VX [18]. Being that a "dry" decontaminant is advantageous for the battlefield and logistically favourable due to the lack of water needed for use, the decision was made to move forward with zirconium powder. Zirconium type C was taken forward over type B mainly due to the improved efficacy observed for GD. Furthermore, type C has increased terminal hydroxyls that provide increased reactivity for acid and base hydrolysis of the agents. There are advantages to developing a novel personnel decontaminant that is "dry", i.e. not requiring water for decontaminant preparation or use. Studies have advocated the use of performing "dry" decontamination during emergency civilian decontamination (as a method to remove the majority of contamination) as a lifesaving intervention while waiting for specialised forms of decontamination [29–31]. Furthermore, water is a scarce commodity in certain environments, and as such, it is useful to provide efficacious products to the warfighter that provide utility in the field. A "dry" decontaminant would also be useful in colder climates where any available water is most likely frozen or pose a risk of frostbite and potentially hypothermia. The results from the pig skin studies provide a basis for $Zr(OH)_4$ to be considered for maturation as a novel skin decontaminant. The $Zr(OH)_4$ performance on CWA contaminated full thickness pig skin is similar to that of the currently fielded RSDL.

Further work is necessary in order to fully evaluate the suitability of $Zr(OH)_4$ as a skin decontaminant. Generally, when evaluating skin decontaminants, a rigorous scientific approach is necessary to ensure the products are safe and effective [32]. Primarily, further efficacy studies are required which compare $Zr(OH)_4$ against currently fielded products using a test system which conforms to OECD 428 procedures [33]. This will provide further experimental endpoints to assess decontamination efficacy. These endpoints can include the amount of CWA penetrating the skin over time, the rate of absorption, the proportion of the applied dose remaining on the skin surface, the amount absorbed in the skin and the proportion that has evaporated from the skin surface. Using a robust test system will serve as a platform to fully assess a range of scenarios such as assessment over various exposure durations and decontaminant dwell times, in addition to assessing the retention of agent within the decontaminant over time.

A further consideration for developing a skin decontamination is the final form factor of the product, i.e. to be administered as a dry power or incorporated into a glove/mitt. This could affect the overall decontamination efficacy and safety profile of the product. For example, how would we expect a warfighter to use the product, and are there any potential contraindications to consider, i.e. rubbing of the powder may improve decontamination efficacy but how can the contaminated powder be removed from the skin and does it pose any further hazards? In contrast, the use of a mitt filled with $Zr(OH)_4$ may limit the amount of powder deposited onto the skin surface, thus potentially increasing the safety profile of the product, but may reduce decontamination efficacy. Furthermore, future research will focus on determining optimal application and use parameters by developing a standardised test system. A robotic arm will be programmed to exert a set pressure and perform various motions reproducibly, such as blotting, wiping and a combination of motions, to (1) assess decontamination efficacy, (2) limit intra- and interlaboratory variability and (3) assess the impact of contaminant spreading.

Initial in vitro dermal toxicology tests will also be performed to ensure $Zr(OH)_4$ does not elicit any adverse effects to the skin. Where applicable, skin irritation and sensitisation potential will be assessed, and depending on the outcomes of rigorous evaluation processes, the product will undergo all requisite testing to ensure it complies with all US Food and Drug Administration (FDA) safety requirements.

References

1. Simon J. Stratagems, combat, and "chemical warfare" in the siege mines of Dura-Europos. Am J Archaeol. 2011;115:69–101.
2. Chauhan S, Chauhan S, D'cruz R, Faruqi S, Singh KK, Varma S, Singh M, Karthik V. Chemical warfare agents. Environ Toxicol Pharmacol. 2008;26:113–22.
3. Chilcott RP, Brown RF, Rice P. Non-invasive quantification of skin injury resulting from exposure to sulphur mustard and Lewisite vapours. Burns. 2000;26:245–50.
4. Chilcott RP. Initial management of mass casualty incidents. In: Arora R, Arora P, editors. Disaster management: medical preparedness, response and homeland security. Oxford: CABI; 2013.

5. Chan HP, Zhai H, Hui X, Maibach HI. Skin decontamination: principles and perspectives. Toxicol Ind Health. 2013;29:955–68.
6. Yang YC, Baker JA, Ward JR. Decontamination of chemical warfare agents. Chem Rev. 1992;92:1729–43.
7. Hurst CR. Decontamination. In: Sidell FR, Takafuji ET, Franz DR, editors. Medical aspects of chemical and biological warfare. Washington, DC: Office of the Surgeon General United States Army; 1997.
8. Roberts G, Maynard RL. Responding to chemical terrorism: operational planning and decontamination. In: Marrs TT, Maynard RL, Sidell F, editors. Chemical warfare agents: toxicology and treatment. 2nd ed. Chichester: Wiley; 2007.
9. Gordon RK, Clarkson ED. Decontamination of chemical warfare agents. In: Gupta RC, editor. Handbook of toxicology of chemical warfare agents. London: Academic Press; 2009.
10. Thors L, Koch M, Wigenstam E, Koch B, Hagglund L, Bucht A. Comparison of skin decontamination efficacy of commercial decontamination products following exposure to VX on human skin. Chem Biol Interact. 2017;273:82–9.
11. Gold MB, Bongiovanni R, Scharf BA, Gresham VC, Woodward CL. Hypochlorite solution as a decontaminant in sulfur mustard contaminated skin defects in the euthymic hairless guinea pig. Drug Chem Toxicol. 1994;17:499–527.
12. Gordon RK, Feaster SR, Russell AJ, Lejeune KE, Maxwell DM, Lenz DE, Ross M, Doctor BP. Organophosphate skin decontamination using immobilized enzymes. Chem Biol Interact. 1999;119:463–70.
13. Gerecke DR, Gray JP, Shakarjiam MP, Casillas RP. Dermal toxicity of sulphur mustard. In: Gupta RC, editor. Handbook of toxicology of chemical warfare agents. San Diego: Elsevier; 2009.
14. Taysse L, Daulon S, Delamanche S, Bellier B, Breton P. Skin decontamination of mustards and organophosphates: comparative efficiency of RSDL and Fuller's earth in domestic swine. Hum Exp Toxicol. 2007;26:135–41.
15. Wagner GW, Bartram PW, Koper O, Klabunde KJ. Reactions of VX, GD, and HD with nanosize MgO. J Phys Chem B. 1999;103:3225–8.
16. Wagner GW, Procell LR, O'connor RJ, Munavalli S, Carnes CL, Kapoor PN, Klabunde KJ. Reactions of VX, GB, GD, and HD with nanosize Al_2O_3. Formation of aluminophosphonates. J Am Chem Soc. 2001;123:1636–44.
17. Wagner GW. Decontamination of chemical warfare agents with nanosize metal oxides. Nanoscale materials in chemistry: environmental applications. Washington, DC: American Chemical Society; 2010.
18. Bandosz TJ, Laskoski M, Mahle J, Mogilevsky G, Peterson GW, Rossin JA, Wagner GW. Reactions of VX, GD, and HD with $Zr(OH)_4$: near instantaneous decontamination of VX. J Phys Chem C. 2012;116:11606–14.
19. Mogilevsky G, Karwacki CJ, Peterson GW, Wagner GW. Surface hydroxyl concentration on $Zr(OH)_4$ quantified by 1H MAS NMR. Chem Phys Lett. 2011;511:384–8.
20. Balow RB, Lundin JG, Daniels GC, Gordon WO, Mcentee M, Peterson GW, Wynne JH, Pehrsson PE. Environmental effects on zirconium hydroxide nanoparticles and chemical warfare agent decomposition: implications of atmospheric water and carbon dioxide. ACS Appl Mater Interfaces. 2017;9:39747–57.
21. Peterson GW, Karwacki CJ, Feaver WB, Rossin JA. Zirconium hydroxide as a reactive substrate for the removal of sulfur dioxide. Ind Eng Chem Res. 2009;48:1694–8.
22. Peterson GW, Rossin JA. Removal of chlorine gases from streams of air using reactive zirconium hydroxide based filtration media. Ind Eng Chem Res. 2012;51:2675–81.
23. Peterson GW, Rossin JA, Karwacki CJ, Glover TG. Surface chemistry and morphology of zirconia polymorphs and the influence on sulfur dioxide removal. J Phys Chem C. 2011;115:9644–50.

24. Wagner GW, Peterson GW, Mahle JJ. Effect of adsorbed water and surface hydroxyls on the hydrolysis of VX, GD, and HD on titania materials: the development of self-decontaminating paints. Ind Eng Chem Res. 2012;51:3598–603.
25. Uchida T, Kadhum WR, Kanai S, Todo H, Oshizaka T, Sugibayashi K. Prediction of skin permeation by chemical compounds using the artificial membrane, Strat-M™. Eur J Pharm Sci. 2015;67:113–8.
26. Karadzovska D, Riviere JE. Assessing vehicle effects on skin absorption using artificial membrane assays. Eur J Pharm Sci. 2013;50:569–76.
27. Barbero AM, Frasch HF. Pig and guinea pig skin as surrogates for human in vitro penetration studies: a quantitative review. Toxicol In Vitro. 2009;23:1–13.
28. Scott RC, Walker M, Dugard PH. A comparison of the in vitro permeability properties of human and some laboratory animal skins. Int J Cosmet Sci. 1986;8:189–94.
29. Josse D, Barrier G. Emergency decontamination in low-resource settings. In: Arora R, Arora P, editors. Disaster management: medical preparedness, response and homeland security. Oxford: CABI; 2013.
30. Kassouf N, Syed S, Larner J, Amlot R, Chilcott RP. Evaluation of absorbent materials for use as ad hoc dry decontaminants during mass casualty incidents as part of the UK's initial operational response (IOR). PLoS One. 2017;12:e0170966.
31. Larner J, Durrant A, Hughes P, Mahalingam D, Rivers S, Matar H, Thomas E, Barrett M, Pinhal A, Amer N, Hall C, Jackson T, Catalani V, Chilcott RP. Efficacy of different hair and skin decontamination strategies with identification of associated hazards to first responders. Prehosp Emerg Care. 2020;24:355–68.
32. Josse D. Effectiveness of chemical, biological, radiological, and nuclear (CBRN) skin decontaminants: toward tests standardization. In: Zhu H, Maibach HI, editors. Skin decontamination: a comprehensive clinical research guide. Cham: Springer International; 2020.
33. OECD. Test no. 428: Skin absorption: in vitro method. Paris: OECD; 2004.

Chapter 11
Findings from the PHOENIX Project: 'Protocols for Hair and the Optimisation of Existing and Novel Decontamination Interventions Through Experimentation'

Tim Marczylo, Tom James, Richard Amlot, and Samuel Collins

Introduction

The global production, transport and use of chemicals, including toxic industrial chemicals, continue to increase [1]. Consequently, the risk of a chemical incident leading to public exposure and potential injury from hazardous chemicals is also increasing. These chemical incidents may be accidental (e.g. chemical spillages, fires) or deliberate (e.g. terrorist) and could lead to preventable exposure of tens of thousands of people every year [1, 2]. Recent accidents include the 2013 Lac-Mégantic rail disaster [3] and the 2015 Tianjin explosion [4]. Deliberate uses of chemical agents have also been reported including acid attacks [5], use of sarin in Syria [6], VX attacks in Malaysia [7] and Novichok use in both the UK and Russia [8, 9]. These highlight the varied chemical threats posed by these incidents.

Whether accidental or deliberate, a chemical incident may expose the public via multiple routes including inhalation or deposition on skin, hair and eyes either from the air or by direct contact [1, 8]. The principal public health intervention following a chemical incident is to use decontamination (reduction, removal or neutralisation of chemical) processes to reduce harm by reducing the exposure of exposed persons

T. Marczylo (✉) · T. James
Radiation, Chemical and Environmental Hazards, United Kingdom Health Security Agency, Chilton, Oxon, UK
e-mail: Tim.Marczylo@ukhsa.gov.uk; Tom.James@ukhsa.gov.uk

R. Amlot
Emergency Response Department Science and Technology, Health Protection Directorate, United Kingdom Health Security Agency, London, UK
e-mail: Richard.Amlot@ukhsa.gov.uk

S. Collins
Global Operations, United Kingdom Health Security Agency, London, UK
e-mail: Samuel.Collins@ukhsa.gov.uk

© The Author(s), under exclusive license to Springer Nature Switzerland AG 2022
A. M. Feschuk et al. (eds.), *Dermal Absorption and Decontamination*, https://doi.org/10.1007/978-3-031-09222-0_11

183

and reducing the potential for transfer of contamination to additional people including emergency responders or to equipment and healthcare facilities.

Mass casualty incidents refer to any incident involving numbers of casualties beyond the normal capacity of emergency and healthcare services (NHS England) [10]. They require first responders to implement appropriate and structured decontamination interventions. Research conducted predominantly in the UK and the USA has recently led to substantive changes to how mass casualty decontamination for chemical incidents is conducted.

UK first responders to a chemical incident were historically advised to stand off and wait for specialist Fire and Rescue Services (FRS) capability including mass decontamination units (MDUs) (see Fig. 11.1). However, delayed intervention increases the potential for harm following exposure to hazardous chemicals. Consequently, informed by the research outputs including the ORCHIDS programme [11–15], the UK operational response moved away from a reliance on specialist operational response (SOR) incorporating MDUs, to more rapidly deployable interventions including emergency evacuation, disrobe and to decontamination strategies that incorporate improvised dry, improvised wet [rinse-wipe-rinse (RWR)] and interim wet methods, known collectively as the initial operational response (IOR) [16]. IOR aims to decontaminate casualties as soon as possible after exposure. In 2015, the USA introduced the Federal Primary Response Incident Scene Management (PRISM) guidance [17]. PRISM incorporates an initial 'disrobe and decontaminate' response to chemical incidents, emphasising the requirement for speed to improve casualty survival and reduce morbidity. In 2019 [18], PRISM was extended to include a triple decontamination protocol (the combination of dry,

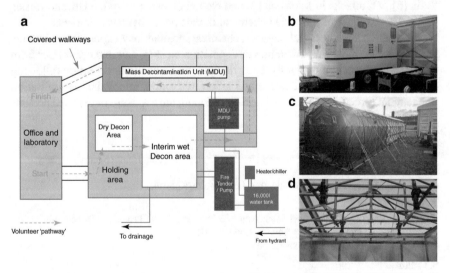

Fig. 11.1 PHOENIX trial site for conducting human volunteer decontamination studies. (**a**) Flow diagram showing route taken by volunteers. (**b**) The Mobile Image Analysis Unit (MIAU). (**c**) The mass decontamination unit (MDU). (**d**) Branch assembly for interim wet decontamination showing four branches

'ladder pipe' (interim) and technical (mass) decontamination), the decontamination of hair and principles for scene decision-making.

These mass casualty chemical decontamination approaches have been systematically optimised and evaluated through a combination of in vitro and human volunteer trials, and the evidence generated has highlighted some common observations.

Speed Is Critical

The estimated time to establish SOR at an incident site in the UK or the USA is 1 h, whereas a time delay of >20 min is predicted for the FRS to conduct gross wet decontamination using a 'ladder pipe system' [15]. Delays in initiating decontamination are suboptimal, especially for toxicants that act following rapid dermal absorption or inhalation. A review of the UK model response in light of conclusions from the ORCHIDS projects [15] concluded that a more rapid intervention was required to minimise the risk of morbidity and mortality. The rapid intervention was named the initial operational response (IOR) and incorporates the removal of casualties from the site of gross contamination, disrobing of casualties to remove potentially contaminated clothing and improvised dry or wet decontamination with any readily available absorbent materials and water. Following this improvised decontamination, interim decontamination is conducted, using fire service vehicles to create a shower corridor (known as the 'ladder pipe' system in the USA) for casualties to walk through. IOR significantly reduced the time between exposure and intervention. Informed by studies funded by the Biomedical Advanced Research and Development Authority (BARDA) [18], the USA has similarly adopted a rapid intervention approach incorporating evacuation, disrobe and improvised decontamination. While IOR and interim procedures may not be as effective as SOR in removing surface contamination, the speed of removal is preferable to delaying removal.

The Importance of Disrobing

Emergency disrobe forms part of the IOR and is recommended within 15 min of exposure to prevent the penetration of the chemical to the skin, transfer to emergency responders and to reduce inhalation exposure from volatile chemicals. Removal of 80–90% of chemicals by disrobing has been suggested [19], but there is little to no published evidence to support this [18]. Initially, clothing is both a barrier preventing contact with skin and a source of inhalation exposure for volatile through off-gassing dependent upon the type of material [20]. Once the chemical has penetrated to skin, clothing may increase the absorption by trapping it as has been demonstrated for chlorine [21]. A survey of US key responders reported that the situation including the degree of contamination, the identity of the chemical agent and the ambient temperature would determine whether they initiate disrobe immediately [22]. In both the UK and the US guidance, responders should consider hypothermia and modesty concerns by making alternative clothing or blankets available [16, 18] and to limit exposure by wearing gloves and to cut off clothing instead of removing clothes over the head. Use of scissors to cut off clothing is particularly useful for non-ambulant casualties [23].

Dry Decontamination of Skin Is an Effective Intervention When Initiated in a Timely Manner

Most decontamination strategies use water (with or without detergents or bleach) to rinse and remove chemicals from skin and hair [24]. Establishing wet decontamination for mass casualties however takes time which delays decontamination [16–18]. Dry decontamination is 'the topical application of absorptive materials to passively remove liquid contaminants from the skin surface' [25] and is a more rapid, 'ad hoc' intervention that can be performed before the arrival of specialist resources [26]. Dry decontamination can utilise any available absorbent material [14] and is more effective than improvised wet decontamination for a range of simulants of chemical warfare agents and toxic industrial chemicals. An exception was dried residues of potassium cyanide, suggesting that wet decontamination is still required for particulate contamination. Amlôt et al. [11] demonstrated 'blue roll' and incontinence pads (two readily available absorbent materials on frontline response vehicles) were equally effective in removing methyl salicylate (MeS, a simulant for sulphur mustard) from volunteers' forearms. Similar observations are reported for non-ambulant casualties [24]. The speed of initiation and the ease of self-decontaminate ensured dry decontamination is now the default method of decontamination (following disrobe) for non-caustic chemicals in both UK and US Federal IOR guidance [16–18].

There Are Optimised Parameters for Mass Decontamination Showering

Structured decontamination using MDUs is an important provision of SOR. These units can supply heated water and a system for introducing detergent for specific periods during the decontamination cycle. The ORCHIDS projects [12, 15, 27] identified optimal parameters for mass decontamination showering known as the 'ORCHIDS protocol' (Table 11.1) with demonstrated efficacy in field trials [19]. Active washing using cloths can increase decontamination efficacy by >20% [12]. Chilcott et al. [18, 28] suggested a maximum 'ORCHIDS protocol' duration of 90 s to partly offset the 'wash-in' effect where skin penetration of chemicals can be temporally increased by washing [29].

Table 11.1 The 'ORCHIDS' protocol for mass casualty decontamination using MDUs

Parameter	Conditions
Temperature	35 °C
Duration	90 s
Active washing	Provision of cotton wash cloths
Detergent	0.5% Detergent solution

Decontamination Methods Have Variable Efficacy for Contaminated Hair

Hair and scalp are relatively unprotected areas of the body and are likely to be significant sites of exposure during and after a chemical incident. Hair can also bind chemical contaminants [29–36]. While hair is a protective barrier for the scalp [26, 28], certain chemicals diffuse rapidly through hair sebum to the follicles and can be absorbed [31, 33]. In vitro studies of the efficacy of hair decontamination following exposure to VX [26, 30, 37] and MeS and 2-chloroethyl ethyl sulphide (CEES, sulphur mustard simulant) [35] revealed that showering alone was the least effective decontamination protocol, and although the application of Fuller's earth (FE) or Reactive Skin Decontamination Lotion (RSDL) up to 45 min post-exposure but prior to showering substantially improved decontamination efficacy, VX and MeS persisted in hair (up to 27% and 57% of the contaminating doses, respectively). Subsequently, Spiandore et al. [35, 36] demonstrated that MeS and CEES trapped in hair rapidly desorb into the surrounding atmosphere. MeS in hair decreased by a twofold factor in the first 2 h following exposure. After 24 h, 8.6% of the initial dose remained in the hair. These findings demonstrate ongoing risks to the contaminated casualty, first responders and other members of the public.

Chilcott et al. [18] demonstrated high hair decontamination efficacy for MeS during a field exercise in the USA. A later, more controlled, volunteer study [25] showed efficacy of dry, ladder pipe system and technical decontamination methods at removing MeS from hair. Hair was not removed in either study which swabbed the hair surface limiting recovery. Significant contamination remaining in the hair may require further action dependent upon toxicity of chemical and rate of off-gassing.

Decontamination Must be Casualty Focused to Facilitate Compliance

Studies examining casualty experiences and behaviour during decontamination [19, 38–42] suggest how emergency responders manage an incident will influence how members of the public behave [19, 41, 42] affecting the outcomes from the incident. Effective incident managements enable members of the public to identify with responders around a shared goal of decontamination [42–44] increased public cooperation and compliance during the decontamination process [42–45]. It is essential to foster a shared identification between emergency responders and the public, to facilitate public compliance. To achieve a shared identification requires effective communication and respect for casualties' needs [38, 41, 42, 46]. Communication should be open and honest, provide regular updates about the nature of the incident and the actions being taking and focus on the health benefits of decontamination [47]. Decontamination exercises and field trials [11, 19, 41] reveal that provision of sufficient practical information is required to ensure that decontamination is undertaken efficiently. Finally, responders should respect members of vulnerable groups that may make them either more susceptible to the effects of the contaminant or put them at increased risk while undergoing decontamination [39].

The PHOENIX Project

The PHOENIX project was a 3-year, multidisciplinary applied research project exploring the effectiveness of emergency decontamination protocols for chemical incidents, funded by the UK Department of Health and Social Care (DHSC) Policy Research Programme. The project aimed to address certain knowledge gaps with respect to mass decontamination: whether current best practice approaches are sufficiently effective for decontamination of hair, whether IOR and SOR in series are advantageous for decontamination of hair and skin and whether these approaches are also effective for the decontamination of novel, more persistent simulants than MeS which has been used in the majority of volunteer studies to date. The specific objectives of the project were to identify solutions for the decontamination of hair using existing or novel decontamination protocols; provide an assessment of the effectiveness of improvised dry and wet decontamination options against chemical simulants; and provide a systematic and holistic assessment of the cumulative benefit of IOR and SOR conducted in sequence. To achieve this work, five human volunteer trials were undertaken.

The aim of the volunteer trials was to compare the effectiveness of different combinations of UK mass casualty decontamination procedures to remove chemical simulants from human volunteers in controlled studies. PHOENIX provided an assessment of the effectiveness of improvised forms of decontamination (dry and wet), interim wet decontamination, and assessed the benefit of conducting IOR and SOR decontamination protocols in sequence. The protocols used mirrored those used by UK emergency services. To assess the effectiveness of decontamination, we used two simulants: a mixture of methyl salicylate (MeS), Invisible Red S (IRS, Chemox Pound Ltd.) and vegetable oil, and a mixture of benzyl salicylate (BeS) and Invisible Green S (IGS, Chemox Pound Ltd.). BeS was developed for use here because it is more persistent/has a lower vapour pressure than MeS and therefore is more suitable for assessing decontamination interventions conducted at longer time points where previous studies have struggled to detect the low levels of MeS remaining on skin. Simulants were applied to discreet areas of the skin (trials 1–3) or hair (trials 4 and 5) of volunteers prior to decontamination (Fig. 11.2). Each trial followed a randomised within subject ($n = 11$–12) design that meant each volunteer completed each decontamination protocol under examination including a 'no-decontamination' control in a randomised order to negate the effects of inter-individual variation and improved performance from habitualisation. The amount of simulant remaining on volunteers' skin or hair was assessed via the recovery and quantitative measurement of MeS and BeS from skin, hair and urine samples using gas chromatography-mass spectrometry [46, 48, 49] and from semi-quantitative fluorescence imaging of IRS and IGS from UV-illuminated images of volunteers.

A research site was established, incorporating a small office space and laboratory to act as point of arrival for study volunteers. The larger enclosure housed the interim wet decontamination corridor and a Mobile Image Analysis Unit (MIAU) for the UV-illuminated photography (Fig. 11.1). A fire tender providing water for

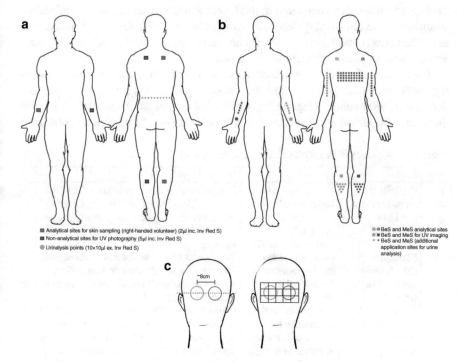

Fig. 11.2 Simulant application sites for volunteers' skin and hair. (**a**) Sites for trials 1 and 2 showing application sites for arms, shoulder and legs. Analytical and non-analytical sites shown are for a right-handed volunteer and were reversed for left-dominant volunteers so that analytical sites were always decontaminated with the weaker hand. Urinalysis points represent simulant application sites without fluorescent markers required to achieve sufficient dose to clearly detect simulant levels in urine. (**b**) Application sites for BeS and MeS in trial 3 for analytical (⊠) UV imaging (■) and sites without fluorescent markers (■) to increase dose for urinalysis. (**c**) Sites targeted for spraying of simulants onto hair and sampling grid utilised for hair retrieval and allowing for simulant spreading during the decontamination process. Eight to ten hairs were removed by cutting as close to the scalp as possible, from each of the grid positions

the interim and specialist decontamination was positioned alongside the main structure (Fig. 11.1a) as was a MDU for trials 3 and 5 (Fig. 11.1c). Operation of the tender and MDU followed a standard operating procedure established in consultation with UK Fire and Rescue Services specialists.

Trial 1 compared the efficacy of improvised dry and wet decontamination procedures, both alone and in sequence, for decontaminating skin [50]. A combination of MeS and IRS was applied to predetermined areas of volunteer's skin at the beginning of each experimental session (Fig. 11.2). These locations were chosen based on their relative perceived difficulty at being decontaminated: the forearm (easy), calf (medium) and upper back (hard). Volunteers were asked to remove the simulant using one of the three improvised decontamination protocols or did not decontaminate in a 'no-decontamination' control (Table 11.2). Each intervention began at 15 min following simulant application, as the estimated time UK first responders would arrive and begin administering decontamination. Both improvised decontamination protocols lasted 3 min in total, yet for improvised dry decontamination, volunteers were able to stop decontaminating once they felt they had finished. The combined intervention involved dry decontamination followed by RWR. The latter was initiated at 18 min after simulant application.

The amount of simulant recovered from the skin of volunteers was lower following each of the improvised decontamination protocols compared to the no-decontamination control (Fig. 11.3a). Combined decontamination further reduced the levels of simulant recovered from skin at all three sites. More simulant remained

Table 11.2 Summary of PHOENIX human volunteer trials 1–5

Trial	Study design	Simulant	Interventions
1	Controlled cross-over study $n = 12$ (4 females, 8 males) Simulants (21 µL total) applied to skin (shoulder, forearm, calf) Intervention initiated at 15 min	MeS mixed 1:1 with vegetable oil and containing IRS (4 mg/mL). For analytical recovery sites 2 µL added on the dominant side of the body, 5 µL on the non-dominant side for UV analysis To increase the chance of detection in urine, 20 × 10 µL simulant without IRS added to the lower back	*Improvised dry*: Pieces of white roll (2-Ply 25 cm × 25 cm) were individually folded in half twice. Participants were instructed to use one piece at a time and to blot and rub their skin working down the body from the shoulders. Participants were instructed to continue until they felt they had finished or until 3 min had elapsed. Participants could use as many pieces of white roll as required *Improvised wet*: Three buckets containing 5 L of ambient temperature water were provided, with one bucket containing 0.5% detergent solution. Decontamination was in three stages lasting 1 min each. Participants were instructed to: • Rinse the body using clean water and a 1 L jug provided • Wipe themselves down using a sponge and the detergent solution, in a downward motion from the shoulders • Rinse using clean water and a 1 L jug *Combined*: Improvised dry followed by improvised wet *No-decontamination control*

Table 11.2 (continued)

Trial	Study design	Simulant	Interventions
2	Controlled cross-over study $n = 12$ (5 females, 7 males) Simulants applied to skin (shoulder, forearm, calf) Improvised initiated at 15 min and interim at 25 min, post application	As for trial 1	*Improvised dry*: As for trial 1 *Improvised wet*: As for trial 1 *Improvised dry and interim*: Following improved dry, 25 min after simulant application, volunteers were directed to a 'ladder pipe' shower system comprising four hose reels and branches to create two shower positions. Decontamination lasted 90 s in two stages lasting 45 s each. Participants were instructed to: • Enter the first shower position and actively wash themselves from the shoulders downwards using their hands • Move to the second shower position and complete a slow 360° turn with their arms held out to the side at shoulder height and rinse their hands in the water once the turn was complete *Improvised wet and interim*: Interim as described above following improvised wet as in trial 1 *No-decontamination control*
3	Controlled cross-over study $n = 11$ (6 females, 6 males) Simulants applied to skin (shoulder, forearm, calf) Improvised initiated at 15 min, interim at 25 min and SOR at 60 min, post application	As for trials 1 and 2 Also, BeS with 4 mg/mL IRS Additional MeS (100 μL) and BeS (300 μL) applied to the back, forearm and calf	*Improvised dry and interim*: As for trial 2 *Improvised wet and interim*: As for trial 2 *Improvised dry, interim and SOR*: As above then at 60 min, volunteers entered the MDU and followed the 'ORCHIDS' protocol *Improvised wet, interim and SOR*: As above then at 60 min, volunteers entered the MDU and followed the 'ORCHIDS' protocol *No-decontamination control*
4	Controlled cross-over study $n = 12$ (4 females, 8 males) Simulants applied to hair	1:1 mix of MeS and vegetable oil and 4 mg/mL IRS BeS with 4 mg/mL IGS Each (500 μL) applied to the back of the head at the level of ears using an airbrush	*Improvised dry*: White roll folded in half twice. Participants completed the process using as many sheets of white roll as they saw fit but only using one sheet at a time up to a maximum of 3 min *Improvised wet*: As described for skin in trial 1 *Improvised dry and interim*: As above with interim as described for trial 2 *Improvised wet and interim*: As above with interim as described for trial 2 *No-decontamination control*
5	Controlled cross-over study $n = 11$ (6 females, 5 males) Simulants applied to hair	As for trial 4	*Improvised dry*: As described above *Improvised dry and interim*: As above with interim as described for trial 2 *Improvised dry, interim and SOR*: As above then at 60 min, volunteers entered the MDU and followed the 'ORCHIDS' protocol *No-decontamination control*

on the upper back following decontamination compared to the arms and legs (Fig. 11.3b, c), indicating that improvised decontamination procedures are less effective for decontaminating areas of the body that are difficult for casualties to reach on their own. There was no significant effect of decontamination on levels of MeS excreted in urine collected over 24 h (Fig. 11.3d).

For both the dry decontamination arm of this study and the combined dry and wet, it was found that the number of sheets of white roll used [1–18, 20, 21] in decontamination was significantly ($p = 0.034$ and $p = 0.032$, respectively) inversely correlated ($r = -0.614$ and $r = -0.645$, respectively) with the amount of MeS remaining on skin. One important conclusion from this trial therefore is that in the event of a chemical incident, exposed members of the public should be provided with free access to suitable absorbent materials to continue decontamination until interim showers are available.

Trial 2 explored the efficacy of improvised dry and wet decontamination alone and in combination with an interim shower (Table 11.2). This sequential approach reflects the operational practice of first responders who would use IOR protocols, as resources become available during an incident. In this trial, MeS with IRS was

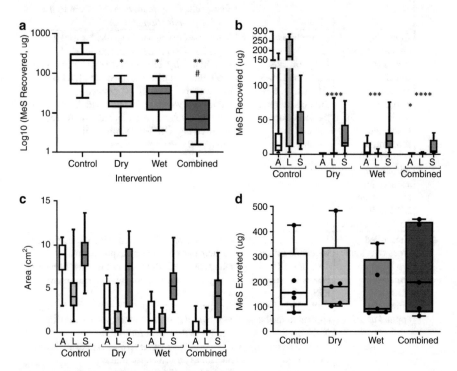

Fig. 11.3 Box and whisker plots of trial 1 results. (**a**) Total MeS recovery from all sites. (**b**) MeS recovery by site (*A* arm, *L* leg and *S* shoulder) and decontamination intervention. (**c**) Area of fluorescence detected by site and decontamination intervention. (**d**) Total MeS excreted in 24 h urine dependent on decontamination intervention. Data are presented as mean and 5–95% range for $n = 12$ participants. Urine data is given for $n = 5$ as other 7 participants missed collecting at least 1 urine sample. *$P < 0.05$, **$P < 0.01$, ***$P < 0.005$, ****$P < 0.0001$ compared to controls, #$P < 0.05$ compared to wet

applied to the same sites as in trial 1 ($n = 12$), and volunteers underwent four decontamination protocols: improvised dry, improvised wet, improvised dry followed by interim, and improvised wet followed by interim, and a no-decontamination control condition (Table 11.2). Interim decontamination comprised a 'ladder pipe' shower system, set up by trained fire service responders using four hose reels and branches, creating two shower positions (Fig. 11.1d). Following a protocol agreed with UK first responders, volunteers were instructed to walk to the first shower position and use their hands to actively wash themselves from the shoulders downwards for 45 s. Next, the volunteers were instructed to move forward to the second shower position where they completed a slow 360° turn and rinsed their hands in the water before exiting the corridor. Interim decontamination began 25 min following simulant application as this is indicative of expected arrival and set up time for FRS frontline appliances following reports of an incident. Alongside skin samples and UV-illuminated images (Fig. 11.4a), urine samples were also collected for 8 h following application of the simulant onto the skin as we observed in trial 1 that the majority of MeS was excreted in this time. Results indicated that conducting interim decontamination after

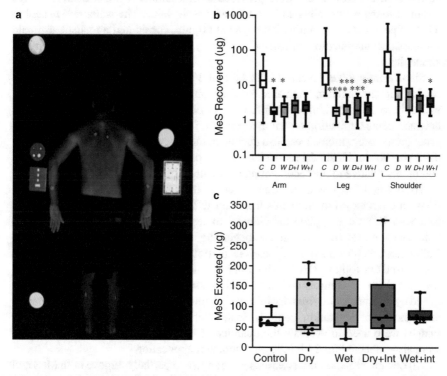

Fig. 11.4 Trial 2 data. (**a**) Volunteer in Mobile Image Analysis Unit showing fluorescent IRS at application sites on the arm, shoulder and leg and calibration used to enable semi-quantitation of data. (**b**) Total MeS recovered from sites dependent upon intervention (*C* control, *D* dry, *W* wet, *D+I* dry and interim, *W+I* wet and interim). (**c**) Total urine excreted in 8 h. Data are presented as mean and 5–95% range for $n = 12$ participants. Urine data is given for $n = 6$ as other 6 participants missed collecting at least 1 urine sample. *$P < 0.05$, **$P < 0.01$, ***$P < 0.005$, ****$P < 0.0001$ compared to controls

improvised decontamination protocols was more effective at removing the simulant from the difficult-to-reach area (shoulder) than either dry or wet improvised decontamination protocols alone (Fig. 11.4b). This supports the operational practice of conducting decontamination protocols in sequence. As observed within trial 1, there was no significant effect of decontamination on total levels of simulant excreted in urine over 8 h (Fig. 11.4c).

Specialist decontamination uses mass casualty decontamination showering facilities that can decontaminate many casualties following a chemical incident and would usually be administered once resources arrive and following IOR protocols. Together, IOR and SOR protocols are designed to allow safe onward transfer of exposed persons to hospitals and rest centres. Trial 3 examined the effectiveness of IOR and SOR decontamination procedures conducted in sequence in line with UK emergency services during a chemical incident [51]. MeS with IRS and BeS with IGS were applied to two predetermined areas on the upper back of volunteers ($n = 12$). Across five study sessions, volunteers underwent sequential decontamination protocols (Table 11.2). Specialist decontamination utilised a mass decontamination unit, and volunteers were provided with a flannel to wash themselves for 2 min in soapy water followed by 1 min with plain water. The water was heated to 37 °C. Specialist decontamination began at 60 min, considered a realistic estimate for mass decontamination unit arrival, assembly and instigation following reports of an incident.

Significantly lower levels of both MeS and BeS were recovered from skin following decontamination compared to no-decontamination controls (Fig. 11.5a, b), while there was no significant difference in either MeS or BeS levels recovered between decontamination conditions (Fig. 11.5). Total area fluorescence data mirrored these observations. Despite a decline in median values with inclusion of SOR, there was no significant decrease observed for urinary BeS for any decontamination conditions relative to no-decontamination control (Fig. 11.5d).

Trials 4 and 5 explored the effectiveness of the different decontamination conditions on the removal of simulants from hair [52]. In both trials, MeS with IRS and BeS with IGS were applied individually to separate locations on the back of the volunteer's heads ($n = 12$) at the beginning of the study session (Fig. 11.2c). Volunteers completed five study sessions in trial 4 (improvised dry, improvised wet, improvised dry followed by interim, improvised wet followed by interim and a 'no-decontamination' control) and three study sessions in trial 5 (improvised dry followed by interim, improvised dry followed by interim and specialist decontamination and a 'no-decontamination' control). Scalp swabs, hair samples and UV-illuminated images were used to evaluate the quantity of simulant remaining. Urine samples were also collected for 24 h following simulant application.

All decontamination interventions were shown to partially remove both MeS and BeS from the hair (Fig. 11.6a, c) and scalp (Fig. 11.6b, d) of participants but to varying extents. Dry decontamination alone, the current default method used in the UK as part of IOR, was shown to reduce the amount of MeS and BeS remaining on the hair of participants (Fig. 11.6a, c). Although results were only significant for the

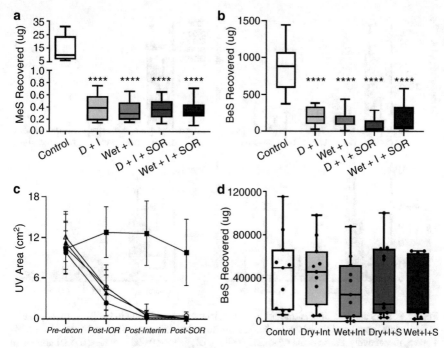

Fig. 11.5 Results from trial 3. (**a**) Total MeS recovered from skin dependent upon intervention (*D+I* dry and interim, *Wet+I* wet and interim, *D+I+SOR* dry, interim and specialist, *Wet + I+SOR* wet, interim and specialist). (**b**) Total BeS recovered from skin dependent upon intervention. (**c**) Area of fluorescence detected by site and decontamination intervention for IGS control (■), D + I (○), Wet + I (●), D + I + SOR (Δ), Wet + I + SOR (▲). (**d**) Total BeS excreted in urine in 24 h. Data are presented as mean and 5–95% range for $n = 12$ participants. Urine data is given for $n = 11$. ****$P < 0.0001$ compared to controls

removal of BeS, these data suggest that dry decontamination, which can be rapidly initiated, is beneficial and should remain the default option for casualty decontamination. Furthermore, the duration of dry decontamination appeared to be more important than the amount of dry decontamination material used; therefore, in an actual incident, it may be prudent for casualties to continue or repeat dry decontamination until interim or mass decontamination interventions become available. Improvised wet decontamination (the rinse-wipe-rinse method) was shown to be more efficacious than dry decontamination but only for BeS.

Trials 4 and 5 demonstrated that current UK decontamination methods (including default dry decontamination) performed in sequence are mostly effective at removing MeS and BeS from hair and underlying scalp. In agreement with studies on skin decontamination, BeS and MeS in 24 h urine were unaltered, raising important considerations with respect to the speed of decontamination and the perceived reduction of risk to the casualty.

Further investigation of dry decontamination found that time spent conducting dry decontamination had an inverse relationship with concentration of MeS

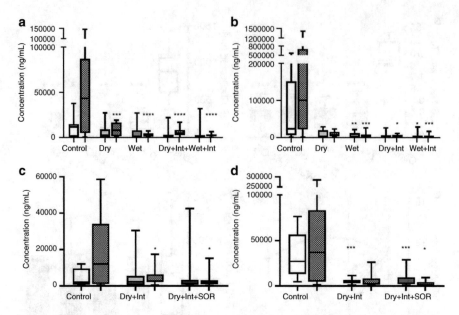

Fig. 11.6 MeS and BeS concentrations in hair (**a**, trial 4; **b**, trial 5) and in swabs (**c**, trial 4; **d**, trial 5). MeS data (open) and BeS data (hashed) are mean and 5–95% range for $n = 12$ and 11 for trials 4 and 5, respectively. Participants $*P < 0.05$, $**P < 0.01$, $***P < 0.005$, $****P < 0.0001$ compared to controls

($r = -0.61$, $p = 0.034$) and BeS ($r = -0.77$, $p = 0.004$) recovered from hair. No correlation was found however for the number of sheets used and simulant remaining on hair. In these studies, we decided not to place any limits on length of hair, and we found recovery of simulants was reduced as the length of hair increased for both MeS (trial 4, $r = -0.82$, $p = 0.002$; trial 5, $r = -0.78$, $p = 0.007$) and BeS (trial 4, $r = -0.74$, $p = 0.01$; trial 5, $r = -0.95$, $p = 0.001$), respectively. Longer hair was also associated with significantly lower simulant recovery in scalp swabs in trial 4 ($r = -0.63$, $p = 0.038$ for MeS; $r = -0.77$, $p = 0.006$ for BeS) but not in trial 5 where recovery of MeS and BeS was much lower.

Overall, results from these human volunteer trials show the initiating decontamination as soon as possible following exposure in a chemical incident and demonstrate some benefits of decontamination interventions conducted in sequence. Improvised decontamination should be rapidly deployed by emergency responders upon arrival to the scene of a chemical incident, and this should be followed by interim decontamination once resources arrive, to ensure that on-scene decontamination is the most beneficial for casualties. As soon as specialist response equipment and responders arrive at the incident scene, mass decontamination should be conducted to ensure that persistent chemicals and harder-to-reach areas of the body are effectively decontaminated.

Discussion and Conclusions

Use of a Benzyl Salicylate (BeS) as a Novel Simulant and What This Adds to Our Understanding

Prior to PHOENIX, human decontamination studies had been mostly conducted using MeS, a simulant for sulphur mustard [27]. The relatively high vapour pressure of MeS (0.034 mmHg at 25 °C) means that under normal conditions, a high proportion of the applied compound is lost to air during experimental conditions unless skin is occluded in any way, e.g. clothing [53]. Loss of MeS increases the variability of recovery from skin, making it difficult to obtain statistically significant differences between decontamination interventions. BeS has a vapour pressure three orders of magnitude lower (7.8×10^{-5} mmHg at 25 °C) than MeS, and consequently recoveries from skin (Fig. 11.5) and hair (Fig. 11.6) were greater. The reduced uncertainty in the recovery of simulants increases the potential to identify statistical differences between decontamination interventions. This is especially true for longer studies such as trials 4 and 5 where uncertainty from simulant loss is exacerbated.

Overall, PHOENIX provides good evidence that established decontamination procedures are effective at removing chemical simulants from skin in line with previous studies [50, 51], including chemicals that are more persistent. Casualties that have passed through IOR and/or SOR therefore can be expected to have an order of magnitude or lower levels of surface chemical contamination remaining. However, it is noticeable that, for BeS which is more persistent than MeS, absolute levels of simulant remaining on skin are considerably higher than for MeS (Fig. 11.5). Further work is required to investigate the roles of simulant physicochemical characteristics to determine whether current best practice would be sufficiently protective of both casualties and first responders.

Hair-Wicking and the Protective Effect of Longer Hair

Prior to PHOENIX, little work had been undertaken to investigate efficacy for the removal of simulants or live agents from hair [26, 30, 33, 35, 36, 54]. What work had been done had largely been conducted in vitro [30, 33, 35, 36] or investigated simulant remaining on the surface of hair [24]. The former studies highlighted the potential hazard from the tendency of hair to release simulant over time which would avoid detection in the latter study. We therefore chose to determine extracted simulant levels following the removal of the hair from volunteers. As with skin analyses, there was more uncertainty for MeS data because of greater variability compared to BeS which demonstrated significantly decreased levels following all intervention protocols (Fig. 11.6). During these studies, we noted that simulant rapidly wicks along hair once applied and therefore decided to also take swabs of scalp. These also demonstrated significant reductions in simulant following decontamination. As with skin, more significant reductions in simulant levels were observed in trial 4 using

BeS than MeS. A side observation was that hair length was inversely correlated with scalp levels confirming that longer hair is protective against chemical penetration to scalp.

Urine Analysis Raises More Questions Than Answers

At the outset of PHOENIX, the hope was that measuring levels of simulant in urine rather than that remaining on skin would not only show a clear decline in concentration with interventions but also give a clear measure of the decline in systemic exposure that could relatively easily be used to estimate health outcomes from performing the different decontamination interventions [46]. What we repeatedly observed was that levels of MeS and BeS excreted in urine were not significantly altered by any decontamination intervention, despite urine levels repeatedly being greater than baseline levels, implying that urinary levels are elevated following skin application. There are two major concerns raised by these data: (1) decontamination interventions may reduce skin contamination, but this does not impact systemic availability, and (2) background exposures to salicylates may be more prevalent than expected. In these studies, decontamination interventions were initiated at 15 min in line with current operational expectations. By this time, it is possible that the simulants have already penetrated skin and most of the applied simulant is beyond the influence of decontamination interventions. Alternatively, the act of decontamination may enhance penetration, the so-called wash-in effect or a combination of these two effects. Studies initiating decontamination at earlier time points would help to address this uncertainty. As part of our studies, volunteers were instructed to avoid foods rich in MeS such as root beer and consumer products that use oil of wintergreen such as muscle rubs and mouthwashes and to not use consumer products that may contain BeS as an adjuvant. Foods are rich in salicylates, and because of this, we chose to look at parent compounds in urine and not salicylic acid and salicyluric acid metabolites common to all salicylates. However, it is possible that MeS is more widely distributed in diet than is known from the published literature. We tested a small number of foodstuffs for MeS and found that tea and coffee contained significant amounts of MeS (unpublished data). It is possible that use of BeS is also more widespread in consumer products but at levels not requiring listing as an ingredient. Future studies would benefit from use of simulants that are not only safe to use but which also have very low background exposures.

Future Directions for Mass Decontamination

Much of the existing data on mass casualty decontamination is based upon studies with MeS. PHOENIX has broadened this to include BeS, but uncertainties around exposure from consumer products and diet together with a desire to understand the applicability of existing decontamination strategies to a broader range of chemicals with varied physicochemical characteristics mean further expanding these studies to encompass a wider range of chemical simulants is desirable. This work would demonstrate whether current best practice is appropriate for all chemical incidents.

Both MeS and BeS are liquids at room temperature which is advantageous for application to volunteers but does not adequately reflect all chemicals being transported in bulk that may include powders or corrosive liquids. Guidance on the removal of powders during IOR differs between the UK and the USA with recommendations of dry and wet decontamination, respectively, whereas both recommend treatment of corrosives with wet decontamination and continuous application of running water [16–18]. Data on decontamination of both powders and corrosives is limited and requires optimisation.

Whenever water-based decontamination methods are recommended, there is often reference to the 'wash-in' effect whereby skin penetration is temporally enhanced by mechanisms including skin hydration [55]. This may be particularly relevant for powders which cannot cross intact skin unless solubilised. Evidence of a wash-in effect comes from in vitro data with the limited in vivo data being inconclusive. Existing data mostly involves study designs non-aligned to mass decontamination, and therefore, there is a need to better understand whether a wash-in effect can be observed in human volunteers undergoing mass decontamination in line with national guidelines including decontamination of powders. To undertake this, the first thing that needs to be done is to identify suitable simulant powders that can be utilised in volunteer studies [56].

For first responders, the outputs from PHOENIX support the initiation of decontamination as soon as is possible. For improvised decontamination, this can be dry decontamination, but it should be noted that even able-bodied casualties struggle to decontaminate less accessible parts of their body. As such, consideration of buddy systems to improve decontamination of inaccessible areas could be included. The longer duration and the more materials used in dry decontamination, the more effective the intervention; therefore, first responders should continue to supply these materials where possible until an interim corridor or MDU can be established. Sequential decontamination protocols improve the removal of chemicals from skin and hair, making onward journey of casualties to hospitals safer for clinical staff. Time to clinical intervention may be critical as PHOENIX suggests that current methods do not effectively decrease systemic availability; however, further investigations are required. Several of these aspects will be targeted within the CHIMERA (chemicals including powders and corrosives decontamination and emergency response assessment) project currently underway.

References

1. World Health Organization. WHO manual for the public health management of chemical incidents. Geneva: World Health Organization; 2009.
2. Bos P, Ruijten M, Gundert-Remy U, Bull S, Nielsen E, Tissot S, et al. Human risk assessment of single exposure in chemical incidents: present situation and emerging chemical incident scenarios. Amersfoort: National Institute for Public Health and the Environment; 2013.

3. Genereux M, Petit G, Maltais D, Roy M, Simard R, Boivin S, et al. The public health response during and after the Lac-Mégantic train derailment tragedy: a case study. Disaster Health. 2014;2(3–4):113–20.
4. Wang HY, Wu HY. Problems in the management of mass casualties in the Tianjin explosion. Crit Care. 2016;20:47.
5. Ahmed F, Maroof H, Ahmed N, Sheridan R. Acid attacks: a new public health pandemic in the west? Int J Surg. 2017;48:32–3.
6. United Nations Mission to investigate allegations of the use of chemical weapons in the Syrian Arab Republic. Final report. 2013.
7. OPCW. Report on the use of a chemical weapon in the death of a DPRK National. 2017.
8. Vale JA, Marrs TO, Maynard RC. Novichok: a murderous nerve agent attack in the UK. Clin Toxicol (Phila). 2018;56(11):1093–7.
9. OPCW. Summary of the report on activities carried out in support of a request for technical assistance by Germany (Technical Assistance Visit–TAV/01/20). 2020.
10. NHS England. Emergency preparedness, resilience and response. Concept of operations for managing mass casualties. London: NHS England; 2017.
11. Amlôt R, Carter H, Riddle L, Larner J, Chilcott RP. Volunteer trials of a novel improvised dry decontamination protocol for use during mass casualty incidents as part of the UK'S initial operational response (IOR). PLoS One. 2017;12(6):e0179309.
12. Amlot R, Larner J, Matar H, Jones DR, Carter H, Turner EA, et al. Comparative analysis of showering protocols for mass-casualty decontamination. Prehosp Disaster Med. 2010;25(5):435–9.
13. Egan JR, Amlôt R. Modelling mass casualty decontamination systems informed by field exercise data. Int J Environ Res Public Health. 2012;9(10):3685–710.
14. Kassouf N, Syed S, Larner J, Amlôt R, Chilcott RP. Evaluation of absorbent materials for use as ad hoc dry decontaminants during mass casualty incidents as part of the UK's initial operational response (IOR). PLoS One. 2017;12(2):e0170966.
15. Optimisation through Research of Chemical Incident Decontamination Systems. http://www.orchidsproject.eu/project.html.
16. Home Office. Initial operational response to a CBRN incident. 2015.
17. Chilcott RP, Amlôt R. Primary Response Incident Scene Management (PRISM) guidance for chemical incidents. Ann Emerg Med. 2015;73(6):671–84.
18. Chilcott RP, Larner J, Durrant A, Hughes P, Mahalingam D, Rivers S, et al. Evaluation of US Federal Guidelines (primary response incident scene management [PRISM]) for mass decontamination of casualties during the initial operational response to a chemical incident. Ann Emerg Med. 2018;73(6):671–84.
19. Carter H, Weston D, Betts N, Wilkinson S, Amlôt R. Public perceptions of emergency decontamination: effects of intervention type and responder management strategy during a focus group study. PLoS One. 2018;13(4):e0195922.
20. Chilcott RP. Managing mass casualties and decontamination. Environ Int. 2014;72:37–45.
21. Matar H, Price S, Chilcott RP. Temporal effects of disrobing on the skin absorption of chemical warfare agents and CW agent simulants. Toxicology. 2010;278(3):344–5.
22. Gaskin S, Pisaniello D, Edwards JW, Bromwich D, Reed S, Logan M, et al. Chlorine and hydrogen cyanide gas interactions with human skin: in vitro studies to inform skin permeation and decontamination in HAZMAT incidents. J Hazard Mater. 2013;262:759–65.
23. Power S, Symons C, Carter H, Jones E, Amlôt R, Larner J, et al. Mass casualty decontamination in the United States: an online survey of current practice. Health Secur. 2016;14(4):226–36.
24. Chilcott RP, Mitchell H, Matar H. Optimization of nonambulant mass casualty decontamination protocols as part of an initial or specialist operational response to chemical incidents. Prehosp Emerg Care. 2018;23(1):32–43.
25. Chilcott RP, Wyke SM. CBRN incidents. In: Sellwood C, Wapling A, editors. Health emergency preparedness and response. Wallingford: CABI; 2016. p. 167–80.

26. Rolland P, Bolzinger MA, Cruz C, Josse D, Briançon S. Hairy skin exposure to VX in vitro: effectiveness of delayed decontamination. Toxicol In Vitro. 2013;27(1):358–66.

27. James T, Wyke S, Marczylo T, Collins S, Gaulton T, Foxall K, et al. Chemical warfare agent simulants for human volunteer trials of emergency decontamination: a systematic review. J Appl Toxicol. 2018;38(1):113–21.

28. Commission E. Evaluation, optimisation, trialling and modelling procedures for mass casualty decontamination [ORCHIDS] [2007203]—Project. 2008. Contract No.: 2007203.

29. Amlôt R, Riddle L, Chilcott RP. Minimum practical showering duration for mass patient decontamination; chemical toxicology report no. 23. Porton Down: Health Protection Agency; 2011.

30. Josse D, Wartelle J, Cruz C. Showering effectiveness for human hair decontamination of the nerve agent VX. Chem Biol Interact. 2015;232:94–100.

31. Grams YY, Whitehead L, Lamers G, Sturmann N, Bouwstra JA. On-line diffusion profile of a lipophilic model dye in different depths of a hair follicle in human scalp skin. J Investig Dermatol. 2005;125(4):775–82.

32. Joseph RE, Tsai W-J, Tsao L-I, Su T-P, Cone EJ. In vitro characterization of cocaine binding sites in human hair. J Pharmacol Exp Ther. 1997;282(3):1228–41.

33. Matar H, Amer N, Kansagra S, Pinhal A, Thomas E, Townend S, et al. Hybrid in vitro diffusion cell for simultaneous evaluation of hair and skin decontamination: temporal distribution of chemical contaminants. Sci Rep. 2018;8(1):16906.

34. Oxley JC, Smith JL, Kirschenbaum LJ, Shinde KP, Marimganti S. Accumulation of explosives in hair. J Forensic Sci. 2005;50(4):826–31.

35. Spiandore M, Piram A, Lacoste A, Prevost P, Maloni P, Torre F, et al. Efficacy of scalp hair decontamination following exposure to vapours of sulphur mustard simulants 2-chloroethyl ethyl sulphide and methyl salicylate. Chem Biol Interact. 2017;267:74–9.

36. Spiandore M, Souilah-Edib M, Piram A, Lacoste A, Josse D, Doumenq P. Desorption of sulphur mustard simulants methyl salicylate and 2-chloroethyl ethyl sulphide from contaminated scalp hair after vapour exposure. Chemosphere. 2018;191:721–8.

37. Rolland P, Bolzinger MA, Cruz C, Briancon S, Josse D. Human scalp permeability to the chemical warfare agent VX. Toxicol In Vitro. 2011;25(8):1974–80.

38. Carter H, Amlôt R. Mass casualty decontamination guidance and psychosocial aspects of CBRN incident management: a review and synthesis. PLoS Curr. 2016;8:5.

39. Carter H, Amlôt R, Williams R, Rubin GJ, Drury J. Mass casualty decontamination in a chemical or radiological/nuclear incident: further guiding principles. PLoS Curr. 2016;8:52.

40. Carter H, Drury J, Amlôt R. Social identity and intergroup relationships in the Management of Crowds during mass emergencies and disasters: recommendations for emergency planners and responders. Policing J Policy Pract. 2018;14(4):931–44.

41. Carter H, Drury J, Amlot R, Rubin GJ, Williams R. Effective responder communication improves efficiency and psychological outcomes in a mass decontamination field experiment: implications for public behaviour in the event of a chemical incident. PLoS One. 2014;9(3):e89846.

42. Carter H, Drury J, Amlôt R, Rubin GJ, Williams R. Effective responder communication, perceived responder legitimacy, and group identification predict public cooperation and compliance in a mass decontamination visualization experiment. J Appl Soc Psychol. 2015;45(3):173–89.

43. Carter H, Drury J, Rubin GJ, Williams R, Amlôt R. The effect of communication during mass decontamination. Disaster Prevention and Management: An International Journal. 2013;22(2):132–47.

44. Carter H, Drury J, Amlôt R, Rubin G, Williams R. Perceived responder legitimacy and group identification predict cooperation and compliance in a mass decontamination field exercise. Basic Appl Soc Psych. 2013;35(6):575–85.

45. Carter H, Drury J, Amlôt R, Rubin G, Williams R. Effective responder communication, perceived responder legitimacy, and group identification predict public cooperation and compliance in a mass decontamination visualization experiment. J Appl Soc Psychol. 2015;45(3):173–89

46. James T, Collins S, Amlot R, Marczylo T. Analysis of chemical simulants in urine: a useful tool for assessing emergency decontamination efficacy in human volunteer studies. Prehosp Disaster Med. 2020;35(5):482–7.
47. Carter H, Drury J, Rubin GJ, Williams R, Amlôt R. Applying crowd psychology to develop recommendations for the management of mass decontamination. Health Secur. 2015;13(1):45–53.
48. James T, Collins S, Amlot R, Marczylo T. GC-MS/MS quantification of benzyl salicylate on skin and hair: a novel chemical simulant for human decontamination studies. J Chromatogr B Analyt Technol Biomed Life Sci. 2019;1129:121818.
49. James T, Collins S, Amlot R, Marczylo T. Optimisation and validation of a GC-MS/MS method for the analysis of methyl salicylate in hair and skin samples for use in human-volunteer decontamination studies. J Chromatogr B Analyt Technol Biomed Life Sci. 2019;1109:84–9.
50. Southworth F, James T, Davidson L, Williams N, Finnie T, Marczylo T, et al. A controlled cross-over study to evaluate the efficacy of improvised dry and wet emergency decontamination protocols for chemical incidents. PLoS One. 2020;15(11):e0239845.
51. Collins S, Williams N, Southworth F, James T, Davidson L, Orchard E, et al. Evaluating the impact of decontamination interventions performed in sequence for mass casualty chemical incidents. Sci Rep. 2021;11(1):3547.
52. Collins S, James T, Southworth F, Davidson L, Williams N, Orchard E, et al. Human volunteer study of the decontamination of chemically contaminated hair and the consequences for systemic exposure. Sci Rep. 2020;10:20822.
53. Chilcott RP. Dermal aspects of chemical warfare agents. In: Marrs T, Maynard R, Sidell F, editors. Chemical warfare agents: toxicology and treatment. 2nd ed. New York: Wiley; 2007. p. 409–22.
54. James T, Collins S, Amlot R, Marczylo T. GC-MS/MS quantification of benzyl salicylate on skin and hair: a novel chemical simulant for human decontamination studies. J Chromatogr B. 2019;1129:121818.
55. Moody RP, Maibach HI. Skin decontamination: importance of the wash-in effect. Food Chem Toxicol. 2006;44(11):1783–8.
56. James T, Collins S, Marczylo T. Identification of novel simulants for toxic industrial chemicals and chemical warfare agents for human decontamination studies: a systematic review and categorisation of physicochemical characteristics. Int J Environ Res Public Health. 2021;18(16):8681.

Chapter 12
Twenty Clinically Pertinent Factors/ Observations for Percutaneous Absorption in Humans

Rebecca M. Law, Mai A. Ngo, and Howard I. Maibach

Key Points
- Percutaneous absorption of drugs and chemicals is affected by multiple factors.
- Clinical implications include enhanced or reduced efficacy and/or toxicity.

Introduction

Clinicians routinely use the topical route to administer medications with minimal consideration of details: If there is an approved topical formulation, then obviously absorption through the skin should work. But is percutaneous absorption that simple? What factors are involved for a medication—or for that matter, for any chemical—to be percutaneously absorbed? What can enhance or reduce topical absorption? We consider these factors when using the topical administration route as they may affect drug efficacy and/or toxicity and hence patient outcome. What follows is evidence based; the interested reader is encouraged to access the 62 reference citations for the evidence behind this discussion of skin absorption (not mucous membranes). Furthermore, textbooks providing in-depth discussions of percutaneous absorption are available as reference sources. The reader is referred to the extensive literature on percutaneous penetration enhancers in the five-volume series edited by

R. M. Law (✉)
School of Pharmacy, Memorial University of Newfoundland, St. John's, NL, Canada
e-mail: Rebecca.law@ucsf.edu

M. A. Ngo
California Department of Toxic Substances Control, Sacramento, CA, USA

H. I. Maibach
Department of Dermatology, University of California San Francisco, San Francisco, CA, USA

© The Author(s), under exclusive license to Springer Nature
Switzerland AG 2022
A. M. Feschuk et al. (eds.), *Dermal Absorption and Decontamination*,
https://doi.org/10.1007/978-3-031-09222-0_12

Dragicevic N. and Maibach H. I. (Percutaneous Penetration Enhancers Chemical Methods in Penetration Enhancement. Springer. ISBN 978-3-662-47039-8).

Factors in Percutaneous Absorption

What questions should we ask when using a topical medication? Consider at least 20 factors. In 1983, we suggested a 10-factor guide in percutaneous absorption based on observations from in vitro and in vivo comparisons [1] which was expanded to 15 [2] in 2012, modified in 2013 [3, 4], with clinical relevance and complexities added in 2017 [5]. To aid the clinician or student, 20 factors affecting topical absorption are presented here in practical terms, including clinical implications. Questions relating to the 20 factors follow:

1. What are the relevant physicochemical properties of the medication/chemical?

Particle size/molecular weight: Smaller molecules are often more easily absorbed; most topical medications are less than or around 500 Da in size/molecular weight with few exceptions. Topical calcineurin inhibitors are efficacious despite larger particle sizes (tacrolimus (Protopic) at MW 822 Da and pimecrolimus (Elidel) at MW 810 Da) [3].

Lipophilicity: Corneocytes are the outer skin layer (stratum corneum) with cell membranes consisting of lipids, with proteins and water. Lipophilic drugs (and lipophilic chemicals) will be more readily absorbed than hydrophilic substances [6]. However, highly lipophilic substances may be less well absorbed than moderately lipophilic compounds.

pH: The pH of the environment will determine the proportion of drug or chemical that is ionized versus unionized. Skin membrane proteins are basic in nature. It is the unionized form of a drug or chemical that passes through membranes. Thus, drugs and chemicals which are primarily in their unionized form in a basic pH environment will be optimally absorbed. Since basic drugs will have a greater proportion in unionized form than acidic drugs, in a basic environment, therefore, basic drugs will be absorbed better than acidic drugs. Less ionization leads to increased lipid solubility and passage through membranes [7].

pKa: pKa is a measure of a chemical's acid strength and provides details of the dissociation of an acid in aqueous solution. Since there is a specific pKa for each substance which relates to pH, knowing the pKa of a drug becomes a useful predictor of percutaneous drug absorption [7].

Partition coefficient (P): The partition coefficient is the ratio of concentrations of a substance in a mixture of two immiscible phases at equilibrium. This ratio is therefore a measure of the difference in solubility of the substance in these two phases. There are two partition coefficients of relevance to percutaneous absorption: the oil-to-water partition coefficient (i.e., octanol/water P) and the partition coefficient for cream or ointment to the stratum corneum (i.e., formulation/skin P). Hydrophobic drugs or chemicals will have a high octanol/water P and will be mainly distributed to hydrophobic areas such as the lipid bilayers of cell membranes, whereas hydrophilic drugs or chemicals (with low octanol/water Ps) will be mainly distributed to aqueous areas such as serum. The partition coefficient between a cream/ointment and the stratum corneum will depend on the product formulation. Thus, knowing the partition coefficients of a drug or chemical for various immiscible phases may be a useful predictor of percutaneous drug absorption and/or drug partitioning between biologic systems, which can include solids such as bone (i.e., blood/bone P).

2.   What effects do the vehicle/formulation of the product have on drug absorption?

Occlusive vehicles often aid absorption by increasing hydration [8]. *Water-based* vehicles are nonocclusive and are less helpful for topical drug absorption, but they allow water-soluble drugs to dissolve in higher concentrations, which may offset the nonocclusive aspect.

Oil-based vehicles provide occlusion and act as humectants to enhance drug penetration. Thus, for example, a betamethasone dipropionate 0.1% ointment will generally have greater potency than a betamethasone dipropionate 0.1% cream. (Note that changing salt forms may affect potency—e.g., betamethasone dipropionate 0.1% cream is more potent than betamethasone valerate 0.1% cream.) Although *alcohol-based or acetone-based* vehicles are less occlusive and have a skin-drying effect, they may enhance solubility of some drugs and thereby augment dermal absorption.

The *pH of the vehicle* may alter the unionized/ionized drug ratio, thus affecting drug absorption, since it is the unionized form of the drug which most efficiently crosses through the skin. Other *excipients* (i.e., inactive ingredients) in the vehicle such as surfactants may have been purposely added to enhance solubility and hence drug absorption.

3.   What effects do the conditions of drug exposure (dose, duration, surface area, and frequency of exposure) have on drug absorption?

Intuitively, greater *dose*, longer *treatment duration*, larger *surface area of application*, and greater *frequency of reapplication* (once up to three or four times a day) should all increase the amount of drug absorbed, and they generally do. However (although the experimental data remains sparse), with corticosteroids, a high single exposure (hydrocortisone 40 µg/cm^2) substantially increases absorption over one-third of the dose (13.3 µg/cm^2) applied either once or three times in 1 day—there was no statistically significant difference seen with increasing frequency of reapplication [9]. With multiple dosing over many days, there is currently insufficient experimental data to provide a general predictive statement.

In addition, the *body surface area-to-body weight ratio* (*BSA/BW*) is important as this may affect drug toxicity, since drug doses are usually based on body weight (with a few exceptions such as in oncology). In particular, newborns have a BSA/BW ratio at least twice that of adults, so that topical drug doses—even when adjusted for body weight—will still cover a larger % BSA than in adults. Thus, newborns are at greater risk of systemic drug toxicity from topical application of drugs or chemicals. It is partially for this reason that sun protection in newborns less than 6 months of age *does not* include the use of sunscreens/sunblocks, even the physical (mineral-based) sunblocks like titanium dioxide. (Recommendations by the American Academy of Pediatrics for sun protection in this population include sun avoidance, using a stroller cover, wearing lightweight long pants, long-sleeve shirts, and hats with wide brims that shade the neck, etc.)

Also, note (a) there may be residual drug remaining on and in the skin even if the dose is wiped off—i.e., treatment duration may be unknowingly extended; (b) repeated exposure over time may lead to chronic toxicity manifestations, such as corticosteroid-induced skin atrophy; and (c) inadvertent chemical/drug exposure may occur via transfer from one person to another, for example, a mother wearing sunscreen and holding her infant with bare arms (further discussed in #14 below).

4. Do the skin appendages (hair follicles, sebaceous glands, apocrine and eccrine sweat glands) have a role in topical drug absorption?

Yes they do. Skin appendages which originate in the dermis are *sub-anatomical pathways* whereby drugs and chemicals can be transported through the skin. Diffusion of chemicals through skin appendages is termed *shunt diffusion*. Hair follicles can contribute to the total skin surface area for drug absorption. Skin appendages are especially important for the penetration and skin storage of larger molecules (e.g., proteins), as discussed in #9 below. Little data exists regarding transport through the eccrine, apocrine, and sebaceous glands.

5. How do the skin sites of application affect absorption?

There is marked *regional variability* in absorption: absorption rates vary at different anatomical skin sites—in general, faster if hair follicles are present in large numbers and somewhat slower if the stratum corneum is thick. More specifically, the scrotum has the highest rate of topical absorption due to having both a very thin stratum corneum and a rich blood supply. The next highest body areas for absorption are the forehead, scalp, and neck. These regional differences may partially relate to skin thickness and the number of cell layers in the stratum corneum. Body areas with the lowest topical absorption rates include the palms and soles.

6.   What population variability factors affect topical absorption?

Ethnicity/Pluralistic Societies: Although the skin is approximately equally thick in persons of different pluralistic societies, the stratum corneum in blacks has more cell layers and a higher lipid content than in whites [10]. These differences may lead to absorption differences. In addition, blacks and Hispanics have stronger irritant reactions than whites to sodium lauryl sulfate [11, 12], a surface-active agent often found in non-medicated and medicated shampoos. Skin irritation may lead to inflammation and enhanced absorption of topical agents. (Note that experimental data in comparing blacks and Hispanic skin is limited, and there is conflicting data.) The interested reader can obtain more information from two textbooks detailing these points: Berardesca E, Leveque J-L, Maibach HI. Ethnic Skin and Hair first ed. CRC Press. Dec 2019. ISBN 9780367389994; and earlier edition Nov 2006 ISBN 978-0849330889.

   Age can significantly affect topical absorption. Aged skin is drier with less skin surface lipids [13]. It is also thinner and more friable—skin aging is associated with progressive dermal atrophy including atrophy of the skin's capillary network, resulting in a gradual reduction of blood supply to the skin [13]. All of these changes may potentially affect topical absorption. Overall, it paradoxically appears that the *permeability barrier function* of the skin is increased as we age. In particular, percutaneous absorption of less lipophilic substances (e.g., hydrocortisone, benzoic acid, acetylsalicylic acid, caffeine) is reduced, while more lipophilic substances (e.g., testosterone, estradiol) are not [13]. However, increased friability may result in broken skin, resulting in the loss of permeability barrier function and increased percutaneous absorption.

   At the other end of the age spectrum, i.e., infants and children, topical absorption may be increased. In the preterm baby, the permeability barrier function of the skin is not yet intact. Prenatal skin undergoes developmental stages in utero (including permeability barrier development, e.g., proteolipid layer and pilosebaceous units), but some functions are not fully developed even in the neonate [14]. Importantly, the acid mantle is developed in the first 4 weeks after birth, and skin surface pH of both term newborns and premature neonates is less acidic than that of children and adults [15]. Newborn skin has higher permeability to topical agents. Pediatric skin is thinner, potentially allowing for an increase in the rate and amount of drug absorbed. In fact, pediatric and in particular neonatal and infant skins have skin surface conditions different from adult skin surface conditions, which may enhance absorption [16].

Skin hydration naturally differs with age. Although at birth the skin surface is rougher and drier compared with older children, within the first 30 days, the skin smoothens and skin hydration increases [16, 17]. During the next 3 months, skin hydration continues to increase and then exceeds that found in adults [17–19]—perhaps relating to sweat gland maturation in function [20]. The stratum corneum in infants 3–12 months of age is significantly more hydrated compared to adult skin [16, 17]. These factors may increase the potential for drug and chemical toxicities in neonates, infants, and children, and this should be kept in mind whenever the topical route is used. For example, increased topical absorption and toxicity have been reported in infants with the use of rubbing alcohol [21, 22], boric acid powders [23], and hexachlorophene baths, emulsions, and soaps [24, 25]—thus, their use should be minimized. The evidence that rubbing enhances percutaneous penetration has recently been reviewed [26]. The preterm infant may be at even greater risk—even medications which are not normally administered topically due to their physicochemical characteristics may be absorbed enough to be efficacious or cause toxicity. For example, a theophylline gel (17 mg spread over an area 2 cm in diameter) applied to the abdomens of premature infants produced therapeutic serum theophylline concentrations [27].

7. How do skin surface conditions affect topical drug absorption?

Hydration is crucial (as discussed above with age comparisons). Well-hydrated skin often promotes topical absorption, and it is for this reason that occlusion is often intentional in product formulation, e.g., ointments are often more potent than creams or lotions, also mentioned earlier, since occlusion creates a humectant effect. Formulation or application changes resulting in potency differences should be remembered when prescribing (e.g., clobetasol or hydrocortisone). For example, a tenfold increase in hydrocortisone absorption was seen when occlusion was applied for 24 h after topical administration [2, 28].

Skin temperature also affects topical absorption: an increase in skin temperature—such as a febrile state or sometimes even when a heating pad is present—may increase topical absorption. For example, skin temperature at 40 °C increases the transdermal delivery of testosterone and fentanyl [29].

The *skin pH* may affect topical absorption: a less acidic skin pH may enhance absorption. The normal stratum corneum is typically acidic and hence favors transport of chemicals and drugs whose pKas allow for greater unionized forms in an acidic environment. Abnormal stratum corneum frequently has higher pH (i.e., a more basic environment), and this would favor the penetration of chemicals and drugs whose pKa allows for greater unionized forms in a basic environment. Thus, the acid mantle of the intact adult skin (pH 4–5) would be an absorption barrier to most basic drugs and some acidic drugs.

Skin pH elevations can occur with occlusion [30] or with a change in the skin microbiome (e.g., caused by prolonged occlusion [30]). Even 1 day of occlusion (with plastic wrap) can cause a 10^4 increase in bacterial count (most significantly with coagulase-negative *Staphylococci*), resulting in a corresponding increase in skin pH [30]. With 4 days of occlusion, the skin pH can change from acidic to neutral (4.38–7.05) [30].

The *skin surface topography* can also affect topical absorption, since it affects lateral spread of drug or chemical (see #19).

8.   How does skin health and skin integrity affect topical absorption?

Be cognizant that *any skin damage or trauma*—be it mechanical, chemical, biocidal, or clinical disease—may potentially enhance topical absorption [5, 31]; and the effects may be more significant for hydrophilic (water-soluble) substances than lipophilic (oil-soluble) substances [31]. These effects are not only demonstrated in in vivo human studies measuring penetration through damaged or diseased skin [31]; enhanced absorption has also been shown in in vitro studies using human models of damaged or diseased skin [32]. Even mild skin trauma such as adhesive tape stripping (which removes stratum corneum layers) may significantly enhance absorption. For example, penciclovir absorption was increased by 1300-fold and acyclovir absorption by 440-fold through tape stripping (to glistening but not broken skin) [33]. Skin compromised by sodium lauryl sulfate (a surfactant) was more permeable to various polyethylene glycols (of different molecular weights) [34].

Skin diseases (e.g., psoriasis, atopic dermatitis [35]) also compromise skin integrity; and topical drugs and chemicals may be absorbed faster and in greater amounts. There is some complexity though. For example, in atopic dermatitis (AD) patients (when compared to healthy individuals), increased absorption occurred not only through lesional skin but also through non-lesional skin [35–37]. Although non-lesional AD skin is "normal-appearing," it still responds to petrolatum applied to it—by increasing stratum corneum thickness, reducing T-cell infiltrates, upregulating antimicrobial peptides, etc. [35]. Also, both lesional and non-lesional skins of AD patients have higher *Staphylococcus aureus* levels than healthy controls, which correlates with AD disease severity [38]. However, it is AD patients with clinically active disease who demonstrated increased skin absorption (in both lesional and non-lesional skins)—patients with clinically inactive disease did not [36, 39, 40]. Furthermore, skin absorption increases significantly with the severity of AD [36, 41, 42]. Practically, this means that topical medications are better absorbed during dermatologic disease flare-ups—thus (a) becoming more effective at that time—a useful phenomenon; (b) being potentially less effective when used as maintenance therapy, especially if intermittent (twice weekly) regimens are used—thus, patient monitoring and follow-up during periods of inactive disease would be important; (c) systemic toxicity from topical medications may be significantly increased during disease flare-ups, especially if higher potency agents within a class of medications are used (e.g., corticosteroids). Furthermore, absorption of and potential systemic toxicity of *any* chemical touching the skin may be similarly increased during a skin disease flare-up, such as in AD.

9. How does substantivity and binding to the different skin components affect topical absorption?

Substantivity can be defined as the adherence of chemicals to the stratum corneum, i.e., more like adsorption. In practical terms, the substantivity of a sunscreen (as an example) would be that sunscreen's ability to remain effective during prolonged exercise, sweating, or swimming; and this may be a property of the active ingredient, the vehicle, or both. Obviously, the greater the substantivity, the greater the potential efficacy and systemic toxicity of a topical formulation that is meant for local/topical treatment or prevention (e.g., sunscreens, antibacterials, antifungals).

Binding can occur to various other skin proteins, lipids, or other substances, which have differing binding sites and chemical affinities [3]. Thus, binding is drug or chemical specific. Bindings to different skin components (such as eccrine and apocrine sweat glands and hair follicles) are also important to consider as the bound drug or chemical may serve as a skin reservoir. Further, drugs or chemicals stored in skin reservoirs may be absorbed systemically, potentially causing prolonged pharmacologic effect or toxicity. This is an area of current decontamination research, as bound substances may not be easily washed off or otherwise removed [3, 4]. (Washing is further discussed in #12).

10. How does topical application result in systemic distribution of the drug or chemical?

Systemic distribution: First, drugs or chemicals are adsorbed to the superficial skin surface (substantivity being an issue here). Second, drugs or chemicals may penetrate and bind to various skin proteins, lipids, skin appendages, and other substances (binding affinity being an issue here). Third, drugs or chemicals penetrate deeper into the lower dermis where there is a vascular blood supply, and partition into the bloodstream for systemic circulation [7]. The important issues here are affinity for blood components such as albumin or other plasma proteins (plasma protein binding) and local blood flow [7]. Vasodilatation enhances blood flow and may promote systemic distribution of a topically administered medication. Of note, some medications may have vasodilating properties—for example, transdermal nitroglycerin (a venodilator) acts within minutes and may be a temporary measure to provide sustained nitroglycerin blood concentrations before intravenous (IV) line insertion can be done to administer an IV nitroglycerin infusion. The converse should also be noted—some medications have vasoconstrictive effects (such as corticosteroids) and may inhibit systemic absorption. In addition to skin surfaces, drugs or chemicals may be applied to (or otherwise be in contact with) mucosal surfaces such as the eyes or nose—the nose has a highly vascular mucosa that almost guarantees systemic absorption.

Thus, there is potential for *systemic toxicity* from topical administration. As exposure from use of ophthalmic drops is to both the eye and surrounding skin, ophthalmic beta-blockers have caused bronchospasm, congestive heart failure and pulmonary edema, bradyarrhythmias and sinus arrest, CNS toxicity, impotence, and dyslipidemias [43–45]. Ophthalmic sulfonamides have induced Stevens–Johnson syndrome [46]. Topical corticosteroids have caused systemic side effects including HPA axis suppression and adrenal insufficiency, Cushing's syndrome, and hypertension [43]. Topical salicylates have caused a refractory hypoglycemia [47] by increasing glucose metabolism and reducing gluconeogenesis [43]. Significant systemic absorption of topical salicylates has resulted in systemic salicylate toxicity: tinnitus, hearing loss, blurred vision, sweating, tachypnea, diarrhea, nausea/vomiting, and weakness [43]. Topical minoxidil 2% applied to the scalp may have caused cardiovascular adverse effects including palpitations, dizziness, hypotension, tachycardia, paroxysmal atrial fibrillation, and sinus arrhythmia [43]. There are many other drugs and chemicals applied topically which may have increased systemic toxicity as skin barrier properties change.

Inadvertent systemic toxicity from cosmeceuticals and other products have occurred. For example, phenol can be cardiotoxic: a phenol and croton oil solution used in deep chemical peels caused cardiac arrhythmias including atrial and ventricular tachycardia, premature ventricular beats, and bigeminy; people with diabetes mellitus, hypertension, and depression may be at higher risk [43]. There is also concern about mercury-containing skin care products (such as skin-lightening creams and soaps, local antiseptics, etc.) and their potential to cause neurotoxicity or nephrotoxicity with enough systemic absorption [43]. Arsenic is another toxic metal that is used (or is a contaminant) in cosmetics, medications, pigments, and natural health products, that when applied onto skin over time or in sufficient amounts can result in systemic toxicity effects including psychoses, seizures, multiorgan failure, and death [43]. Be cognizant that *any* drug or chemical that touches the skin has the potential for percutaneous absorption that may result in systemic distribution and possible systemic toxicity.

11. How, if at all, does exfoliation affect topical absorption?

Exfoliation is part of a natural skin cell renewal process: keratinocytes begin as box-like basal cells at the base of the epidermis, then migrate up towards the skin surface, flattening out to become a layer of overlapping corneocytes which have no nuclei—thus termed dead skin cells—which are then "sloughed off," i.e., exfoliated. Drugs or chemicals bound to skin cells could either be *lost by the exfoliation process* or be *absorbed deeper into the dermis*; thus, exfoliation can affect drug bioavailability after topical administration. Urea, which is minimally absorbed topically, can be used as an exfoliation marker [48].

12.   Does washing affect topical absorption?

There are two opposing wash effects which can affect topical absorption of drugs and chemicals. Loss by exfoliation can be enhanced by washing [2] even hours after application [48] if there is drug remaining in the stratum corneum; and this would be a *washing-off* effect. Note that for highly lipid-soluble drugs or chemicals (e.g., pesticides), washing with soap and water may not be sufficiently effective in removing them [49].

In fact, the opposite may happen: washing the site of application in between doses may actually enhance topical absorption/penetration; and this would be a *washing-in* effect [50–52] (see also #13 below). Be aware that washing may promote drug or chemical penetrance through the skin leading to toxicity—for example, with insect repellents [50–52]. Care should be taken when insect repellents are used, especially in children. The US Environmental Protection Agency (EPA) recommends that instructions on the label be followed [5] for insect repellent products, and they should be used according to the time of day when mosquitoes are most active—which may vary for the species and type of diseases transmitted [5]. Care should also be taken in the work environment if there is occupational exposure to chemicals: workers should be counselled to wear protective clothing and use protective equipment, and warned about the "wash-in" phenomenon [5]. They should be aware that the mechanical friction from handwashing may increase percutaneous absorption in particular of inorganic compounds [50].

13.   Does rubbing or massaging affect topical absorption?

There are two important concepts here: *rub enhancement* and *rub resistance*, both of which occur with rubbing/massaging. One example of *rub enhancement* relates to sunscreen application and washing: the mechanical stress of skin washing can massage the sunscreen deeper into the hair follicle [53]; and this washing/massaging may enhance transfollicular sunscreen absorption [50]. Massaging may also increase the follicular penetration depth of liposomes (used as drug carriers) [54, 55]. Massaging/rubbing reduces skin barrier function to facilitate penetration [55]. However, this effect differs between hydrophilic and lipophilic substances—lipophilic/organic substances are less affected, if at all.

With regard to *rub resistance*, this is a term used to describe whether a substance applied topically will still be effective after being rubbed with a textile (clothing, towel, etc.). Rub resistance would be an important factor for a sunscreen or a topical medication to possess, and a rub resistance factor (RRF) can be calculated to allow comparisons between products of the same class (e.g., sunscreens) [56]. Parameters that influence RRF include rubbing pressure, rubbing duration, rubbing speed, and the textile (composition, thickness, etc.) [56]. Obviously, the higher the RRF, the greater the amount of drug or chemical remaining on the skin, and the greater the likelihood for percutaneous absorption.

14. Can medications or chemicals be transferred from one person to another through skin contact, clothing, or contact with an inanimate surface?

Yes. As briefly mentioned in #3 above, inadvertent drug or chemical exposure can occur via transfer from one person to another—such as a mother wearing sunscreen and holding her baby with bare arms. Drug transfer can sometimes have serious consequences: a father who used testosterone cream without routine handwashing after application transferred enough testosterone over time to his infant son to cause precocious puberty—pronounced virilization in a 2-year-old boy [57]. The skin-to-skin contact time need not be lengthy: a controlled 15 min ventral forearm to ventral forearm rub/contact time transferred sufficient estradiol from donor volunteers to recipient volunteers for estradiol to be detected in the recipients' urine [58]. There was also enough estradiol left on the sleeve of the donors for the possibility of transfer from clothing to occur [58]. Using a hair follicle drug screening test, a Department of Human Services detected methamphetamine in newborns and young children—postulating that "sweat glands glom onto meth which can then be transferred through skin-to-skin contact, like coddling an infant" [59]. However, besides sweat, other possibilities were children picking it up "from the environment, from the smoke or residue" [59]. Other examples include additional controlled studies confirming that skin-to-skin drug transfers exist [60, 61]. Skin-to-skin transfer can also occur in the same individual [61].

Practically, what does this mean? Anytime that a topical medication or chemical substance is used, we should be aware that transfer may occur from one person to another, including to infants who may be at greater risk of systemic toxicity—unless the substance is inert. Obviously, the other factors of percutaneous absorption would also apply to the transferred drug or chemical, and those factors would ultimately determine the clinical significance of the drug or chemical transfer.

15. How is topical absorption affected if a drug or chemical is volatile?

Volatility means that a substance has the ability to spontaneously vaporize into the air or, in the case of a topical agent applied on skin, to evaporate from skin over time. Medications or chemicals applied to skin are often in product formulations that are a mixture of active and inactive ingredients, some of which may be volatile while others are not. For volatile substances, the degree of volatility may vary from substance to substance and may be affected by other factors such as formulation (pH, etc.), environment (humidity, temperature, etc.), and skin characteristics (pH, hydration, skin temperature, etc.). Some substances may be volatile only when certain conditions are met. For example, methamphetamine HCl (a basic drug with a pKa of 9.9) in aqueous solution can change from a nonvolatile salt to a volatile free base when the pH of the solution exceeds 4 or 5 [62].

What implications does volatility of a drug or chemical have on percutaneous absorption? Important issues include the following: (a) For a multi-ingredient product, the contents of what is left behind may alter the function of the applied product, which may have implications for efficacy and safety [63]. (b) If the vehicle and not the active ingredient is volatile, over time there will be a concentrating effect as more and more of the vehicle evaporates, potentially increasing the potency and/or toxicity of the active ingredient. This is important as volatile solvents are commonly used in drug and other formulations (cosmetic, patch test [64], etc.), for example, an acetone-based benzoyl peroxide product or an acetone-based patch test chemical [64]. (c) Skin patch testing detects contact irritants and allergens, and volatility can lead to false positives and false negatives—test vehicle evaporation leading to too high a test chemical concentration causing a false-positive result [64], and test chemical evaporation leading to too low a test chemical concentration causing a false-negative result [64, 65]. For example, fragrance chemicals are usually volatile substances and are common contact allergens often patch tested as "Fragrance mix 1" and "Fragrance mix 2." A study of two radiolabeled fragrance chemicals (geraniol and citronellol) detected that, due to evaporation, within 40 min geraniol lost up to 39% of its dose and citronellol up to 26% of its dose [65]. (d) Rapid volatilization reduces the dose and prevents oversaturation of skin's absorptive capacity. This allows for a direct relationship between dose and percutaneous absorption for volatile substances that is calculable (i.e., predictable). Two equations have been developed to correlate the relationship between volatilization and absorption for a small dose vs. a large dose [66]. These equations may be useful in assessing the risk of topical products and their pharmacokinetics/pharmacodynamics/toxicities. An in-depth discussion of these equations is beyond the scope of this chapter, and the interested reader should review the reference indicated [66].

Volatility is important in other ways. Mosquito repellents depend on volatility for their effects, and volatility remains a limiting efficacy factor (i.e., in providing sufficient biting protection from mosquitoes). Traditional contact repellents such as *N,N*-diethyl-*meta*-toluamide (DEET) applied on human skin require frequent reapplication and may carry a risk of systemic absorption [67]. However, spatial repellents may prevent mosquito entry into particular areas or into a home and may be particularly useful in mosquito-borne disease endemic areas [67]. For example, metofluthrin-impregnated latticework plastic strips were capable of preventing the resting of *Aedes Aegypti* (L.) within residences in Vietnam for a minimum of 8 weeks after they were introduced [67, 68].

16. Does metabolic transformation occur during topical absorption, and if so, how and what? Does cutaneous metabolism occur?

Depending on the drug or chemical, *metabolic transformation* can occur in skin prior to systemic absorption, since there are metabolizing enzymes in skin. Both phase I (e.g., CYP450 enzymes) and phase II (e.g., N-acetyltransferase) enzymes have been found in skin—the mRNA and protein being detected more often than the quantified enzyme activity (being much lower than in the liver and often at the limit of detection) [69]. Sometimes, UV light is required for transformation (see #17). Biotransformation changes the drug or chemical. This change can be in the drug's physicochemical properties or in its pharmacodynamic activity, or it may be both. This can result in (a) an active agent becoming inactive (a degradation process); (b) an inactive agent becoming active (an activation process for a prodrug); and (c) a lipophilic agent becoming more water soluble (via various metabolic pathways, e.g., oxidation, hydroxylation, acetylation, etc.). These changes can affect the drug's penetration through the skin. For example, highly lipophilic compounds, often large, do not penetrate through the skin well (a good thing). However, the highly lipophilic preservative butylparaben (one example) can be metabolized to *p*-hydroxybenzoic acid in skin—this metabolite is less lipophilic and thus more readily penetrates through the skin [2, 70]. Cutaneous metabolism of endogenous substrates such as vitamin A and vitamin D also occurs [2].

17. Does photochemical transformation occur during topical absorption, and if so, how and what?

Similar to #16, the effect of UV light on a drug or chemical applied to the skin can cause a *photochemical transformation* (degradation or activation, etc.). In particular, photochemical changes to a drug or chemical can induce a phototoxic or photoallergic reaction. A *phototoxic* reaction is caused by a drug or chemical absorbing UVA and causing direct damage to sun-exposed skin, whereas a *photoallergic* reaction requires the drug or chemical to be changed by UVA into an allergen—with skin damage occasionally spreading beyond the sun-exposed skin areas. *Photosensitivity*—an adverse cutaneous response to normally harmless doses of UV radiation—is a property related to the drug chemistry and can be seen with topical or systemic administration. Examples of phototoxic agents include amiodarone, tetracyclines (e.g., doxycycline), coal tar, psoralens, and sulfonamides. Examples of photoallergic agents include sulfonamides, sulfonylureas, thiazides, chloroquine, carbamazepine, etc. Practically, if a drug or chemical is known to cause photosensitivity, sun protection is recommended if used during the day; application/dosing at night rather than in more sunlit hours may minimize photosensitivity.

Table 12.1 Clinically pertinent factors of percutaneous absorption

1	Relevant physicochemical properties (particle size/molecular weight, lipophilicity, pH, pKa, partition coefficient)
2	Vehicle/formulation
3	Conditions of drug exposure (dose, duration, surface area, exposure frequency)
4	Skin appendages (hair follicles, glands) as sub-anatomical pathways
5	Skin application sites (regional variation in penetration)
6	Population variability (prematurity, infants, and aged)
7	Skin surface conditions (hydration, temperature, pH)
8	Skin health and integrity (trauma, skin diseases)
9	Substantivity and binding to different skin components
10	Systemic distribution and systemic toxicity
11	Exfoliation
12	Washing-off and washing-in
13	Rubbing/massaging
14	Transfer to others (from human to human and hard surface to human)
15	Volatility
16	Metabolic biotransformation/cutaneous metabolism
17	Photochemical transformation and photosensitivity
18	Excretion kinetics
19	Lateral spread
20	Chemical method of determining percutaneous absorption

18.   How does metabolism affect excretion kinetics of the drug or chemical? and how does excretion kinetics relate to topical absorption?

A drug or chemical can be excreted from the body unchanged, or it may undergo metabolic changes before excretion. Thus, the discussions in #16 and #17 regarding biotransformation in the skin will affect excretion kinetics. For example, a highly lipophilic drug or chemical that is biotransformed into a more water-soluble metabolite will not only be more easily absorbed through the skin, but it will also be more easily excreted in the urine. Water-soluble drugs often do not require metabolic changes for urinary excretion, and a greater proportion of the administered dose may be excreted unchanged.

Metabolism and excretion are two mechanisms for elimination of a drug or chemical, which can be affected by numerous factors [7]. Note that metabolism and excretion pharmacokinetics can differ greatly between structurally similar drugs or chemicals. Thus, depending on the substance, elimination (i.e., *drug clearance*) may or may not be in proportion to the dose absorbed. For researchers conducting in vivo studies, the clearance rate of the drug or chemical must be considered when estimating percutaneous absorption from blood or tissue samples [7].

19.   How does lateral spread affect percutaneous absorption?

Lateral spread is the ability of a topical agent to spread beyond the site of application, i.e., the drug or chemical "flows" laterally on the skin surface from the application area to outside of it [71]. (Note that lateral spread is also more commonly used in describing earthquake phenomena.) Lateral spread of a topically applied drug or chemical is a competitive process to drug or chemical penetration into the stratum corneum [71, 72]. The spreading can reduce the amount of drug substance within the area of application which can modify the desirable effect expected in the treated area [71]. *Time* is a factor: for example, a 10% urea in water solution applied to skin provided a 90.4% recovery rate at the site of application after 1 h versus a 79.6% recovery rate after 6 h [71]. Why is there less urea remaining at the site of application after 6 h than after 1 h? The cause is lateral spread and not percutaneous absorption as less than 1% of urea penetrates in vivo in man [73]. Thus, lateral spread is time dependent. Furthermore, *skin surface topography* can affect the degree of lateral spread: primary furrow networks such as fingerprints and palm prints can function as pathways for lateral spreading [72], whereas follicles and wrinkles can be reservoirs for drugs or chemicals, and little is known about lateral spread in these areas. Although there is no difference in lateral spread between forearm and back [72], little is known about other anatomical sites. Practically, we should be aware that lateral spread happens, and the lengthier the time from the time of application, the greater the effect of lateral spread, resulting in less and less drug or chemical remaining at the site of application for percutaneous absorption.

20.   For investigators, does the method of determining percutaneous absorption influence the results and the interpretation of study results?

Based on what has been discussed from the 19 factors above, many issues can influence percutaneous absorption and, if not controlled for, can be confounders to study results. In particular, in vivo studies would be subject to many more confounding variables than in vitro studies. In vitro experiments can sometimes be better controlled than in vivo studies. Also, differences in experimental parameters such as animal species, anatomical site, vehicle, preparation of skin samples (in vitro studies), and other exposure conditions may affect the interpretation of and comparison between studies [2]. Furthermore, there are limits of quantification and limits of detection which must be kept in mind when interpreting study results.

Summary

In summary, percutaneous absorption is complex and requires more thought than just simply applying a topical formulation on the skin and assuming that it works. Many factors—at least the 20 that have been discussed here (Table 12.1)—need to be considered as they may affect the efficacy and/or toxicity of the medications and hence patient outcome.

Acknowledgements There are no conflicts of interest from any of the authors, and there are no sources of funding for this manuscript.

Author Contributions R. Law had the idea to provide a practical and clinically relevant version of M. Ngo and H. Maibach's pivotal 15 steps of percutaneous absorption paper—for practitioners—and in the process expanded to 20 factors with contribution from H. Maibach; R. Law performed the literature search—with additional sources from H. Maibach's vast experience; R. Law drafted the work; R. Law and H. Maibach critically revised the work at several time points, and M. Ngo critically revised the work twice.

References

1. Wester RC, Maibach HI. Cutaneous pharmacokinetics: 10 steps to percutaneous absorption. Drug Metab Rev. 1983;14(2):169–205.
2. Ngo MA, Maibach HI. Chapter 6: 15 Factors of percutaneous penetration of pesticides. In: Knaak JB, Timchalk C, Tornero-Velez R, editors. Parameters for pesticide QSAR and PBPK/PD models for human risk assessment. Washington, DC: American Chemical Society; 2012. p. 67–86.
3. Hui X, Lamel S, Qiao P, Maibach HI. Isolated human/animal stratum corneum as a partial model for 15 steps in percutaneous absorption: emphasizing decontamination, part I. J Appl Toxicol. 2013;33:157–72.
4. Hui X, Lamel S, Qiao P, Maibach HI. Isolated human and animal stratum corneum as a partial model for the 15 steps in percutaneous absorption: emphasizing decontamination, part II. J Appl Toxicol. 2013;33:173–82.
5. Li BS, Ngo MA, Maibach HI. Clinical relevance of complex factors of percutaneous penetration in man. Curr Top Pharmacol. 2017;21:85–107. http://www.researchtrends.net/tia/title_issue.asp?id=11&in=0&vn=21.
6. Keurentjes AJ, Maibach HI. Percutaneous penetration of drugs applied in transdermal delivery systems: an in vivo based approach for evaluating computer generated penetration models. Regul Toxicol Pharmacol. 2019;18:104428.
7. Burton ME, Schentag JJ, Shaw LM, Evans WE. Applied pharmacokinetics and pharmacodynamics: principles of therapeutic drug monitoring. 4th ed. Baltimore: Lippincott Williams & Wilkins; 2006.
8. Marechal Y. The water molecule in (bio)macromolecules. In: The hydrogen bond and the water molecule: the physics and chemistry of water, aqueous and bio media. Amsterdam: Elsevier; 2007. p. 249–75. https://doi.org/10.1016/B978-044451957-3.50011-1.
9. Wester RC, Noonan PK, Maibach HI. Frequency of application on percutaneous absorption of hydrocortisone. Arch Dermatol. 1977;113:620–2.
10. Berardesca E, Mariano M, Cameli N. Biophysical properties of ethnic skin. In: Vashi NA, Maibach HI, editors. Dermatoanthropology of ethnic skin and hair. Cham: Springer International Publishing AG; 2017.

11. Berardesca E, Maibach HI. Racial differences in sodium lauryl sulfate induced cutaneous irritation: black and white. Contact Dermat. 1988;18:65–70.
12. Berardesca E, Maibach HI. Sodium-lauryl-sulfate-induced cutaneous irritation. Comparison of white and Hispanic subjects. Contact Dermat. 1988;19:136–40.
13. Roskos KV, Maibach HI, Guy RH. The effect of aging on percutaneous absorption in man. J Pharmacokinet Biopharm. 1989;17(6):617–30.
14. Hoath SB, Maibach HI. Neonatal skin: structure and function. 2nd ed. Boca Raton: CRC Press; 2003.
15. Mauro TM, Behne MJ. Chapter 3: Acid mantle. In: Hoath SB, Maibach HI, editors. Neonatal skin: structure and function. 2nd ed. Boca Raton: CRC; 2003.
16. Nikolovski J, Stamatas GN, Kollias N, et al. Barrier function and water-holding and transport properties of infant stratum corneum are different from adult and continue to develop through the first year of life. J Investig Dermatol. 2008;128:1728–36.
17. Oranges T, Dini V, Romanelli M. Skin physiology of the neonate and infant: clinical implications. Adv Wound Care. 2015;4(10):587–95.
18. Hoeger PH, Enzmann CC. Skin physiology of the neonate and young infant: a prospective study of functional skin parameters during early infancy. Pediatr Dermatol. 2002;19:256–62.
19. Visscher MO, Chatterjee R, Munson KA, et al. Changes in diapered and non-diapered infant skin over the first month of life. Pediatr Dermatol. 2000;17:45–51.
20. Saijo S, Tagami HJ. Dry skin of newborn infants: functional analysis of the stratum corneum. Pediatr Dermatol. 1991;8:155–9.
21. Brayer C, Micheau P, Bony C, et al. Neonatal accidental burn by isopropyl alcohol. Arch Pediatr. 2004;11(8):932–5.
22. DeBellonia RR, Marcus S, Shih R, et al. Curanderismo: consequences of folk medicine. Pediatr Emerg Care. 2008;24(4):228–9.
23. George AJ. Toxicity of boric acid through skin and mucous membranes. Food Cosmet Toxicol. 1965;3:99–101.
24. Martin-Bouyer G, Toga M, Lebreton R, et al. Outbreak of accidental hexachlorophene poisoning in France. Lancet Public Health. 1982;319(8263):91–5.
25. Mullick FG. Hexachlorophene toxicity—human experience at the Armed Forces Institute of Pathology. Pediatrics. 1973;51(2):395–9.
26. Li BS, Cary JH, Maibach HI. Should we instruct patients to rub topical agents into skin? The evidence. J Dermatol Treat. 2018;19:1–5.
27. Evans NJ, Rutter N, Hadgraft J, et al. Percutaneous administration of theophylline in the preterm infant. J Pediatr. 1985;107(2):307–11.
28. Zhai H, Maibach HI. Effects of skin occlusion on percutaneous absorption: an overview. Skin Pharmacol Appl. 2001;14(1):1–10.
29. Shomaker TS, Zhang J, Ashburn MA. A pilot study assessing the impact of heat on the transdermal delivery of testosterone. J Clin Pharmacol. 2001;41(6):677–82.
30. Aly R, Shirley C, Cunico B, Maibach HI. Effect of prolonged occlusion on the microbial flora, pH, carbon dioxide and transepidermal water loss on human skin. J Investig Dermatol. 1978;71(6):378–81.
31. Gattu S, Maibach HI. Modest but increased penetration through damaged skin: an overview of the in vivo human model. Skin Pharmacol Physiol. 2011;24(1):2–9.
32. Gattu S, Maibach HI. Enhanced absorption through damaged skin: an overview of the in vitro human model. Skin Pharmacol Physiol. 2010;23:171–6.
33. Morgan CJ, Renwick AG, Friedmann PS. The role of stratum corneum and dermal microvascular perfusion in penetration and tissue levels of water-soluble drugs investigated by microdialysis. Br J Dermatol. 2003;148:434–43.
34. Jakasa I, Verberk MM, Bunge AL, et al. Increased permeability for polyethylene glycols through skin compromised by sodium lauryl sulfate. Exp Dermatol. 2006;15:801–7.
35. Jacob SE. Percutaneous absorption risks in atopic dermatitis. Br J Dermatol. 2017;177:11–2.

36. Halling-Overgaard AS, Kezic S, Jakasa I, et al. Skin absorption through atopic dermatitis skin: a systematic review. Br J Dermatol. 2017;177(1):84–106.
37. Garcia OP, Hansen SH, Shah VP, et al. Impact of adult atopic dermatitis on topical drug absorption: assessment by cutaneous microdialysis and tape stripping. Acta Derm Venereol. 2009;89:33–8.
38. Tauber M, Balica S, Hsu CY, et al. *Staphylococcus aureus* density on lesional and nonlesional skin is strongly associated with disease severity in atopic dermatitis. J Allergy Clin Immunol. 2016;137:1272–4.
39. Jakasa I, de Jongh CM, Verberk MM, et al. Percutaneous penetration of sodium lauryl sulfate is increased in uninvolved skin of patients with atopic dermatitis compared with control subjects. Br J Dermatol. 2006;155:104–9.
40. Jakasa I, Verbek MM, Esposito M, et al. Altered penetration of polyethylene glycols into uninvolved skin of atopic dermatitis patients. J Investig Dermatol. 2007;127:129–34.
41. Hata M, Tokura Y, Takigawa M, et al. Assessment of epidermal barrier function by photoacoustic spectrometry in relation to its importance in the pathogenesis of atopic dermatitis. Lab Invest. 2002;82:1451–61.
42. Mochizuki J, Tadaki H, Takami S, et al. Evaluation of out-in skin transparency using a colorimeter and food dye in patients with atopic dermatitis. Br J Dermatol. 2009;160:972–9.
43. Alikhan FS, Maibach HI. Topical absorption and systemic toxicity. Cutan Ocul Toxicol. 2011;30(3):175–86.
44. Lewis PR, Phillips TG, Sassani JW. Topical therapies for glaucoma: what family physicians need to know. Am Fam Physician. 1999;59:1871–9.
45. Goldberg I, Moloney G, McCluskey P. Topical ophthalmic medications: what potential for systemic side effects and interactions with other medications? Med J Aust. 2008;189:356–7.
46. Rubin Z. Ophthalmic sulfonamide-induced Stevens–Johnson syndrome. Arch Dermatol. 1977;113:235–6.
47. Raschke R, Arnold-Capell PA, Richeson R, et al. Refractory hypoglycemia secondary to topical salicylate intoxication. Arch Intern Med. 1991;151:591–3.
48. Zheng Y, Vieille-Petit A, Chodoutard S, Maibach HI. Dislodgeable stratum corneum exfoliation: role in percutaneous penetration? Cutan Ocul Toxicol. 2011;30(3):198–204.
49. Zhu H, Maibach HI. Skin decontamination. Heidelberg: Springer; 2019.
50. Rodriguez J, Maibach HI. Percutaneous penetration and pharmacodynamics: wash-in and wash-off of sunscreen and insect repellent. J Dermatol Treat. 2016;27:11.
51. Moody RP. Letter to the editor: the safety of diethyltoluamide insect repellents. JAMA. 1989;262:28–9.
52. Moody RP, Benoit FM, Riedel R, Ritter L. Dermal absorption of the insect repellent DEET (*N,N*-diethyl-*m*-toluamide) in rats and monkeys: effect of anatomical site and multiple exposure. J Toxicol Environ Health. 1989;26:137–47.
53. Lademann J, Patzelt A, Schanzer S, et al. In vivo laser scanning microscopic investigation of the decontamination of hazardous substances from the human skin. Laser Phys Lett. 2010;7:884–8.
54. Trauer S, Richter H, Kuntsche J, et al. Influence of massage and occlusion on the ex vivo skin penetration of rigid liposomes and invasomes. Eur J Pharm Biopharm. 2014;86:301–6.
55. Phuong C, Maibach HI. Effect of massage on percutaneous penetration and skin decontamination: man and animal. Cutan Ocul Toxicol. 2016;35(2):153–6.
56. Delamour E, Miksa S, Lutz D, Guy C. How to prove 'rub-resistant' sun protection. Cosmet Toilet Sci Appl. 2016. https://www.cosmeticsandtoiletries.com/testing/efficacyclaims/How-to-Prove-Rub-resistant-Sun-Protection-373779591.html.
57. Franklin SF, Geffner ME. Precocious puberty secondary to topical testosterone exposure. J Pediatr Endocrinol Metab. 2003;16:107–10.
58. Wester RC, Hui X, Maibach HI. In vivo human transfer of topical bioactive drug between individuals: estradiol. J Investig Dermatol. 2006;126:2190–3.

59. Linck M. Screens detect all: Mom, dad, kids, newborns all test positive for meth. Sioux City J. 2003. https://siouxcityjournal.com/news/screens-detect-all-mom-dad-kids-newborns-all-test-postive/article_5c9a48cf-4855-5308-ba83-c11bf1b44239.html.
60. Dmochowski RR, Newman DK, Sand PK, et al. Pharmacokinetics of oxybutynin chloride topical gel. Clin Drug Investig. 2011;31(8):559–71.
61. Isnardo D, Vidal J, Panyella D, Vilaplana J. Nickel transfer by fingers actas dermo-Sifiliográficas (English Edition). Acad Esp Dermatol Venereol. 2015;106:5. https://doi.org/10.1016/j.adengl.2015.04.011.
62. Salocks CB, Hui X, Lamel S, et al. Dermal exposure to methamphetamine hydrochloride contaminated residential surfaces: surface pH values, volatility, and in vitro human skin. Food Chem Toxicol. 2012;50(12):4426–40.
63. Rouse NC, Maibach HI. The effect of volatility on percutaneous absorption. J Dermatol Treat. 2016;27(1):5–10.
64. Bruze M. Thoughts on how to improve the quality of multicentre patch test studies. Contact Dermat. 2016;74:168–74.
65. Gilpin SJ, Hui X, Maibach HI. Volatility of fragrance chemicals: patch testing implications. Dermatitis. 2009;20(4):200–7.
66. Kasting GB, Miller MA. Kinetics of finite dose absorption through skin 2: volatile compounds. J Pharm Sci. 2006;95:268–80.
67. Norris EJ, Coats JR. Current and future repellent technologies: the potential of spatial repellents and their place in mosquito-borne disease control. Int J Environ Res Public Health. 2017;14(2):124–68.
68. Kawada H, Temu EA, Minjas JN, et al. Field evaluation of field repellency of metofluthrin impregnated latticework plastic strips against *Aedes aegypti* (L.) and analysis of environmental factors affecting its efficacy in My Tho City, Tien Giang, Vietnam. Am J Trop Med Hyg. 2006;75:1153–7.
69. Kazem S, Linssen EC, Gibbs S. Skin metabolism phase I and phase II enzymes in native and reconstructed human skin: a short review. Drug Discov Today. 2019;24(9):1899–910.
70. Bando H, Mohri S, Yamashita F, et al. Effects of skin metabolism on percutaneous penetration of lipophilic drugs. J Pharm Sci. 1997;86(6):759–61.
71. Vieille-Petit A, Blickenstaff N, Coman G, Maibach H. Metrics and clinical relevance of percutaneous penetration and lateral spreading. Skin Pharmacol Physiol. 2015;28:57–64.
72. Jacobi U, Schanzer S, Weigmann H-J, et al. Pathways of lateral spreading. Skin Pharmacol Physiol. 2011;24:231–7.
73. Feldman RJ, Maibach HI. Absorption of some organic compounds through the skin in man. J Investig Dermatol. 1970;54:399–404.

Chapter 13
Lateral Spread and Percutaneous Penetration: An Overview

Rebecca M. Law and Howard I. Maibach

Introduction

Lateral spread is one of at least 20 observed factors affecting percutaneous penetration of drugs and chemicals. Unlike some of the other factors such as physicochemical properties, vehicle/formulation, drug exposure conditions (dose, duration, surface area, exposure frequency), and potential for systemic distribution and systemic toxicity, the phenomenon of lateral spread is sometimes overlooked in quantitation of drug research. However, lateral spread may affect or be affected by the above or other factors affecting percutaneous penetration, including skin appendages (hair follicles, glands) serving as sub-anatomical pathways, regional variation in penetration between skin application sites, population variability (premature, infants, and aged), skin surface conditions (hydration, temperature, pH), skin health and integrity (trauma, skin diseases), substantivity and binding to different skin components, stratum corneum (SC) exfoliation, washing-off and washing-in, rubbing/massaging, transfer to others (human to human and hard surface to human), volatility, metabolic biotransformation/cutaneous metabolism, photochemical transformation and photosensitivity, excretion kinetics, and chemical method of determining percutaneous absorption [1]. Lateral spread—even when modest—may alter pharmacologic and toxicologic effects of drugs and chemicals.

R. M. Law (✉)
School of Pharmacy, Memorial University of Newfoundland, St. John's, NL, Canada
e-mail: Rebecca.law@ucsf.edu

H. I. Maibach
Department of Dermatology, University of California San Francisco,
San Francisco, CA, USA

© The Author(s), under exclusive license to Springer Nature
Switzerland AG 2022
A. M. Feschuk et al. (eds.), *Dermal Absorption and Decontamination*,
https://doi.org/10.1007/978-3-031-09222-0_13

Definition

Lateral spread is a term most commonly used in describing earthquake phenomena—landslides radiating out from an epicenter. In 1970, the phenomenon of epidermal surface loss rate implying lateral spread was seen and described for topical application of organic compounds [2]. An early use of the term "lateral spread" as it relates to percutaneous application occurred in 1988, when the lateral spread of clobetasol 17-propionate was quantified and compared for two formulations [3]. *Lateral spread* has been defined as the ability of a topical agent or formulation to spread beyond application site. In essence, the drug or chemical "flows" laterally on the skin surface from the application area to outside of it [4]. Other terminologies describing the same phenomenon include *lateral diffusion* [5–9] and *transverse diffusion* [10]. Note that lateral spread may be occurring not only on the skin surface but within the stratum corneum (SC), i.e., an inward diffusion and lateral spread within the SC layers rather than penetration [2–4, 6, 8]. Furthermore, we know little about deeper lateral spread which may be occurring in the viable epidermis, dermis, and subcutaneous fat.

The phenomenon of lateral spread has been used medically in other ways—for example, in the clinical evaluation of adequate cryosurgical treatment of skin cancer, the predictable relationship between lateral spread of freeze and the depth of freeze is a key concept [11]. Lateral spread is also commonly used to describe the local expansion of carcinomas [12].

Consequences of Lateral Spread

Lateral spread of a topically applied drug or chemical is a competitive process to drug or chemical penetration into SC and beyond [2, 4]. Spreading can reduce the amount of drug substance within the area of application which can modify the desirable effect expected for the topically treated area [2, 3]. In addition, if the desired effect is systemic, and topical application is just a convenient route of administration, lateral spread can possibly lead to significant drug loss and hence reduced bioavailability. Thus, a drug's pharmacologic and toxicologic effects may potentially be altered—even with modest lateral spread.

Lateral spread would also affect the determinations of minimal effective dose (MED), median lethal dose (LD_{50}), maximum tolerated dose (MTD), or the no observable adverse effect level (NOAEL) for drugs, and the no observable/observed effect level (NOEL) for toxicity of chemicals on skin.

The effect of a drug—whether pharmacologic or toxicologic—is usually dose dependent, whether administered topically or systemically. This is also generally true for chemicals humans are exposed to—unless, of course, if inert. The potential for toxicity (e.g., to an individual organ system such as kidney or liver) is usually quantified using animal studies. How is this done for topical agents? By establishing the threshold known as NOEL.

NOEL is a method where a known topical dose (X amount of mass/Y application area) is consistently increased (e.g., doubling, tripling, quadrupling, etc., the X amount of mass while maintaining the identical Y application area) until an organ effect is observed. The NOEL is the dose limit that has *not* affected the organ, which defines the maximum dose that can be tolerated before toxicity happens. This concept is used when first doses are considered, with the units in mass/surface area, often as mg/cm^2.

Thus, lateral spread, which affects drug and chemical penetration, would need to be considered as, even if imprecisely, a "correction factor" for percutaneous drug dosing or chemical toxicity considerations. As mentioned earlier, the potential for renal, hepatic, or other toxicities is usually quantified using animal studies. This quantified data is then estimated for humans using "correction factors" such as adding one logarithm to convert from the animal species to humans. This is already imprecise and is an area of research. How to include lateral spread as an additional "correction factor" is another area of future research.

Consequences of lateral spread may vary depending on the formulation, the chemical or drug involved, the condition of the skin, the site of application, and even environmental factors such as heat and humidity causing sweating. These consequences may potentially include less drug absorbed systemically or reduced rate of absorption. The clinical consequences, if any, will be drug-specific and vary with the particular drug's therapeutic index. A drug which has a wide therapeutic index will be less likely to show a clinical consequence (such as a reduced therapeutic effect) due to lateral spread. An example is topical hydrocortisone which has a wide therapeutic index.

Evidence for the Lateral Spread Phenomenon

The lateral spread/lateral diffusion phenomenon has been investigated for many years, and there is ongoing research.

Spread Pattern

The spread pattern is characteristic. Lateral diffusion/lateral spread occurs on the surface of the SC, along the plane of the lipid bilayers within the SC, and goes deeper from bilayer to bilayer, spreading via adjacent lipid channels between corneocytes (overlapping flattened dead keratinocytes which serve a barrier function) (Fig. 13.1). This may be occurring through the tail group region or the head group region or both, and the process is characterized by a lateral diffusion coefficient D_{lat} [8].

In greater detail, lateral diffusion coefficients are typically measured in phospholipid bilayer systems and for fluorescently labeled lipids (>600 Da) and proteins as large as 10^5 Da, using the fluorescence recovery after photobleaching (FRAP) technique and data-fitting to Fick's second law [8]. Lateral diffusion obeys Fick's second law which is the diffusion equation, with the steady-state diffusion flux along a given bilayer described by Fick's first law. Diffusion coefficient values ranged from 2.68×10^{-9} (for fentanyl) to 2.62×10^{-6} cm^2/h (for nicotine) in one in vitro human

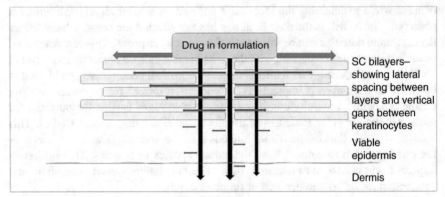

Horizontal arrows = potential pathways of lateral spread (on skin surface and along SC bilayers, possibly in viable epidermis and dermis)
Vertical arrows = percutaneous penetration (a competitive process)

Fig. 13.1 Lateral spread and percutaneous penetration after topical drug application

cadaver skin study [8]. For more discussion about lateral diffusion coefficients, please refer to Johnson et al. [8].

Note that lateral diffusion/lateral spread does not involve diffusing between different phases [8].

Meanwhile, skin penetration directly down from the central application site through the bilayers of the SC then through the layers of skin occurs simultaneously (Fig. 13.1).

Factors Affecting Lateral Spread

Molecular Weight

In 1996, lateral diffusion of several small organic compound-fluorescent probes in human SC extract (from human cadaver skin from the back, chest, and abdomen) was investigated by Johnson et al., and lateral diffusion coefficients were calculated. Results showed a decrease in diffusion coefficients with increasing probe molecular weight (MW) [7]. In 2012, Gee et al. compared caffeine (MW 194.19 g/mol), ibuprofen (MW 206.28 g/mol), and hydrocortisone (MW 362.46 g/mol) and found differences in lateral spread: by 3 min after application, caffeine and ibuprofen (with similar MW) had already demonstrated wider lateral spread than hydrocortisone (with a much higher MW) [6].

Time

Vieille-Petit et al. [4] applied a 10% urea in water solution to in vitro abdominal human skin, collected no later than 24 h after death, and noticed a 90.4% recovery rate at the 5 cm² application site after 1 h, versus a 79.6% recovery rate after 6 h.

Why is there less urea remaining at the site of application after 6 h than after 1 h? The cause is lateral spread and not percutaneous absorption as less than 1% of urea penetrated forearm skin in vivo in man [2]. Thus, lateral spread is time dependent.

Time-Dependent Redistribution

Redistribution of drug/chemical concentration can happen over time which alters drug or chemical concentrations at any one site. In 2004, Schicksnus and Muller-Goymann applied a 5% ibuprofen cream (crème) in vitro to human abdominal surgery clippings and measured the drug concentration below the application site and in the surrounding skin. Results showed lateral spread and time-dependent changes in drug concentration at different areas. Initially, the central area (cream applied) had the highest ibuprofen concentration, the areas alongside the central area had lower drug concentration, and there was little drug in the outer areas. However, later on, after the central area drug concentration reached a maximum, from then on, a redistribution of ibuprofen was observed, resulting in a decline of drug concentration in the central area, while the outer areas continued to show an increase in drug concentration [9].

The following figure of ibuprofen amount per skin area at the central area of drug application (0 mm) and at 4 mm, 6 mm, and 8.5 mm from the central site describes the varying drug concentrations at each area during a drug accumulation phase (at 1.3–4.3 h) and a drug redistribution phase (at 5–6.3 h). Redistribution over time as lateral spread happens is evident (Fig. 13.2).

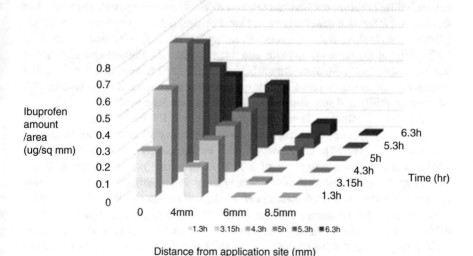

Fig. 13.2 Lateral diffusion of ibuprofen over time

An in vivo study in humans by Gee et al. [13] using an ibuprofen 5% w/v etha-nolic solution also demonstrated the time dependency of lateral spread and depth of penetration. Eight participants (4M, 4F) aged 24–29 years with no history of skin disease participated in a 6 h study. Standard doses of ibuprofen solution (1.8 µL) were applied to participants' left and right flexor forearms, and the appli-cation sites were tape stripped either at 3 min, 3 h, or 6 h after application, using one application site per time point per participant for tape stripping. (Application sites were left unoccluded and participants wore short-sleeve clothing to minimize the potential of transfer and drug loss.) Tape stripping was done using concentric tape of known diameter, and the amount of ibuprofen adhering to the adhesive tape was determined by HPLC with a limit of quantification of 0.5 ng. The amount of SC protein removed by tape stripping was also quantified and used to normalize the amount of ibuprofen, in order to minimize intersubject variability. Normalized drug amounts representing ibuprofen recovery at 3 min, 3 h, and 6 h were pre-sented as percentage of the initial dose. The distance of surface lateral spread was measured as between 0–4 mm, 4–8 mm, 8–12 mm, and 12–16 mm. Results showed rapid surface lateral spread to about 12 mm which was evident at 3 min, with simi-lar spread but deeper penetration at 3 h, and less spread and less depth at 6 h. Additional evaluations in the same study using other formulations are discussed later [13].

Physicochemical Properties

In 2012, Gee et al. compared the extent of lateral spread for caffeine vs. hydrocorti-sone vs. ibuprofen—three substances with very different physicochemical proper-ties including partition coefficients (P) and MW (discussed earlier). Ibuprofen has an ideal log P for skin penetration (3.51) and formed a deep (penetration) and wide (lateral spread) drug reservoir soon after application [13]. Caffeine is the most hydrophilic of the three compounds and demonstrated the highest spreadability of the three, seen on the SC skin surface both at 3 min and 3 h later. Gee surmised that this may relate to the moisture (i.e., aqueous) layer formed on the skin surface [13, 14]. Spreadability and spreading behavior is discussed later [15].

Jacobi et al. studied lateral spread using the UV-filter substances butyl methoxydibenzoyl-methane (BMM) and 4-methylbenzylidene camphor (4-MC) in o/w emulsions [16, 17]. They studied both substances in 2004 and focused on BMM at a higher concentration of 3.72% in the same o/w emulsion in 2011. Spreading of both substances took place mainly on the surface of the SC. It was unusual that they noted no differences in the lateral spreading and distribution between the two substances, since BMM is more polar and lipophilic than 4-MC. They surmised that the emulsion (or some of its components) might be mainly responsible for the transport/movement of these two substances within the SC and on its surface [17]. Later researchers have identified formulation as a factor as discussed below.

Formulation

As mentioned earlier, the lateral spread of clobetasol 17-propionate was quantified and compared for two formulations: propylene glycol (PG) and di-*n*-butyl adipate (BA) [3]. This was an in vivo human study where 6 square test areas were mapped out on the upper back of ten normal male volunteers. PG-based ointment was applied to three test areas and BA-based ointment applied to the other three sites. Radioactive samples of tritium-labeled clobetasol 17-propionate (dose = 12 MBq/g ointment over 1.5 cm^2 test area) were spread evenly over each test area; then test sites were protected by applying a small Perspex box to ensure no rub or loss of drug due to touching.

Eight hours after application, the protective coverings were removed and five successive skin surface biopsies were taken from each of the six sites of application and from each of six immediately adjacent sites (with the immediately adjacent sites each having one lateral edge approximately 1 mm from the lateral edge of the marked site of application). Radioactivity of the biopsy samples was prepared using an identical procedure for all samples, and any radioactive ointment adhering to the Perspex boxes was recovered again using an identical procedure for all samples.

The radioactive label applied per volunteer was approximately 0.9 MBq. Twenty-eight test sites were assessed for each ointment (two covers were dislodged and measurements not taken). Differences in radioactivity were seen in the test areas versus the adjacent sites and between the five SC layers. In the test areas, differences were seen between the five SC layers: the radioactivity levels for both PG and BA ointments were similar in the two outermost SC layers; however, in the inner three layers, the radioactivity levels of the PG ointments were significantly higher. The *reverse* was seen in the areas adjacent to the test sites, as follows: even though the mean radioactivity levels were generally less than 10% at each site, the BA ointment formulation gave significantly higher radioactivity levels than the PG formulation in the three outermost SC layers ($p < 0.0002$), with no significant difference seen in the inner two layers [3].

Lateral spread was evident for both ointments, as 5–12% had spread out from the application site after 8 h. Formulation differences led to (1) greater lateral spread for the BA formulation, accounting for the increased radioactivity level in the upper three SC layers in the adjacent area, and (2) greater inward diffusion/percutaneous penetration for the PG formulation, accounting for the increased radioactivity in the inner three layers of the test site. The lower viscosity of BA likely accounted for the greater lateral spread of clobetasol 17-propionate in this ointment base as compared to the PG base [3].

The 2014 study by Gee et al. (described in section "Time-Dependent Redistribution" as showing time dependency of lateral spread) not only looked at ibuprofen over time but also compared the ibuprofen ethanolic solution alone versus ibuprofen + PG + PEG200 versus ibuprofen + octisalate (OS) versus ibuprofen + PG + PEG200 + OS. Ibuprofen applied alone or together with OS undergoes lateral diffusion within the SC relatively rapidly and spreads to a higher degree than when applied in formulations containing PG and PEG200 [13].

Viscosity

Is viscosity the reason accounting for the difference in lateral spread in the clobeta-sol 17-propionate study discussed in the section "Formulation" above? A recent study [15] compared five o/w emulsions, with the oil phase consisting of varying percentages of isohexadecane (IHD) and stearic acid (SA) from 0 to 20%, holding all other components constant (in the oil phase, aqueous phase, and preservatives). Emulsions with IHD are less viscous than those with SA as demonstrated by differences in flow and viscoelastic properties analyzed using a stress-controlled rheometer, with the emulsion with 20% IHD/0% SA being least viscous and 0% IHD/20% SA being most viscous. The spreading behavior of the emulsions was assessed by 18 expert women assessors focusing on the "ease of spreading" attribute with a protocol designed to mimic the spreading speed of skin care products. Emulsions with IHD have higher ease of spreading, with 20% IHD/0% SA being highest and 0% IHD/20% SA being lowest [15].

Skin Surface Topography

Skin surface topography can affect the degree of lateral spread: primary furrow networks such as fingerprints and palm prints can function as pathways for lateral spreading. This was confirmed by Jacobi et al. [16] using scanning microscopy and photography using dye to show lateral spreading. However, follicles and wrinkles can be reservoirs for drugs or chemicals and retard lateral spreading. This was also confirmed by Jacobi et al. using scanning microscopy and photography which showed dye in follicle orifices with a reduced amount of dye in the surrounding area—both at 1 h and 24 h after application—the remaining dye in the follicle orifices at 24 h was faint but still noticeable [16]. Not much else is known about lateral spread in follicles and wrinkles.

Anatomical Sites

The skin site of application may be a factor in lateral spread. Although there appears to be no significant difference in lateral spread between forearm and back [16], however, little is known about other anatomical sites.

Natural Lateral Spread Phenomena

Lateral spread happens with natural substances such as cholesterol too (i.e., non-drug and nonchemical), which is consistent with the free volume theory. In 1992, Almeida et al. investigated the diffusion process of dimyristoylphosphatidylcholine (DMPC)/cholesterol mixtures using prepared lipid multibilayers to simulate the stratum corneum [5]. This *in vitro* study used various molar ratios of DMPC/cholesterol at temperatures between 22 and 58 °C. They found that cholesterol concentrations reach a critical mass/concentration that fills up the small free volumes, followed by area expansion in the plane of the bilayer. In other words, the free volume is saturable. When this free area is occupied, accommodation of more cholesterol is only possible by a lateral expansion of the lipid bilayer [5].

In more detail, when cholesterol is added (to the Ld phase) beyond the concentration which saturates the small free volumes, a transition occurs, from the disordered to the ordered phase. The free volume in the bilayer is reduced, and consequently the fraction of *trans* conformers in the acyl chain of the phospholipid molecules is increased. Each cholesterol molecule spans only one of the two monolayers as do the phospholipid molecules. Adding more cholesterol results now in an expansion in the plane of the bilayer and in better packing, i.e., a more ordered structure [5].

Summary and Future Needs

Knowledge-wise, we have some understanding of lateral spread and some information about various factors affecting lateral spread as discussed above. There is *in vitro* and *in vivo* research, and it is generally assumed for *in vitro* penetration studies that the area in the *in vitro* chamber (as stated in ug or mg/cm^2) is representative of the *in vivo* situation. Furthermore, it is also assumed that a small sample (as may be used in the studies) would be representative of a larger sample (e.g. the size of the skin area).

However, we need more data on anatomical site differences in lateral spread as we have but one observation so far. More data on rheology, viscosity, etc. and the types of vehicles and formulations are also needed. Vehicle formats and vehicle ingredients, which clearly affect percutaneous penetration, require additional study with respect to the competing effect of lateral spread. In addition, even though there is some information, more data on the effects of physicochemical properties on lateral spread, such as MW, solubility, charge, pKa, hydrophilicity, partition coefficients, possibly hydrogen bonding, and even substantivity, will be useful. Additional research on the likelihood of further spread in the epidermis, dermis, subcutaneous fat, and deep tissue would enhance our understanding of this phenomenon. Furthermore, research into the clinical effects of lateral spread - with respect to systemic absorption, efficacy and toxicity - would enhance our understanding of the consequences of lateral spread.

Practically, we should be aware that lateral spread happens, and the lengthier the time from the time of application, the greater the effect of lateral spread, resulting in less and less drug or chemical remaining at the site of application for percutaneous absorption. We believe that taking lateral spread into account will enhance the quality of the interpretation of toxicologic and pharmacologic studies, including in the determination of bioequivalence.

Conclusions

In conclusion, why is lateral spread of relevance to percutaneous penetration?

1. It may result in less drug or chemical being absorbed systemically, potentially reducing bioavailability.
2. It may reduce the rate of absorption of drug or chemical, potentially prolonging the onset of action.
3. It may result in less drug or chemical remaining at the original site of application. This may affect the accuracy of quantification studies of the drug or chemical's penetration into skin.
4. It may be a key factor in determining bioequivalence between innovator and generic topical formulations.
5. Percutaneous penetration research of drugs or chemicals should incorporate a "correction factor" to estimate the effect of lateral spread on the results of quantitation studies.

Author Contributions Rebecca Law performed the literature search, wrote the manuscript, drew the figures, and critically reviewed the manuscript multiple times. Howard Maibach reviewed the references, provided insightful input and comments, and critically reviewed the manuscript multiple times.

Declaration of Conflict of Interest Rebecca Law and Howard Maibach declare that they have no conflict of interest.

Funding This research did not receive any specific grant from funding agencies in the public, commercial, or not-for-profit sectors.

References

1. Law RM, Ngo M, Maibach HI. Twenty clinically relevant factors/observations for percutaneous absorption in humans. Am J Clin Dermatol. 2020;21(1):85–95. https://doi.org/10.1007/s40257-019-00480-4.
2. Feldman RJ, Maibach HI. Absorption of some organic compounds through the skin in man. J Investig Dermatol. 1970;54:399–404.
3. Ashworth J, Watson WS, Finlay AY. The lateral spread of clobetasol 17-propionate in the stratum corneum in vivo. Br J Dermatol. 1988;119:351–8.
4. Vieille-Petit A, Blickenstaff N, Coman G, Maibach H. Metrics and clinical relevance of percutaneous penetration and lateral spreading. Skin Pharmacol Physiol. 2015;28:57–64.
5. Almeida PFF, Vaz WLC, Thompson TE. Lateral diffusion in the liquid-phases of dimyristoylphosphatidylcholine/cholesterol lipid bilayers—a free-volume analysis. Biochemistry. 1992;31(29):6739–47.
6. Gee CM, Nicolazzo JA, Watkinson AC, Finnin BC. Assessment of the lateral diffusion and penetration of topically applied drugs in humans using a novel concentric tape stripping design. Pharm Res. 2012;29(8):2035–46.

7. Johnson ME, Berk DA, Blankschtein D, et al. Lateral diffusion of small compounds in human stratum corneum and model lipid bilayer systems. Biophys J. 1996;71(5):2656–68.
8. Johnson ME, Blankschtein D, Langer R. Evaluation of solute permeation through the stratum corneum: lateral bilayer diffusion as the primary transport mechanism. J Pharm Sci. 1997;86(10):1162–72.
9. Schicksnus G, Muller-Goymann CC. Lateral diffusion of ibuprofen in human skin during permeation studies. Skin Pharmacol Physiol. 2004;17:84–90.
10. Lieb WR, Stein WD. Non-Stokesian nature of transverse diffusion within human red-cell membranes. J Membr Biol. 1986;92(2):111–9.
11. Torre D. Understanding the relationship between lateral spread of freeze and depth of freeze. J Dermatol Surg Oncol. 1979;5(1):51–3.
12. Kanno Y, Koshita S, Ogawa T, et al. Peroral cholangioscopy by SpyGlass DS versus CHF-B260 for evaluation of the lateral spread of extrahepatic cholangiocarcinoma. Endosc Int Open. 2018;6(11):E1349–54. https://doi.org/10.1055/a-0743-5283.
13. Gee CM, Watkinson AC, Nicolazzo JA, Finnin BC. The effect of formulation excipients on the penetration and lateral diffusion of ibuprofen on and within the stratum corneum following topical application to humans. J Pharm Sci. 2014;103:909–19.
14. Gloor M, Willebrandt U, Thomer G, et al. Water content of the horny layer and skin surface lipids. Arch Dermatol Res. 1980;268(2):221–3.
15. Gore E, Picard C, Geraldine S. Complementary approaches to understand the spreading behaviour on skin of O/W emulsions containing different emollients. Colloids Surf B Biointerfaces. 2020;193:111132. https://doi.org/10.1016/j.colsurfb.2020.111132.
16. Jacobi U, Schanzer S, Weigmann H-J, et al. Pathways of lateral spreading. Skin Pharmacol Physiol. 2011;24:231–7.
17. Jacobi U, Weigmann H-J, Baumann M, et al. Lateral spreading of topically applied UV filter substances investigated by tape stripping. Skin Pharmacol Physiol. 2004;17(1):17–22.

Chapter 14
Regional Variation in Percutaneous Absorption: Evidence from In Vitro Human Models

Aileen M. Feschuk, Nadia Kashetsky, Chavy Chiang, Anuk Burli, Halie Burdick, and Howard I. Maibach

Introduction

Percutaneous absorption can be defined as the passage of a topically applied substance into the bloodstream [1]. This may occur via the transepidermal pathway, which is diffusion across skin layers, or the appendageal pathway, which is entry through hair follicles or sweat ducts [2]. Percutaneous absorption is of importance given its role in topical medicaments, transdermal drug systems, and dermatotoxicology [3–8]. The importance of percutaneous absorption is not a new concept. For instance, dermally penetrating agents were used in both the First World War (e.g., phosgene, sulfur mustard, and lewisites) and the Second World War (e.g., hydrogen cyanide gas) [9]. However, there is evolving evidence for its role in cosmetics, lotions, and sunscreens and occupational chemical exposure evaluation [10–18].

Law et al. [19] identified over 20 factors which influence percutaneous absorption, including skin application sites, and skin appendages such as hair follicles and glands. The importance of considering the anatomical site of exposure when assessing percutaneous absorption is well established. This is because contaminants may be absorbed differently depending on the anatomical site of contact [20]. In fact, the European Food Safety Authority (EFSA) has "site of application" on their list of

A. M. Feschuk (✉) · N. Kashetsky
Faculty of Medicine, Memorial University of Newfoundland, St. John's, NL, Canada
e-mail: amfeschuk@mun.ca

C. Chiang · A. Burli
School of Medicine and Dentistry, University of Rochester, Rochester, NY, USA

H. Burdick
University of South Dakota Sanford School of Medicine, Sioux Falls, SD, USA

H. I. Maibach
Department of Dermatology, University of California San Francisco, San Francisco, CA, USA

© The Author(s), under exclusive license to Springer Nature Switzerland AG 2022
A. M. Feschuk et al. (eds.), *Dermal Absorption and Decontamination*, https://doi.org/10.1007/978-3-031-09222-0_14

"minimum information on dermal absorption studies to be presented in assessment reports" [21]. The presence and importance of regional variation in percutaneous absorption has also been acknowledged by public health agencies other than the EFSA and EPA, including the Organisation for Economic Co-operation and Development (OECD) and the World Health Organization (WHO) [22, 23].

Regional variation in hair follicle density is a commonly postulated basis underlying regional variation in percutaneous absorption. First, hair follicles contribute to an increased surface area of skin available for drug absorption [19]. Illel et al. [24] noted that hair follicles play an important role in percutaneous absorption. Lademann et al. [25] demonstrated that hair follicles provide an efficient pathway for absorption of topically applied substances in addition to intercellular route. The storage reservoir capacity of the hair follicle is tenfold longer than that of the stratum corneum [26]. The density of hair follicles differs depending upon the anatomical location [27]. For example, there is a high density of small hair follicles on the forehead, while there is a small density of larger follicles in the lower leg [27]. It is of interest that Otberg et al. [28] showed that hair follicles are considered weak spots in providing protection against hydrophilic drugs and thus enable rapid delivery of topically administered drugs. Indeed, nanotechnological approaches to delivering drugs to the hair follicles, and subsequent rapid absorption via percutaneous absorption, is used to treat alopecia and acne [29–32].

In addition to hair follicle density, some other factors postulated to yield regional variation of percutaneous absorption include the thickness of the stratum corneum, which is the outermost layer of the epidermis and is considered the main barrier to absorption [21]. The density of sweat and sebaceous glands can influence dermal absorption as well [21]. Additionally, areas with richer blood supplies are generally more permeable [19]. In fact, some penetrants may not penetrate through the entire scalp, but rather are absorbed into the bloodstream just below the hair follicles [33], and this should be taken into consideration when conducting in vitro percutaneous absorption experiments.

Studies investigating regional variation in percutaneous absorption in humans in vivo were summarized by Bormann and Maibach [34]. However, there is little known regarding regional variation in percutaneous absorption in humans in vitro. Hence, the aim of this review was to summarize and analyze existing data on this important topic of regional variation in percutaneous absorption in in vitro human models.

The first in vitro model for skin penetration was developed in the 1940s (in response to chemical warfare during the Second World War), and it greatly resembles contemporary static and flow-through diffusion cells [35]. The static diffusion cell, also known as the Franz diffusion cell [36], has been extensively used since 1975 [35], and the flow-through diffusion cell has been used since the mid-1980s [35, 37]. The flow-through apparatus mimics the vascularization of the skin because the continuous flow of the receptor chamber removes penetrant once it has permeated [35, 37]. However, the flow-through system is also more expensive and more technically challenging than the static diffusion system [35].

The two most commonly used methods to evaluate percutaneous absorption in in vitro models are the finite method and infinite method [20, 38]. The finite method involves mounting skin in the donor chamber of a diffusion cell and bathing it in receptor fluid with known amount of the chemical [20, 38]. The amount of chemical is then measured in the receiving chamber to indicate the amount penetrated [20, 38]. The infinite dosing technique involves mounting skin between two chambers of fluid, and a large of chemical in an aqueous solution is added to one side [20, 38]. Penetration is quantified by determining the concentration of the penetrant in the receptor fluid, as a function of time [20, 38]. Sampling of the receptor fluid is continued until steady state is reached [20, 38].

Infinite dosing is the more commonly used method of the two [20], and because it provides continuous replacement medium necessary to maintain physiological conditions, it is recommended for metabolism studies [37]. However, a major limitation of infinite dosing is that it does not mimic the common situation in which a penetrant would be encountered, where a relatively small amount (a finite dose) of the penetrant is in contact with the skin [38]. A drawback of finite dosing includes that it can result in "pseudo steady-state" where the amount penetrated is transiently linear and then plateaus [38]. Beyond the plateau, the amount penetrated remains constant due to depletion of the penetrant [38]. An additional drawback of finite dosing methodology includes that applying small finite doses evenly across the skin is difficult [38]. The bioavailability of penetrants applied in finite doses is dependent on the amount of penetrant applied per unit area, and therefore, even distribution over the whole area is necessary to minimize variation in results [38].

Theoretical models are used to describe transport of a penetrant through the skin and are recognized as highly important for estimating exposure levels [23]. Flux is defined as "the amount of material crossing a defined area in a set time," and chemicals with higher dermal flux are absorbed more readily than those with lower flux [21]. The lag time is defined as "the time taken for the absorption of a chemical across the skin to reach a linear flux" [21]. Lag time can be obtained by taking the line of linear flux on an absorption: time plot and extrapolating back to X-intercept [21]. Therefore, lag time is a function of flux, making them good parameters for comparison. Flux and lag time are important for predicting absorption based on a set of circumstances. For example, a short exposure to a substance with a short lag time and medium flux can result in higher total absorption than a short period of exposure to a compound with a higher maximal flux but a longer lag time [39]. Additionally, knowledge of lag time is important because if sampling is performed quickly following exposure to a substance with a long lag time, it may appear like the substance does not penetrate the skin at all [39].

Methods

This systematic review follows guidelines outlined by the Preferred Reporting Items for Systematic Reviews and Meta-Analyses (PRISMA) [40].

Search Strategy

A literature search utilizing Embase, PubMed, and Web of Science databases was conducted in May 2021. The search strategy employed was as follows: ("percutaneous absorption" or "percutaneous penetration" or "dermal absorption" or "dermal penetration" or "skin absorption" or "skin penetration") and ("regional difference" or "regional variation" or "regional location" or "anatomical location" or "anatomical variation" or "anatomy" or "anatomical site" or "anatomical region" or "body site" or "body location"). Temporal, geographical, and/or language filters were not applied. An additional search of the patent literature was performed in January 2022 using uspto.gov. The search terms "transdermal" and "regional variation" were used.

Eligibility

Articles were considered eligible for inclusion if these (1) included quantitative data on regional differences in percutaneous absorption, (2) included human in vitro study models, and (3) were written in English. Articles containing quantitative data on regional differences in percutaneous absorption in vivo were excluded, as these were already summarized within a year prior to writing this manuscript [34].

Data Screening

Title/abstract screening was completed by two independent researchers (A.F. and H.I.M.). Full-text review was completed independently by two researchers (A.F., N.K.) and conflicts resolved by a third (H.I.M.). Relevant article references were manually searched to identify any additional studies that fit inclusion criteria.

Data Extraction and Analysis

Data extractions were completed by five independent researchers (A.F., N.K., C.C., A.B., H.B.) and verified by one independent researcher (H.I.M). Data on (1) study characteristics, (2) human skin samples, (3) test chemicals and physicochemical properties, (4) amount of test chemical, (5) method of application, (6) method of analyzing results, and (7) main results and conclusions were collected, summarized, and analyzed.

Results

Study Characteristics

Title and abstract screening of 524 studies, followed by full-text review of 73 investigations, yielded 8 studies that fit inclusion criteria (Fig. 14.1). Between the 8 studies, a total of 15 anatomical regions were investigated. These anatomical regions and the number of studies in which they were investigated are as follows: abdomen (6), scalp (5), scrotum (2), breast (2), upper arm (1), palm (1), dorsum of hand (1), cheek (1), neck (1), torso (unspecified) (1), back (1), inguinal region (1), thigh (1), lower leg (1), foot (1). Further study characteristics can be visualized in Table 14.1.

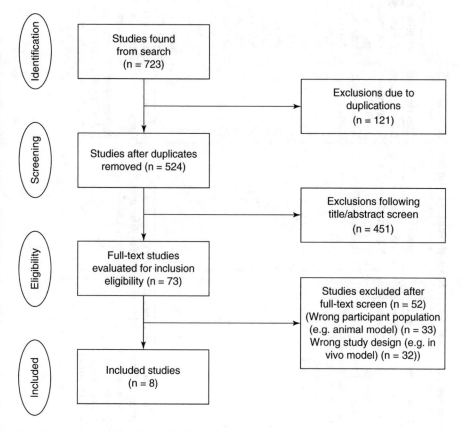

Fig. 14.1 Method of identifying eligible studies

Table 14.1 Summary of study characteristics, methodologies, and results of included studies

Author (year)	Sample size	In vitro model	Anatomical region	Chemical	Chemical class	Percutaneous absorption analysis	Results summary
Smith et al. [41]	NR	Male Caucasian skin samples collected during autopsies (excess fat, subcutaneous tissue, and long protruding hairs were removed)	Abdomen and scrotum	1. Water vapor 2. 5% Salicylic acid in lanolin 3. Hydrogen sulfide	1. Nontoxic gas 2. Keratolytic emollient 3. Flammable, toxic gas	1. Electric hygrometer was sealed to the epidermal side of the sample and detected any water vapor escaping from the epidermal surface 2. Dilute ferric chloride was used as an indicator for the penetration of salicylic acid 3. Lead acetate paper was sealed over the dermal side of the chamber and used to detect the presence of hydrogen sulfide	All the three experiments concluded that scrotal skin is a much less effective barrier than abdominal skin
Ritschel et al. [42]	$n = 5$	Skin samples collected from human cadavers (subcutaneous fat and hypodermis were removed)	Abdomen and scalp	1. ^{14}C-coumarin 2. ^{3}H-griseofulvin 3. ^{3}H-propranolol	Radiolabeled drugs 1. Anticoagulant 2. Antifungal 3. Beta-blocker	Measured using a liquid scintillation counter and steady-state flux, lag times, diffusion coefficients, and permeability of the test drugs calculated	Higher permeation levels in the scalp versus abdomen skin

| Harada et al. [43] | $n = 17$ | Skin samples obtained from surgery (subcutaneous fat was removed) | Cheek, neck, back, lower leg, foot, sole, scrotum, inguinal, thigh, and breast | Salicylic acid | Keratolytic | Receiver fluid samples were analyzed using fluorescence spectrophotometry and penetration rate estimated using cumulative amount of chemical reaching the receiver and time | Least to greatest penetration of salicylic acid: sole, back, breast, lower leg, foot, thigh, inguinal, neck, cheek, and scrotum |
| Ogiso et al. [44] | NR | Skin samples obtained from Japanese men and women (aged 23–60) (hair was trimmed off of scalp skin; adherent fat and visceral materials were removed) | Abdomen and scalp | 1. Ketoprofen 2. Melatonin 3. Fluorouracil 4. Acyclovir | Drugs 1. Nonsteroidal anti-inflammatory 2. Lipophilic hormone 3. Antimetabolite 4. Synthetic nucleoside analogue (antiviral) | Receiver fluid samples analyzed using liquid chromatography and penetration rate, skin/vehicle partition coefficient of the drug, diffusion constant within the skin, and lag time were calculated | Higher permeation in the scalp versus abdomen skin |

(continued)

Table 14.1 (continued)

Author (year)	Sample size	In vitro model	Anatomical region	Chemical	Chemical class	Percutaneous absorption analysis	Results summary
Schmitt et al. [45]	$n = 22$	Skin samples from Caucasian females were taken during plastic surgery (subcutaneous fat was removed)	Upper arm, breast, and abdomen	α-Pinene β-Pinene β-Myrcene Limonene Phenylethanol Linalool *Trans*-rose oxidase *Cis*-rose oxidase Isomenthone β-Citronellol Geraniol Eugenol Methyleugenol	Components of essential rose oil	Acceptor fluid samples analyzed using gas chromatography and steady-state flux, apparent permeability coefficients, and lag times were calculated	The permeability coefficient of abdominal skin was greater than that of upper arm skin for linalool and eugenol, but less than that of upper arm skin for β-myrcene, *trans*-rose oxide, and *cis*-rose oxide. Breast skin had a significantly greater permeability coefficient for linalool than the upper arm. Abdominal skin had a significantly greater permeability coefficient than breast skin for β-pinene and *cis*-rose oxidase. The upper arm skin displayed the greatest lag time for all 13 substances. Breast skin displayed the smallest lag time for each of the 13 substances with the exception of eugenol. Abdominal skin showed the greatest lag time for eugenol

	n	Skin	Site	Compound	Category	Method	Findings
Rolland et al. [46]	n = 11	Skin samples of males and females (aged 23–63) collected during surgery	Abdomen and scalp	VX	Chemical warfare agent	VX equivalents (the sum of VX and its active metabolites) were determined using an enzymatic method, and cholinesterase activity was measured using a microplate reader. The calibration curve determined the VXeq in samples. Maximal flux and lag times were calculated	Faster permeation through scalp skin approximately versus abdominal skin
Trabaris et al. [47]	n = 72	Full thickness human cadaver skin sections	Scalp, palm, torso, and dorsal hand	Dichloroacetonitrile (DCAN), chloral hydrate (CH), trichloroacetonitrile (TCAN), dibromoacetonitrile (DBAN), bromochloroacetonitrile (BCAN), and chloroacetonitrile (CAN)	Disinfection by-products	Dermal flux through the skin samples in diffusion cells by gas chromatography	Increased permeability in the dorsal hand and torso skin versus the palm due to increased thickness in the stratum corneum in the palm and scalp
Elmahdy et al. [48]	n = 54	Skin samples taken from male and female cadavers (aged 18–76) and dermatomed to 600 ± 50 µm	Abdomen and scalp	Dipropylene glycol monomethyl ether (DPGME), diisopropyl methylphosphonate (DIMP), methyl salicylate (MeS)	C-14 Chemical warfare simulants	Receiver fluid samples were assayed for C-14 test penetrant using a liquid scintillation counter	Scalp skin displayed greater total skin absorption than abdominal skin

NR not reported

Study Results

Study 1: Smith et al. (1961)

Smith et al. [41] conducted three experiments investigating regional variation in percutaneous absorption. Experiment A examined differences in diffusion of water vapor through abdominal versus scrotal skin. Skin samples from 5 white males between the ages of 55 and 72 years (sample size $n = 5$) were collected during autopsies. Skin was cut into pieces of approximately 2.5 cm², and excess fat, subcutaneous tissue, and long protruding hairs were removed. Samples were placed over an aperture consisting of a plastic chamber containing physiological saline. An electric hygrometer was sealed to the epidermal side of the sample and detected any water vapor escaping from the epidermal surface.

Experiment B investigated the permeability of scrotal and abdominal skin, taken from two autopsies, to 5% salicylic acid in lanolin which was added to the epidermal surface, and the samples were then incubated in a desiccator at 35 °C. Dilute ferric chloride was used as an indicator for penetration of salicylic acid, measured at 15, 30, 60, and 120 min.

Experiment C examined the permeability of scrotal and abdominal skin to hydrogen sulfide. Lead acetate paper was sealed over the dermal side of the chamber and employed to detect hydrogen sulfide presence. The lead acetate paper was left for 8 min before removal.

Experiment A found that the average water vapor diffusion rates of scrotal skin varied between 1.6- and 22.1-fold higher than abdominal skin, with a mean of 7.4. Experiment B demonstrated that salicylic acid penetrated into the dermis within 15 min (identified by the color change of the ferric chloride indicator), while abdominal skin was not penetrated prior to 2 h postexposure. Results of Experiment C were measured qualitatively by inspection of the lead acetate paper. Scrotal skin enabled greater darkening of the lead acetate paper, indicating increased hydrogen sulfide gas penetration compared to abdominal skin. Overall, Smith et al. [41] concluded that scrotal skin is a markedly less effective barrier than abdominal skin, despite a lack of apparent histological differences found between the epidermis of the two anatomical sites. However, Smith et al. [41] did not comment on differences in hair follicle density between the two areas. This may be because it was previously assumed that stratum corneum layer was the diffusion limiting factor, whereas the hypothesis that hair follicles play a greater role was not applied in 1961 [48].

Study 2: Ritschel et al. (1989)

Ritschel et al. [42] studied the percutaneous penetration of three radiolabeled drugs, ^{14}C-coumarin, ^{3}H-griseofulvin, and ^{3}H-propranolol, and examined differences between various anatomical regions. Skin was taken from the scalp and abdomen of human cadavers (sample size $n = 5$), and subcutaneous fat and hypodermis were removed. Circular sections of skin with a diameter of 2 cm were placed in the glass diffusion cells of a Thomas diffusion cell apparatus. Then, 200 µL drug solution in phosphate buffer (pH 7.4) was applied to the stratum corneum. Five mL pH 7.4 phosphate buffer comprised the receptor fluid. Two hundred µL receptor fluid was collected periodically over 48 h (and immediately replaced with 200 µL buffer solution). Percutaneous absorption was measured using a liquid scintillation counter and steady-state flux, lag times, diffusion coefficients, and permeability of the test drugs calculated. Permeation parameters were obtained by plotting the cumulative amount of substance penetrated per cm^2 versus time (i.e., the steady-state flux was obtained from the slope of these plots, the lag time was the intercepts of the plots, the permeability constant was the steady-state flux divided by the initial concentration, and the diffusion coefficient was the membrane thickness squared, divided by 6 times the lag time).

For abdominal skin, steady-state flux measured in ng/cm²/h for abdominal skin was 130.0 ± 78.2, 10.4 ± 6.1, and 30.4 ± 6.3 for coumarin, griseofulvin, and propranolol, respectively. Steady-state flux through scalp skin was 172.4 ± 64.0, 15.5 ± 7.7, and 42.5 ± 11.0. for coumarin, griseofulvin, and propranolol, respectively. There were significant differences between absorption of coumarin and propranolol in abdominal skin vs. scalp skin. Permeability constants of coumarin, griseofulvin, and propranolol, measured in cm/h for abdominal skin, were 9.1×10^{-3}, 1.3×10^{-3}, and 1.2×10^{-3}, respectively. Permeability constants of coumarin, griseofulvin, and propranolol, measured in cm/h for scalp skin, were 12.05×10^{-3}, 1.94×10^{-3}, and 1.7×10^{-3}, respectively. Therefore, there were no significant differences in permeability constants of the scalp and abdomen. Ritschel et al. [42] noted that the fractional increase in flux from abdominal skin to scalp skin was not constant between the three chemicals (49% for griseofulvin, 40% for propranolol, and 32% for coumarin). Data demonstrated that a potential explanation for higher permeation levels in the scalp is that percutaneous absorption occurs through the pilosebaceous unit rather than through the epidermis. Scalp has more sebaceous glands and follicles than abdominal skin.

Study 3: Harada et al. (1993)

Harada et al. [43] studied the permeability of salicylic acid in in vitro human skin samples of various anatomical regions obtained from surgery (total sample size: $n = 17$; $n = 1$ for cheek, neck, back, lower leg, foot, sole, and scrotum, each; $n = 2$ for inguinal; $n = 3$ for thigh, $n = 5$ for breast). A 0.785 cm^2 circular area of skin mounted on a Franz-type diffusion cell was exposed to 1 mL test solution, equating 500 µg salicylic acid. Fifty µL samples were regularly taken from the receiver cell and replaced with fresh solution over 72 h. Receiver fluid samples were analyzed for salicylic acid content using fluorescence spectrophotometry. Penetration rate was then estimated by plotting the cumulative amount of salicylic acid reaching the receiver against time. In addition, salicylic acid penetration rate through shed snakeskin was determined and utilized as a comparative reference to report human skin penetration rates.

The mean ± standard error of mean salicylic acid penetration from a solution with a pH of 4 through human neck and human breast skin measured 1.97 (only one sample tested) and 0.37 ± 0.09, respectively. Penetration rates of the remaining skin sites were only reported as relative to that of shed snakeskin, and data showed that skin sites yielding least to greatest penetration of salicylic acid were the sole (penetration not detected), back at 1.1×, breast at 1.3×, lower leg at 1.4×, foot at 1.7×, thigh at 1.8×, inguinal at 4.4×, neck at 6.5×, cheek at 7.5×, and scrotum at 60× that of snakeskin.

Study 4: Ogiso et al. (2002)

Ogiso et al. [44] documented in vitro penetration of lipophilic drugs, melatonin (MT) and ketoprofen (KP), and hydrophilic drug, 5-fluorouracil (5FU), through human scalp or abdominal skin samples obtained from Japanese men and women [total sample size not reported (NR); sample size: $n = 3$–14 skin samples per penetration protocol × 3 drugs × 2 anatomical regions]. Skin thickness was not reported. Drugs were dissolved in a mixture of propylene glycol and ethanol, along with distilled water and gentamicin solution, yielding a 1.78% drug in solution concentration. Skin samples were mounted in a Franz diffusion cell, and 0.5 mL of liquid formulation was loaded onto the stratum corneum. Receptor fluid was periodically collected over 32 h for scalp skin and 52 h for abdominal skin and immediately replaced with fresh solution. Drug content in collected solutions was determined by liquid chromatography.

Mean ± standard deviation of MT and 5FU fluxes through scalp skin, measuring 6.79 ± 4.98 and 19.16 ± 14.18 μg/h × cm², respectively, were significantly higher at 27- and 48-fold that through abdominal skin, which measured 0.34 ± 0.17 and 0.40 ± 1.16 μg/h × cm², respectively. Conversely, mean KP flux through scalp skin, measuring 43.62 ± 14.65 μg/h × cm², was only 1.5-fold higher and not significantly more compared to that through abdominal skin, which measured 29.01 ± 10.32 μg/h × cm². However, mean lag time of KP diffusing through the scalp was significantly shorter than that of abdominal skin, measuring 5.98 ± 1.28 and 17.93 ± 5.7 h, respectively. Ogiso et al. [44] noted these data indicated both hydrophilic and lipophilic drugs penetrated through scalp skin more rapidly than abdominal skin. Based upon fluorescence microscopy evaluating the penetration of a separate liquid formulation containing fluorescent probes through scalp skin at various time points, which showed the main pathway of drug penetration to be transfollicular rather than transepidermal, Ogiso et al. [44] concluded that rapid penetration through the scalp for both lipophilic and hydrophilic drugs was related to enhanced hair follicle density on the scalp compared to the abdomen.

Study 5: Schmitt et al. (2010)

Schmitt et al. [45] examined the percutaneous permeation of the main constituents of rose oil including the monoterpenes alpha-pinene, β-myrcene, limonene, linalool, *trans*-rose oxide, *cis*-rose oxide, isomenthone, β-citronellol, and geraniol on abdominal, breast, and upper arm skin. Skin was obtained from Caucasian female patients that underwent plastic surgery (sample size of upper arm $n = 6$ from 59-year-old female, breast skin $n = 4$ with unknown patient age, and abdominal skin $n = 12$ from two patients aged 31 and 39). Experiments were performed in a Franz diffusion cell, and 1000 μL native rose oil was added to the donor compartment. After 0, 3, 6, 9, 12, 24, and 27 h, the acceptor fluid samples were analyzed by gas chromatography. The primary outcomes analyzed included permeability coefficient = (quotient of flux which is calculated by the slope of the cumulative amount penetrated as a function of time and the donor concentration) and lag time calculated as the time intercept, from the cumulative amount penetrated as a function of time plot.

No overarching trend was identified between the permeability of the 13 substances through upper arm, breast, and abdominal skin. However, significant differences between apparent permeability coefficients of abdominal and breast skin were found for the following substances: β-pinene and *cis*-rose oxide. In both cases, the permeability coefficient of abdominal skin was greater than that of the breast. Significant differences between apparent permeability coefficients of abdominal and upper arm skin were noted for the following substances: β-myrcene, linalool, *trans*-rose oxide, *trans*-rose oxidase, and eugenol. Specifically, the permeability coefficient of abdominal skin was greater than that of upper arm skin for linalool and eugenol, but less than that of upper arm skin for β-myrcene, *trans*-rose oxide, and *cis*-rose oxide. Significant differences between apparent permeability coefficients of breast and upper arm skin were detected for linalool. Specifically, the breast exhibited a greater apparent permeability coefficient for linalool than the upper arm.

Lag time of each of the 13 substances was determined for the three anatomical test sites. Upper arm skin displayed the greatest lag time for all 13 substances. Breast skin exhibited the smallest lag time for each of the 13 substances with the exception of eugenol. Abdominal skin showed the greatest lag time for eugenol.

Study 6: Rolland et al. (2011)

Rolland et al. [46] studied the percutaneous penetration of nerve agent VX, a potent chemical warfare agent, through scalp and abdominal skin. Skin samples were purchased from Biopredic International after surgical intervention. Skin with and without a hypodermis was studied. A 5 mg/cm^2 dose was applied to the center of a 1.13 cm^2 skin surface. A Franz diffusion cell was used. Four hundred μL receptor fluid was collected at 2, 4, 6, 8, 10, 12, 22, and 24 h postexposure. Penetration rate, permeated dose, total absorbed fraction, and apparent lag time were determined.

Rolland et al. [46] found that in full thickness skin without a hypodermis, the VX equivalent (VXeq), defined as the sum of VX and its active metabolites, penetrated through human scalp skin approximately 1.5-fold faster than through human abdominal skin, and the apparent lag time was 3.5-fold lower for scalp than abdominal skin. These investigators also found that when the hypodermis was preserved, permeability and skin reservoir capacity of human scalp skin was twofold higher than that of human abdominal skin. Further, when the hypodermis was not preserved, permeability and skin reservoir capacity of human scalp skin was fourfold higher than that of human abdominal skin, indicating that the role of the hypodermis varies regionally.

Specifically, the apparent lag time of VX penetration through scalp skin ($n = 6$) without a hypodermis and with a hypodermis was 2 ± 0.3 vs. 3.3 ± 0.3, respectively. For abdominal skin ($n = 5$) without and with a hypodermis, the lag time was 7 ± 0.7 and 6.1 ± 0.4, respectively. The penetration rate [%Qo/h (%Qo being the total absorbed fraction of VX)] of VX through scalp skin without and with a hypodermis was 1.4 ± 0.32 vs. 0.31 ± 0.13, respectively. The penetration rate (%Qo/h) of VX through abdominal skin without and with a hypodermis was 0.91 ± 0.19 and 0.12 ± 0.03. The permeated dose of VX at 24 h (%Qo) of VX through scalp skin without and with a hypodermis was 29.1 ± 6.9 vs. 7.8 ± 2.9, respectively. The permeated dose of VX at 24 h (%Qo) through abdominal skin without and with a hypodermis was 15.8 ± 3.3 vs. 4.2 ± 1.7, respectively. The %Qo through the scalp without and with a hypodermis was 56.9 ± 10.25 vs. 63.6 ± 4.9, respectively. The total absorbed fraction of VX (%Qo) through abdominal skin without and with a hypodermis was 21.3 ± 4.2 vs. 18.9 ± 6.6, respectively.

Study 7: Trabaris et al. (2012)

Trabaris et al. [47] examined the regional differences in percutaneous absorption of disinfection by-products, including dichloroacetonitrile (DCAN), chloral hydrate (CH), trichloroacetonitrile (TCAN), dibromoacetonitrile (DBAN), bromochloroacetonitrile (BCAN), and chloroacetonitrile (CAN). Skin from the scalp, palm, torso, and dorsal hand of full thickness human cadaver skin sections (epidermis and dermis intact, subcutaneous tissue removed) was collected for experimental use (sample size: $n = 72$, $n = 3$ samples each protocol × 4 locations × 6 chemicals). Experiments were performed through diffusion cells, where whole skin was exposed to test chemicals for 3 h at 37 °C, using 5 mg/L CAN and DCAN, 15 mg/L BCAN, 25 mg/L DBAN, and 100 mg/L TCAN and CH solutions. Percutaneous absorption was measured by dermal flux through the skin samples in diffusion cells by gas chromatography.

Mean dermal flux (± SD) in mg/h-cm^2 for each chemical was significant as follows: CAN ranged from 0.015 ± 0.028 for the scalp to 0.42 ± 0.097 for the dorsal hand. DCAN ranged from not detected for the scalp to 0.32 ± 0.08 for the dorsal hand. TCAN ranged from not detected for the scalp and palm to 0.91 ± 0.2 for the dorsal hand. BCAN ranged from not detected for the scalp to 0.54 ± 0.085 for the torso. DBAN ranged from 0.022 ± 0.0053 for the scalp to 0.97 ± 0.21 for the torso. Finally, CH ranged from 0.0023 ± 0.00044 for the scalp to 0.098 ± 0.014 for the dorsal hand. Trabaris et al. [47] concluded that there was significantly enhanced permeability in the dorsal hand and torso skin versus the palm due to increased thickness in the stratum corneum in the palm and scalp. Evidence indicated that a decrease in thickness of the stratum corneum and an elevated number of epidermal appendages resulted in an increased dermal permeability. It is noteworthy that chemicals enter the bloodstream before traveling through the entire epidermis, and thus, these results may underestimate in vivo effects.

Study 8: Elmahdy et al. (2020)

Elmahdy et al. [48] determined the regional differences in percutaneous absorption of C-14-labeled chemical warfare simulants, including dipropylene glycol mono-methyl ether (DPGME), diisopropyl methylphosphonate (DIMP), and methyl salic-ylate (MeS). Skin from the abdomen and scalp of male and female human cadavers was collected and dermatomed to a thickness of 600 ± 50 μm [sample size: $n = 54$ ($n = 9 \times 3$ chemicals $\times 2$ locations)]. Experiments were performed by mounting the samples onto a flow-through diffusion cell system and applying 10 μL test chemical (10% concentration) to a 0.8 cm^2 area of skin. The flow rate was 4 μL/h. One hundred μL of receptor fluid was sampled at 30, 60, and 120 min and then every 2 h postexposure for 24 h. Scintillation counting was used to determine the penetration of C-14-labeled test penetrant into the receptor fluid. Presence and percent test chemical in the receptor fluid were used to represent the amount of test chemical that might have penetrated through the skin and into the bloodstream if performed in vivo.

The test penetrant, DPGME, showed a maximum penetration rate of $4.7 \pm 1\%$ dose/cm^2/h through the scalp at 2 h postexposure. The amount of DPGME collected in the receptor fluid over the 24 h collection period totaled $16.85 \pm 2.67\%$ for the scalp. DPGME demonstrated a maximum penetration of $0.8 \pm 1\%$ dose/cm^2/h through the abdominal skin at 6 h postexposure. The % applied DPGME collected in the receptor fluid over the 24 h collection period totaled $8.3 \pm 1.57\%$ for abdominal skin. DIMP presented a maximum penetration rate of $4.5 \pm 0.9\%$ dose/cm^2/h through the scalp at 4 h postexposure. The % applied DIMP in the receptor fluid of scalp skin experiments totaled $22.23 \pm 4.44\%$ after 24 h. DIMP showed a maximum penetration rate of $0.7 \pm 0.2\%$ dose/cm^2/h through abdominal skin at 6 h postexposure. There was $7.52 \pm 2.24\%$ of the applied DIMP in the receptor fluid following abdominal skin tests. MeS penetrated through scalp skin at a maximum rate of 0.4 ± 0.1% dose/cm²/h at 2 h postexposure. There was 7.2 ± 0.66% of the applied dose of MeS retrieved from the receptor fluid after 24 h. MeS penetrated through abdominal skin at a maximum rate of 0.1 ± 0.01% dose/cm²/h at 2 h postexposure. There was 1.3 ± 0.36% of the applied dose of MeS retrieved from the receptor fluid after 24 h. Elmahdy et al. [48] concluded that abdominal skin displayed lesser total absorption than the scalp.

Discussion

Conclusions Regarding Regional Variation in Percutaneous Absorption

This systematic review summarized eight articles investigating the regional variation of percutaneous absorption in in vitro human models and found several important conclusions. Comparisons were made based on findings that were consistent between at least two or more studies. First, of the eight articles investigated, four compared percutaneous absorption between scalp and abdominal regions [42, 44, 46, 48]. All four studies comparing the penetration of scalp and abdominal skin concluded that the scalp was more permeable than abdominal skin. In addition, the torso enabled less absorption than the scrotum in both studies in which these sites were compared [41, 43].

Specifically, Ritschel et al. [42] concluded that the scalp displayed increased flux and decreased lag time compared to the abdomen. However, it is important to note that the difference was only significant for two of the three penetrants tested (coumarin and propranolol) and was not significantly different for griseofulvin. Ogiso et al. [44] noted that the permeation of 5FU and MT through the scalp was 48- and 27-fold greater than the permeation through abdominal skin, respectively. The flux of KP was 1.5-fold higher through the scalp than through abdominal skin; however, this difference was not statistically significant. Rolland et al. [46] observed that VX penetrated through scalp skin 1.5-fold greater than through abdominal skin. Elmahdy et al. [48] noted that scalp skin displayed greater total skin absorption than abdominal skin. Therefore, all four studies which compared the penetration of scalp and abdominal skin concluded that scalp samples were more permeable than abdominal ones. This same finding was demonstrated multiple times in vivo [49–51]. Elmahdy et al. [48] postulated this observation to be largely due to increased hair follicle density in scalp than abdominal skin, which offers a larger surface area for absorption, and disruption of the epidermal barrier favors more rapid penetration of substances. Elmahdy et al. [48] found that the scalp had 73 ± 6 hair follicles/cm², whereas the abdomen had only 9 ± 5 hair follicles/cm².

All four studies comparing scalp and abdominal percutaneous absorption concluded that the scalp was more permeable than abdominal skin. Interestingly, each of these four studies tested the absorption of different substances. Generally, the smaller the molecular weight and the more lipophilic a substance, the more it will penetrate the skin [19, 52]. However, at some point, very highly lipophilic substances may be less well absorbed than moderately lipophilic substances [19]. Ten substances were tested within these four investigations which included ^{14}C-coumarin, ^{3}H-propranolol, ^{3}H-griseofulvin, melatonin, ketoprofen (KP), 5-fluorouracil (5FU), VX, dipropylene glycol monomethyl ether (DPGME), diisopropyl methylphosphonate (DIMP), and methyl salicylate (MeS). All of these substances vary greatly in their physical/chemical properties. For example, VX, 5FU, and DPGME are hydrophilic, while the remainder of test substances are lipophilic. Therefore, data suggest that the anatomical location exerts a more prominent role on the rate of percutaneous absorption than the chemical properties of the penetrant as both hydrophilic and hydrophobic substances tended to penetrate scalp skin faster than abdominal skin. However, it is important to note that this finding is specific to the studies included in this review and does not generalize to every compound. For example, due to their chemical properties, some compounds (e.g., those of high volatility or high molecular size) will not penetrate the skin regardless of where they are applied.

Interestingly, Trabaris et al. [47] investigated the penetration of the torso compared to the scalp and concluded that torso skin exhibited a higher dermal flux than the scalp. Although the abdomen is part of the torso, the exact test location of the torso was unspecified and therefore does not necessarily contradict our earlier conclusion that the scalp displays higher dermal absorption than the abdomen. Trabaris et al. [47] attributed their somewhat contradictory findings to the fact that their study examined penetration through full thickness skin. The OECD Guidance Notes on Dermal Absorption [22] noted that human in vitro studies should preferably use split thickness skin. This is partly because split thickness skin is thought to better reflect in vivo conditions where some test chemicals may not penetrate through the entire scalp, but rather are absorbed into the capillaries just below the hair follicles [33].

The abdomen enabled less absorption than the scrotum in both studies in which these sites were compared. Smith et al. [41] found that the scrotum was more penetrable than the abdomen. Harada et al. [43] noted that the scrotum was more penetrable than the inguinal region anatomically defined as the lower border of the abdominal wall. The high penetrability of scrotal skin may be attributed to its thin stratum corneum and vast blood supply [19]. Although not tested, Smith et al. [41] predicted that female genital skin may display enhanced susceptibility to percutaneous absorption similar to scrotal skin.

Study Limitations

This review has limitations to consider. Due to the heterogeneity and small sample sizes of available data, it is difficult to order anatomical regions from most to least permeable. Experimental methods differed between studies where some used static

(Franz) versus flow-through diffusion systems. Studies also used different parameters to represent percutaneous absorption, such as lag time, versus flux rate, versus permeability coefficient which made it difficult to compare results.

Another limitation of data is that not all studies reported the mass balance values, and therefore, some penetrants might be lost to factors other than percutaneous absorption such as evaporation if there are accidental and undiscovered openings within the seal of the apparatus.

Limitations specific to included studies include that Smith et al. [41] employed primitive and unusual methodology (e.g., using lead acetate paper for studying percutaneous absorption and incubating samples in a desiccator at 35 °C, respectively), and therefore their findings should be interpreted with adequate caution. Additionally, Harada et al. [43] used very small sample sizes for each test location ($n = 1$ for cheek, neck, back, lower leg, foot, sole, and scrotum, each; $n = 2$ for inguinal; $n = 3$ for thigh, $n = 5$ for breast). Schmitt et al. [45] received all 6 upper arm skin samples from a single donor, all 4 breast skin samples from a different single donor, and the 12 abdominal skin samples were collected from only two donors.

Due to ethical considerations, in vitro methods are often used as a substitute for in vivo methods. Maibach and Wester [53] stated that in vivo studies are the preferential model for determining the penetration potential of a compound and constitute the most relevant to clinical practice. This is because in vivo studies better explore physiological effects such as metabolism, distribution, and excretion of the test substance [37]. An important in vivo study was conducted by Maibach et al. [51]. They used radioactively labeled parathion, malathion, and carbaryl to contaminate various anatomical sites of human volunteers while keeping all other variables constant. They found that the palm was approximately as penetrable as the forearm, which has been used as a control. The abdomen and dorsum of the hand were twice as penetrable as the forearm. Sites of high follicle density (scalp, jaw angle, postauricular area, and forehead) were four times as penetrable as the control. The highest absorption occurred at the axilla, which demonstrated a four- to sevenfold increase in absorption compared to the control, and the scrotum, which allowed almost total absorption.

This is not to say that in vivo methodology does not have limitations of its own. For example, in vivo methods usually measure absorption rate indirectly (e.g., measuring excretion of the test penetrant from the body) [37]. Metabolism and excretion of penetrants are affected by numerous factors, and substance elimination may or may not accurately indicate the amount absorbed [19], and if this is not properly corrected for, it could lead to large errors. Additionally, indirect methods can only be used for chemicals that are involatile [20], and security of the application is more difficult in vivo.

Lehman et al. [54] reviewed 30 published studies with the aim of determining the in vitro–in vivo correlation for percutaneous absorption in humans and found that so long as methods were kept consistent, there was a less than twofold difference between in vitro and in vivo results for any one compound, and stated that percutaneous absorption data obtained using excised human skin models closely approximated those obtained in vivo. However, a twofold difference in the amount penetrated is still an important consideration when determining important toxico-logical values such as the LD_{50} of a topical drug, as in vitro underestimation may lead to toxic overdoses. However, Bormann and Maibach [34] summarized the regional variation of percutaneous absorption in vivo and reached conclusions simi-lar to ours. This includes that the head and genital areas appear to be highly pene-trable and that more studies are needed to develop a regional model of penetrability in humans.

Practical Application of Results

Therefore, there is a need for more data, both in vitro and in vivo, in order to provide conclusive data on this important topic. In the case of a chemical warfare or an occu-pational exposure to a toxic industrial chemical, prioritizing the decontamination of certain anatomical locations indicates the difference between whether or not contami-nants breach the circulatory system. For example, the scalp is a commonly unpro-tected area which might receive more exposure during chemical warfare or an accident with toxic industrial chemicals, than a less permeable area of the body like the abdo-men, which is also more likely to be protected with clothing. In a study by Wester et al. [18], the percentage dose of a chemical warfare simulant that was absorbed through unclothed skin was 1.78 ± 0.41, but was only 0.29 ± 0.17 for uniformed skin. Additionally, according to Chilcott [55], approximately 50% of contaminant is removed by disrobing following an overhead exposure, and 70% is removed by dis-robing following a face-on exposure. This implies that the clothing itself serves as a brief barrier and reservoir for the contaminants (hence dampening the amount that immediately comes into contact with the skin). Therefore, in the event that a universal decontamination protocol is established, it will need to advise disrobing as quickly as possible and prioritizing decontamination of the scalp, head, and neck over the trunk and limbs. Further, knowledge of regional variation in percutaneous absorption may be harnessed advantageously in order to optimize transdermal delivery of drugs, which often requires the use of absorption enhancers [44, 56, 57].

Conclusions

The scrotum and scalp appear to be areas highly susceptible to percutaneous absorp-tion when compared to other body regions such as the abdomen. However, there is a paucity of conclusive data regarding the absorptivity of other anatomical loca-tions. Experimentation testing and ranking the susceptibility of different anatomical locations is of vital importance, given its relevance in decontamination and trans-dermal drug delivery protocols. Commonly exposed areas, such as the face, neck, chest, and limbs, need to be prioritized, as these loci may be most likely to come into contact with unwanted chemicals. With increasing availability of high-quality in vitro data, it should be possible to estimate relative permeability from one site to another as proposed by Guy and Maibach [58].

Acknowledgements We would like to thank Dr. Howard I. Maibach for his mentorship and guidance throughout the course of completing this manuscript.

The authors of this chapter would like to acknowledge the original source of publication, Taylor & Francis Online, whose website can be accessed via the following link: https://www.tandfonline.com/. The original publication of this chapter can be found via the following link: https://doi.org/10.1080/10937404.2022.2032517.

Declaration of Interest Statement We declare that no financial interest or benefit has arisen from the direct application of this research.

Data Availability Statement The authors confirm that the data supporting the findings of this study are available within the article.

References

1. Idson B. Percutaneous absorption. J Pharm Sci. 1975;64:901–23. https://doi.org/10.1002/jps.2600640604.
2. Sobanska AW, Robertson J, Brzezinska E. Application of RP-18 TLC retention data to the prediction of the transdermal absorption of drugs. Pharmaceuticals. 2021;14:147. https://doi.org/10.3390/ph14020147.
3. Kovacik A, Kopecna M, Vavrova K. Permeation enhancers in transdermal drug delivery: benefits and limitations. Expert Opin Drug Deliv. 2020;17:145–55. https://doi.org/10.1080/17425247.2020.1713087.
4. Luo L, Lane ME. Topical and transdermal delivery of caffeine. Int J Pharm. 2015;490:155–64. https://doi.org/10.1016/j.ijpharm.2015.05.050.
5. Reifenrath WG, Olson JJ, Vedula U, Osimitz TG. Percutaneous absorption of an insect repellent *p*-menthane-2,8-diol: a model for human dermal absorption. J Toxicol Environ Health A. 2008;72:796–806. https://doi.org/10.1080/15287390902800371.
6. Ross JH, Reifenrath WG, Driver JH. Estimation of the percutaneous absorption of permethrin in humans using the parallelogram method. J Toxicol Environ Health A. 2011;74:351–63. https://doi.org/10.1080/15287394.2011.534425.
7. Wester RC, Maibach HI. In vivo percutaneous absorption and decontamination of pesticides in humans. J Toxicol Environ Health. 1985;16:25–37. https://doi.org/10.1080/15287398509530716.
8. Wester RC, Maibach HI, Bucks DAW, Aufrere MB. In vivo percutaneous absorption of paraquat from hand, leg, and forearm of humans. J Toxicol Environ Health. 1984;14:759–62. https://doi.org/10.1080/15287398409530624.
9. Ganesan K, Raza SK, Vijayaraghavan R. Chemical warfare agents. J Pharm Bioallied Sci. 2010;2:166–78. https://doi.org/10.4103/0975-7406.68498.
10. Andersen RM, Coman G, Blickenstaff NR, Maibach HI. Percutaneous absorption from soil. Rev Environ Health. 2014;29:169–74. https://doi.org/10.1515/reveh-2014-0053.
11. Boman A, Maibach HI. Percutaneous absorption of organic solvents. Int J Occup Environ Health. 2000;6:93–5. https://doi.org/10.1179/oeh.2000.6.2.93.
12. Champmartin C, Marquet F, Chedik L, Decret MJ, Aubertin M, Ferrari E, Grandclaude MC, Cosnier F. Human in vitro percutaneous absorption of bisphenol S and bisphe-

nol A: a comparative study. Chemosphere. 2020;252:126525. https://doi.org/10.1016/j.chemosphere.2020.126525.

13. Hamilton M, Hill I, Conley J, Sawyer TW, Caneva DC, Lundy PM. Clinical aspects of percutaneous poisoning by the chemical warfare agent VX: effects of application site and decontamination. Mil Med. 2004;169:856–62. https://doi.org/10.7205/MILMED.169.11.856.

14. Kim J-Y, Im JE, Lee JD, Kim K-B. Analytical method development and percutaneous absorption of propylidene phthalide, a cosmetic ingredient. J Toxicol Environ Health A. 2021;84:811–20. https://doi.org/10.1080/15287394.2021.1944941.

15. Matta MK, Florian J, Zusterzeel R, et al. Effect of sunscreen application on plasma concentrations of sunscreen active ingredients. JAMA. 2020;323:1098. https://doi.org/10.1001/jama.2019.20747.

16. Rehal B, Maibach HI. Percutaneous absorption of vapors in human skin. Cutan Ocul Toxicol. 2011;30:87–91. https://doi.org/10.3109/15569527.2010.534522.

17. Tanojo H, Wester RC, Shainhouse JZ, Maibach HI. Diclofenac metabolic profile following in vitro percutaneous absorption through viable human skin. Eur J Drug Metab Pharmacokinet. 1999;24:345–51. https://doi.org/10.1007/BF03190043.

18. Wester RC, Tanojo H, Maibach HI, Wester RC. Predicted chemical warfare agent VX toxicity to uniformed soldier using parathion in vitro human skin exposure and absorption. Toxicol Appl Pharmacol. 2000;168:149–52. https://doi.org/10.1006/taap.2000.9028.

19. Law RM, Ngo MA, Maibach HI. Twenty clinically pertinent factors/observations for percutaneous absorption in humans. Am J Clin Dermatol. 2020;21:85–95. https://doi.org/10.1007/s40257-019-00480-4.

20. EPA (U.S. Environmental Protection Agency). Dermal exposure assessment: a summary of EPA approaches. Washington, DC: National Center for Environmental Assessment; 2007. http://www.epa.gov/ncea.

21. EFSA (European Food Safety Authority), Buist H, Craig P, Dewhurst I, Hougaard Bennekou S, Kneuer C, Machera K, Pieper C, Court Marques D, Guillot G, Ruffo F, Chiusolo A. Guidance on dermal absorption. EFSA J. 2017;15:487. https://doi.org/10.2903/j.efsa.2017.4873.

22. OECD (Organisation for Economic Co-operation and Development) Environment, Health and Safety Publications. Guidance notes on dermal absorption. 2nd ed. Paris: OECD Development Centre; 2019. https://www.oecd.org/chemicalsafety/testing/Guidance%20Notes%20Dermal%20Absorption%20156_Oct2019_clean.pdf.

23. WHO (World Health Organization). Dermal absorption. Geneva: World Health Organization; 2006. https://apps.who.int/iris/handle/10665/43542.

24. Illel B, Schaefer H, Wepierre J, Doucet O. Follicles play an important role in percutaneous absorption. J Pharm Sci. 1991;80:424–7. https://doi.org/10.1002/jps.2600800505.

25. Lademann J, Otberg N, Jacobi U, Hoffman RM, Blume-Peytavi U. Follicular penetration and targeting. J Investig Dermatol. 2005;10:301–3. https://doi.org/10.1111/j.1087-0024.

26. Lademann J, Richter H, Schaefer UF, Blume-Peytavi U, Teichmann A. Hair follicles—a long-term reservoir for drug delivery. Skin Pharmacol Physiol. 2006;19:232–6. https://doi.org/10.1159/000093119.

27. Otberg N, Richter H, Schaefer H, Blume-Peytavi U, Sterry W, Lademann J. Variations of hair follicle size and distribution in different body sites. J Investig Dermatol. 2004;122:4–19. https://doi.org/10.1046/j.0022-202X.2003.22110.x.

28. Otberg N, Patzelt A, Rasulev U, Hagemeister T, Linscheid M, Sinkgravem R, Sterry W, Lademann J. The role of hair follicles in the percutaneous absorption of caffeine. Br J Clin Pharmacol. 2008;65:488–92. https://doi.org/10.1111/j.1365-2125.2007.03065.x.

29. Al Mahrooqi JH, Khutoryanskiy VV, Williams AC. Thiolated and PEGylated silica nanoparticle delivery to hair follicles. Int J Pharm. 2021;593:120130. https://doi.org/10.1016/j.ijpharm.2020.120130.

30. Fang C-L, Aljuffali IA, Le Y-C, Fang J-Y. Delivery and targeting of nanoparticles into hair follicles. Ther Deliv. 2014;5:991–1006. https://doi.org/10.4155/tde.14.61.

31. Limcharoen B, Toprangkobsin P, Banlunara W, Wanichwecharungruang S, Richter H, Lademann J, Patzelt A. Increasing the percutaneous absorption and follicular penetration of retinal by topical application of proretinal nanoparticles. Eur J Pharm Biopharm. 2019;139:93–100. https://doi.org/10.1016/j.ejpb.2019.03.014.

32. Patzelt A, Lademann J. Drug delivery to hair follicles. Expert Opin Drug Deliv. 2013;10:787–97. https://doi.org/10.1517/17425247.2013.776038z.

33. Bronaugh RL. In vitro diffusion cell studies. In: Riviere JE, editor. Dermal absorption models in toxicology and pharmacology. Boca Raton: Taylor and Francis Group; 2006. p. 21–7.

34. Bormann J, Maibach HI. Effects of anatomical locational on in vivo percutaneous penetration in man. Cutan Ocul Toxicol. 2020;39:213–22. https://doi.org/10.1080/15569527.202 0.1787434.

35. Holmgaard R, Benfeldt E, Nielsen JB. Percutaneous penetration—methodological consideration. Basic Clin Pharmacol. 2013;115:101–9. https://doi.org/10.1111/bcpt.12188.

36. Franz TJ. Percutaneous absorption on the relevance of in vitro data. J Investig Dermatol. 1975;64:190–5. https://doi.org/10.1111/1523-1747.ep12533356.

37. Bronaugh RL, Stewart RF, Congdon ER, Giles AL. Methods for in vitro percutaneous absorption studies I. Comparison with in vivo results. Toxicol Appl Pharmacol. 1982;62:474–80. https://doi.org/10.1016/0041-008X(82)90148-X.

38. Lau WM, Ng KW. Finite and infinite dosing. In: Dragicevic N, Maibach HI, editors. Percutaneous penetration enhancers drug penetration into/through the skin: methodology and general considerations. Berlin: Springer; 2017. p. 35–44. https://doi.org/10.1007/978-3-662-53270-6_3.

39. Nielsen JB, Sorensen JA, Nielsen F. The usual suspects-influence of physiochemical properties on lag time, skin deposition, and percutaneous penetration of nine model compounds. J Toxicol Environ Health Part A. 2008;72:315–23. https://doi.org/10.1080/15287390802529872.

40. Page MJ, McKenzie JE, Bossuyt PM, Boutron I, Hoffmann TC, Mulrow CD, Shamseer L, Tetzlaff JM, Akl EA, Brennan SE, Chou R, Glanville J, Grimshaw JM, Hróbjartsson A, Lalu MM, Li T, Loder EW, Mayo-Wilson E, McDonald S, McGuinness LA, Stewart LA, Thomas J, Tricco AC, Welch VA, Whiting P, Moher D. The PRISMA 2020 statement: an updated guideline for reporting systematic reviews. BMJ. 2021;372:n71. https://doi.org/10.1136/bmj.n71.

41. Smith JG, Fischer RW, Blank H. The epidermal barrier: a comparison between scrotal and abdominal skin. J Investig Dermatol. 1961;36:337–43.

42. Ritschel WA, Sabouni A, Hussain AS. Percutaneous absorption of coumarin, griseofulvin and propranolol across human scalp and abdominal skin. Methods Find Exp Clin Pharmacol. 1989;11:643–6.

43. Harada K, Murakami T, Kawasaki K, Higashi Y, Yamamoto S, Yata N. In-vitro permeability to salicylic acid of human, rodent, and shed snake skin. J Pharm Pharmacol. 1993;45:414–8. https://doi.org/10.1111/j.2042-7158.1993.tb05567.x.

44. Ogiso T, Shiraki T, Okajima K, Tanino T, Iwaki M, Wada T. Transfollicular drug delivery: penetration of drugs through human scalp skin and comparison of penetration between scalp and abdominal skins in vitro. J Drug Target. 2002;10:369–78. https://doi.org/10.108 0/1061186021000001814.

45. Schmitt S, Schafer UF, Dobler L, Reichling J. Variation of in vitro human skin permeation of rose oil between different application sites. Forsch Komplementmed. 2010;17:126–31. https://doi.org/10.1159/000315043.

46. Rolland P, Bolzinger MA, Cruz C, Briancon S, Josse D. Human scalp permeability to the chemical warfare agent VX. Toxicol In Vitro. 2011;25:1974–80. https://doi.org/10.1016/j.tiv.2011.06.021.

47. Trabaris M, Laskin JD, Weasel CP. Effects of temperature, surfactants and skin location on the dermal penetration of haloacetonitriles and chloral hydrate. J Expo Sci Environ Epidemiol. 2010;22:393–7. https://doi.org/10.1038/jes.2012.19.

48. Elmahdy A, Cao Y, Hui X, Maibach H. Follicular pathway role in chemical warfare simulants percutaneous penetration. J Appl Toxicol. 2020;41:964–71. https://doi.org/10.1002/jat.4081.

49. Feldmann RJ, Maibach HI. Regional variation in percutaneous absorption of 14C cortisol in man. J Investig Dermatol. 1967;48:181–3. https://doi.org/10.1038/jid.1967.29.
50. Lev-Tov H, Maibach HI. Regional variations in percutaneous absorption. J Drug Dermatol. 2012;11:e48–51.
51. Maibach HI, Feldman RJ, Milby TH, Serat WF. Regional variation in percutaneous penetration in man. Arch Environ Health. 1971;23:208–11. https://doi.org/10.1080/00039896.197 1.10665987.
52. Fu XC, Wang GP, Wang YF, Liang WQ, Yu QS, Chow MSS. Limitation of Potts and Guy's model and a predictive algorithm for skin permeability including the effects of hydrogen-bond on diffusivity. Pharmazie. 2004;59:282–5.
53. Maibach HI, Wester RC. Percutaneous absorption: in vivo methods in humans and animals. J Am Coll Toxicol. 1989;8:803–13. https://doi.org/10.3109/10915818909018039.
54. Lehman PA, Raney SG, Franz, and T.J. Percutaneous absorption in man: in vitro–in vivo correlation. Skin Pharmacol Physiol. 2011;24:224–30. https://doi.org/10.1159/000324884.
55. Chilcott R. Managing mass causalities and decontamination. Environ Int. 2014;72:37–45. https://doi.org/10.1016/j.envint.2014.02.006.
56. Mathur V, Satrawala Y, Rajput M. Physical and chemical enhancers in transdermal drug delivery systems. Asian J Pharm. 2010;4:173. https://doi.org/10.22377/AJP.V4I3.143.
57. Pathan IB, Setty CM. Chemical penetration enhancers for transdermal drug delivery systems. Trop J Pharm Res. 2009;8:173–9. https://doi.org/10.4314/tjpr.v8i2.44527.
58. Guy RH, Maibach HI. Correction factors for determining body exposure from forearm percutaneous absorption data. J Appl Toxicol. 1984;4:26–8. https://doi.org/10.1002/jat.2550040106.

Chapter 15
Experimental Variability in TEWL Data

Reva P. Peer, Anuk Burli, and Howard I. Maibach

Introduction

Stratum corneum plays critical roles in human survival; one such role is as a barrier against excessive water loss [1]. Transepidermal water loss (TEWL), a widely used and accepted means of quantifying the stratum corneum's effectiveness as a barrier against water loss, quantifies water lost from the body by non-eccrine sweating [2]. TEWL's importance is highlighted by the fact that TEWL in humans has been investigated since the 1960s and remains a major field of research, related to topics ranging from its effect on human aging and skin color on TEWL [3–5].

Although a wide breadth of TEWL research exists, there is much disparity in their conclusions. For example, we reviewed 26 major studies investigating the impact of skin of color on TEWL; results conflicted. Many studies contradicted each other on whether skin of color significantly impacts TEWL or not, and, even if a significant effect was found, studies disagreed on what the significant impact was [6].

In a major review on TEWL and aging, Kottner et al. conducted a meta-analysis comparing TEWL results from 152 studies and found that TEWL is generally lower in older adults; however, this was only for 11 of 21 comparisons, and therefore, they were unable to make clear conclusion regarding age and TEWL [7]. The conflicting results in both large data sets indicate a need to evaluate possible confounding variables.

R. P. Peer (✉) · A. Burli
School of Medicine and Dentistry, University of Rochester, Rochester, NY, USA
e-mail: Reva_Peer@urmc.rochester.edu

H. I. Maibach
Department of Dermatology, University of California San Francisco,
San Francisco, CA, USA
e-mail: Howard.Maibach@ucsf.edu

© The Author(s), under exclusive license to Springer Nature
Switzerland AG 2022
A. M. Feschuk et al. (eds.), *Dermal Absorption and Decontamination*,
https://doi.org/10.1007/978-3-031-09222-0_15

We suggest that one reason there is variation in TEWL data rests with confounding variables that significantly impact TEWL. Many TEWL studies attempt to control for such variables, including room temperature and the consumption of certain foods, etc.; however, TEWL research lacks uniformity regarding which variables to control for, and often only a select few variables are matched for [8, 9].

Here, we identify multiple important confounding variables that can significantly impact TEWL. By matching study subjects for as many of these variables as possible, we can potentially reduce disparity in TEWL metrics.

Materials and Methods

We searched Embase; PubMed; Google; Google Scholar; the Miner Library Online Database of the University of Rochester in Rochester, NY, USA; standard dermatology textbooks; and the Dermatology Library at the University of California, San Francisco, CA, USA. An initial search was conducted using keywords related to TEWL (i.e., TEWL, standardization, evaporimeter, water loss) to generate a list of potential confounding variables. A subsequent search included words pertaining to these variables (i.e., aging, gender, seasons, ambient temperature, obesity, smoking) and words pertaining to TEWL (i.e., TEWL, stratum corneum, skin, skin barrier function, water loss). These references were reviewed, and relevant and representative publications were procured. For every article, only results regarding basal TEWL were analyzed and presented. Both articles independently reviewed cited articles.

Results

Experimental Variables

Sample Size and Power

Sample size is an important aspect of any experimental design. Large sample sizes may identify differences that are not biologically important, while small sample sizes are poorer representatives of a population and may not discern biological differences—even if they are important, i.e., small sample sizes have low power [10]. Power is the probability that the experiment would be able to reject the null hypothesis when it is rightly false. A higher power limits the chance of committing a type II error and is often set at least 0.8. Power is related to interindividual variance, sample size, and the acceptable risk level, α [11]. Therefore, an adequate sample size ensures a study has power and, therefore, has strong evidence to support its conclusion. One can calculate the necessary sample size needed for a study to have accurate power for an acceptable risk level. However, of the articles reviewed here, only one explicitly stated that they used power analysis to determine the minimum sample size required for adequate power [12]. Two other articles did some sample-related calculations as well but did not explicitly state whether they conducted power analysis. Mehta et al. stated they calculated sample size using a software, and Young et al. calculated effect sizes [5, 13]. Without power analysis, one cannot determine if the study included enough subjects to be considered strong evidence. For example, Hillebrand et al. reanalyzed Wilson et al. Wilson et al. investigated the relationship between race and TEWL by measuring TEWL in skin from 12 white subjects and ten African American individuals [14]. Hillebrand et al. used their own data on forearm TEWL in 452 Chinese women of various age groups to calculate the coefficient of TEWL variance forearm. As this data was specific to Chinese women, they also compared their coefficient with studies that investigated other populations and ethnic groups to confirm its accuracy [11]. Wilson et al. observed a significant difference ($p < 0.01$) with African American skin having 10% higher in vitro TEWL versus their white skin counterparts [14]. However, after conducting power analysis, Hillebrand et al. found that to observe a 10% difference between white and African American individuals in vivo with 80% power and statistical significance ($p < 0.05$), one would require at least 172 white and 172 African American individuals. This highlights the importance of taking sample size and power into consideration when planning/conducting and analyzing studies [11].

Evaporimeter Standardization

Evaporimeter standardization is another potential variable. Three major techniques for determining TEWL have been described. The first is a closed chamber method, where a hygroscopic substance inside a glass tube is placed on the skin and the change in the weight of this substance is used to measure TEWL. However, there are drawbacks to this method; this substance is saturable, and therefore, at high relative humidity, this method is ineffective, this method cannot continuously measure TEWL, and one must control for the relative humidity and vapor in the chamber prior to introducing the substance. Another method is via a ventilated chamber that passes gas of a known humidity and velocity through a chamber placed on the skin and then comparing the effluent and affluent air to determine TEWL. Its disadvantage is that it introduces a forced convection factor that increases TEWL by physically removing a layer of more humid air from the skin surface. Finally, the open chamber method, commonly used in many evaporimeters, measures the water gradient at two points in the water gradient boundary of the skin and, therefore, not impacted by this convection factor. Note that it is impacted by local air currents and relative humidity fluctuations [15].

Pinnagoda et al. determined intra-instrumental variability in TEWL in vitro and in vivo recorded with four evaporimeters and determined small standard deviations and therefore a low intra-instrumental variability. There was greater variability between individual instruments. This was hypothesized to be the result of the age of the instrument as older instruments tended to stabilize slower and measured lower

TEWL [16]. Pinnagoda et al. subsequently suggested that aging of instruments may be due to the aging of the probe sensors [17]. This underscores the importance of regularly checking and calibrating the instrument.

In addition, there appears to be variation between instruments made by different manufacturers. De Paepe et al. compared two commonly used evaporimeters made by two manufacturers when measuring forearm skin TEWL. One machine measured significantly higher TEWL values than the other. This illustrates that using more than one brand of machine can cause potential result variation [18]. Another aspect of evaporimeter standardization was the use of probe protection covers. Pinnagoda et al. described how the use of a cover can elevate the probe above the necessary boundary where TEWL measurements must occur. TEWL measurements will thus be lower with a probe cover. Furthermore, the higher the TEWL rate, the greater the difference between the TEWL values when using and when not using the cover [17]. A goal still to be met will be an international standardization method.

Technician Training

Another confounding variable investigated was technician training, as how the instrument is handled and how the measurement process is conducted impacts the resultant TEWL value. Training errors can be minimized by a complete understanding of the equipment and training in the use of the instrument based on the instrument handbook. For example, the ServoMed Evaporimeters handbook discusses zero drift, wherein changes in relative humidity and the temperature of the probe can affect measurements. When conducting a measurement, the probe is exposed to skin's high humidity and temperature. Hence, condensation will remain in the probe, and the instrument will have a nonzero water evaporation value (WE) zero level [19]. Pinnagoda et al. described that having the technician wave the probe vertically up and down speeds up the time for the probe to return to normal, within 2–4 min [16]. Temperature zero drift can occur since contact with human skin can raise probe temperature. This can be due to the subject's skin or the technician's hand. The handbook states that a change in water evaporation zero level $\pm$ 1–2 g/m^2 h can occur due to a 5 min measurement with the technician holding the probe [19]. Pinnagoda discussed accessories for holding the probe, such as insulating gloves, that the technician can use to avoid skin contact [17]. Finally, Nilsson et al. investigated the impact of contact pressure on TEWL. They measured TEWL on the thigh with increasing mechanical load on the probe and observed an increase of about 10% in the evaporation rate for every additional 100 g applied to the probe [20]. These findings highlight the importance of adequate technician training and instrument operation on TEWL measurements.

Room Temperature

The room temperature for TEWL measurement also potentially impacts TEWL. Cravello et al. measured TEWL in six women at three ambient temperatures (20, 25, and 30 °C) and found significant correlation between ambient temperature and TEWL; TEWL increased with increasing temperature [21]. Lamke et al. measured water evaporation from skin in nine men and ten women who spent 30 min in a climate chamber at three temperatures, 15, 28, and 41 °C, and observed a significant increase in mean evaporation between 15 and 28 °C and between 15 and 41 °C and between 28 and 41 °C [22]. Chen et al. investigated the effect of experiencing changes in temperature on TEWL from outside to a temperature-controlled building. A subject may experience the same effect when coming into a temperature-controlled environment for TEWL measurements. Chen et al. measured TEWL in eight male and eight female subjects during three temperature changes (32–24, 28–24 °C, and 20–24 °C). The immediate difference in the TEWL value was significant for all temperature change sets, with TEWL decreasing with the down-steps in temperature [23]. Pinnagoda et al. recommended a room temperature of 20–22 °C to minimize such fluctuations [17].

Environmental Variables

Season

Seasonal changes correspond to climatic changes including changes in temperature, wind, humidity, etc. Therefore, such climatic changes can impact the skin and barrier function and hence TEWL (Table 15.1). Most studies investigating the relationship between TEWL and seasonal fluctuations compared TEWL during winter and summer seasons. Kikuchi et al. examined 39 Japanese females and measured their TEWL on the cheek and forearm during summer and winter. TEWL increased significantly at both sites in winter compared with summer [26]. Similar results were found in other studies. Li et al. measured TEWL in 40 Chinese adults and 40 Chinese children on the elbow, face, décolletage, dorsal hand, outer forearm, lower outer leg, and heel during winter and summer. TEWL was higher during winter at all sites except the heel, which had a lower TEWL in the winter compared to summer [27]. Wei et al. found the same results in 25 females from Ohio on the lower legs, as did Muizzuddin et al. on the cheeks of 40 females from Arizona and New York, and Yang et al. in 72 females from China on the cheek, but not the forearm [28, 30, 31].

However, Song et al. measured TEWL in 100 Korean men during summer and winter on the forehead, cheek, and forearm, and TEWL was significantly higher for the forehead and forearm during the summer. Cheek had a similar trend but did not achieve significance [29]. Black et al. also had contradicting results to the above; they collected TEWL values in 24 women during February, April, July, and December of the same year on their calf, inner forearm, and crow's feet area. For the forearm and calf, there was a significant increase in TEWL in July compared to all other months. Crow's feet area had a similar trend but did not reach significance. Black et al. only described December as winter and July as summer, but did not describe the seasons of the other 2 months [24].

Table 15.1 TEWL (transepidermal water loss): impact of season. All studies found an impact of season on TEWL. Most studies found that TEWL was increased in winter compared to summer; however, two found opposite results and some no significant differences. Conflicting results were also found when investigating four seasons. SD = standard deviation [24–32]

Study	Subjects (age range or mean ± SD, sample size, sex)	Season (months)	Site	Season and TEWL result
Black et al. [24]	18–35 years, $n = 24$, females	February, April, July, December	Calf, inner forearm, crow's foot wrinkle area on the face	Forearm and calf: July > February, April, and December ($p < 0.05$).
				Crow's feet: same trend but not significant
Kikuchi et al. [26]	20s, $n = 9$	Summer (August to October); winter (December to April)	Cheek, mid flexor forearm	Cheek ($p < 0.0001$) and forearm ($p < 0.01$): winter > summer
	30s, $n = \prime\prime$			
	40s, $n = \prime\prime$			
	50s, $n = 5$			
	60s, $n = 4$			
	70s, $n = 3$			
	Japanese females			
De Paepe et al. [25]	21–31 years, $n = 16$, females	Autumn (October); winter (February to March)	Nasolabial area, forehead	Winter > autumn for both sites ($p < 0.01$ for both)
Muizzuddin et al. [28]	18–45 years, $n = 18$ (Tucson, Arizona), $n = 22$ (Long Island, NY)	Summer (June to August); winter (December to February)	Cheek	Baseline TEWL: winter > summer ($p < 0.001$)
	Caucasian females			
Li et al. [27]	"Parents" 40–50 years, $n = 40$	Winter (January); summer (August to September)	Elbow, face, décolletage, dorsal hand, outer forearm, lower outer leg, heel	Winter > summer at all sites except at heel summer < winter
	"Children" 18–25 years, $n = 40$			No statistical significance stated in baseline TEWL
	Chinese males and females			
Song et al. [29]	20–59 years, $n = 100$	Summer (July); winter (January)	Forehead, cheek, forearm	Forehead and forearm: summer > winter ($p < 0.05$)
	Korean males			Cheek: summer > winter but did not reach significance
Wei et al. [30]	23–64 years, $n = 25$ females	Summer and winter[a]	Lower legs	Winter > summer ($p < 0.0001$)

Table 15.1 (continued)

Study	Subjects (age range or mean ± SD, sample size, sex)	Season (months)	Site	Season and TEWL result
Yang et al. [31]	19–28 years, $n = 72$	Spring, summer, autumn, and winter	Cheek, forearm	Cheek: spring > summer ($p < 0.05$), winter > summer ($p < 0.05$)
	Females in China			Forearm: no significant differences
Ye et al. [32]	19–53 years, $n = 24$	Spring (April); summer (July); autumn (October); winter (January)	Forehead, cheek, submaxilla	Forehead: spring and autumn < summer and winter ($p < 0.001$ and $p < 0.05$)
	Chinese females[b]			Submaxilla: spring and autumn < summer and winter ($p < 0.01$)
				Cheeks: autumn < spring and summer and winter ($p < 0.001$)

[a] No months stated, season in Cincinnati, OH
[b] All with a 5% lactic acid stinging test result ≥3 and >3 sensitivity factors

Others compared TEWL values during autumn and spring as well. De Paepe et al. measured TEWL on the nasolabial area and the forehead of 16 females during autumn and winter. TEWL increased significantly in winter compared to autumn [25]. Ye et al. investigated TEWL in 24 individuals from China with 5% lactic acid stinging scores ≥3 and had three sensitivity factors during all four seasons on the forehead, cheeks, and submaxilla. Forehead and submaxilla TEWL was significantly greater during summer and winter compared to spring and autumn. On cheeks, TEWL was significantly greater in spring, summer, and winter seasons compared to autumn. Both studies determined TEWL to be higher in winter compared to autumn [32]. Lastly, Yang et al. had a cohort of 72 women from China and measured TEWL during all four seasons on the cheek and forearm and found no significant difference in TEWL on the forearm between seasons. However, on the cheek, TEWL during spring was significantly higher than in summer and consistent with the previously discussed findings that TEWL in winter was significantly higher than in summer [31].

Altitude

TEWL's potential relationship with altitude has only been recently investigated: Lee et al. measured TEWL in 136 Sudanese females with 49 from Jakarta, with an altitude of 7 m, and the remaining 87 from Bandung, with an altitude of 768 m, on the forehead and cheek and observed no significant effect of altitude on TEWL at both sites [33].

Individual Variables

Age

Physical and biological properties of skin change with age. The effect of age on TEWL has been widely studied (Table 15.2). Several found no significant TEWL effect of age. For example, Rougier et al. studied 23 males in age groups 20–30,

Table 15.2 TEWL (transepidermal water loss): impact of age. While not all the studies agree, most found that older than 60 had significantly lower baseline TEWL compared to younger individuals. SD = standard deviation [5, 34–46]

Study	Subjects (age, sample size, sex) by age strata	Site	Age and TEWL result
Rougier et al. [42]	20–30 years, $n = 8$, males	Upper-outer arm	No significant differences
	45–55 years, $n = 8$, males		
	65–80 years, $n = 7$, males		
Cua et al. [37]	"Young adult" (25.9 ± 1.4 years), $n = 7$, females	Forehead, upper arm, volar and dorsal forearm, postauricular, palm, abdomen, upper back, thigh, ankle	Elderly had significantly lower basal TEWL at the upper arm ($p \leq 0.05$) and abdomen ($p \leq 0.01$). Lower in elderly at all other sites except the postauricular but not significant
	"Elderly" (74.6 ± 1.9 years), $n = 8$, females		
	Caucasians		
Cua et al. [38]	"Young" (24.9 ± 1.1 years), $n = 7$, females	Forehead, postauricular, upper arm, volar and dorsal forearm, palm, abdomen, thigh, ankle, upper back, lower back	Significantly lower baseline TEWL in the older population compared to young at all body regions ($p \leq 0.05$) except the postauricular and palm
	"Old" (75.3 ± 2.4 years), $n = 7$, females		
	"Young" (28.7 ± 0.5 years), $n = 7$, males		
	"Old" (73.8 ± 1.9 years), $n = 8$, males		
	Caucasians		
Wilhelm et al. [45]	"Young adult" (26.7 ± 2.8 years), $n = 14$, males and females	Forehead, dorsal aspect upper arm, dorsal and volar aspect forearm, postauricular, palm, abdomen, upper and lower back, extensor surface of the thigh, ankle	TEWL was significantly lower in aged group compared to young adults at all regions ($p \leq 0.05$) except the postauricular and palm
	"Aged" (70.5 ± 13.8), $n = 15$, males and females		
Conti et al. [36]	12–60 years, $n = 63$, males and females	Forehead, cheek, forearm extensor and flexor, antecubital fossa, abdomen, upper back, lumbar region, buttocks, pretibial, calf, palm, dorsal hand, sole	TEWL significantly higher in younger compared to older group on the epigastrium, buttocks, and calf ($p < 0.05$)
	61–92 years, $n = 24$, males and females		

Table 15.2 (continued)

Study	Subjects (age, sample size, sex) by age strata	Site	Age and TEWL result
Fluhr et al. [40]	"Children" 1–6 years, $n = 44$, males and females	Volar forearm	No significant differences
	"Parent" 21–44 years, $n = 44$, males and females		
Marrakchi and Maibach [41]	24–34 years, $n = 10$, not stated	Forehead, upper eyelid, nose, cheek, nasolabial and perioral areas, chin, neck, volar forearm	No significant differences
	66–83 years, $n = 10$, not stated		
Wen and Jiang [44] [abstract]	$n = 62$	Neck, inner side of flexible forearm	TEWL significantly lower in subjects older than 60 than younger ($p < 0.05$)
Firooz et al. [39]	10–20 years, $n = 10$	Forehead, cheek, nasolabial fold, neck, forearm, dorsal side of the hand, palm, leg	No significant differences
	20–30 years, $n = "$		
	30–40 years, $n = "$		
	40–50 years, $n = "$		
	50–60 years, $n = "$		
	All groups with males and females		
Boireau-Adamezyk et al. [35]	18–30 years, $n = 10$	Face, dorsal forearm, upper inner arm	Linear regression: significant decrease in TEWL with age at the face and upper inner arm ($p < 0.05$); no significant correlation for dorsal forearm
	30–40 years, $n = "$		
	40–55 years, $n = "$		
	55–70 years, $n = "$		
	French females		
Sato et al. [43]	"Elderly" 70–89 years, $n = 41$	Buttocks, back[a], outer side of lower leg[b], inner forearm	No significant differences
	"Middle-aged" 35–45 years, $n = 20$		
	Males and females in Tokyo		
Baumrin et al. [34]	Infants (6 weeks to 12 months)	Dorsal forearm, ventral upper arm	Higher TEWL in infants than adults
	G1: 6 weeks to 3 months, $n = 12$		Linear decrease with age at both sites:
	G2: 3–6 months, $n = 11$		Dorsal forearm
	G3: 6–12 months, $n = 20$		$R = 0.37$
	Adults 18–35 years, $n = 60$, all females		$p = 0.01$
	All South African		Ventral arm
			$R = 0.18$
			$p = 0.23$

(continued)

Table 15.2 (continued)

Study	Subjects (age, sample size, sex) by age strata	Site	Age and TEWL result
Mehta et al. [5]	G1: 5–20 years, $n = 110$	Scalp, forehead, forearm, leg	TEWL significantly higher in G1 and G2 compared to G3 and G4 at all sites ($p < 0.05$) but not significant on the forearm
	G2: 21–35 years, $n = 169$		
	G3: 36–50 years, $n = 126$		
	G4: 51–70 years, $n = 95$		
	Indian males and females		
Xie et al. [46]	G1: 16–20 years, $n = 45$	Midpoint of the connection line between the lower edge of the ear and suprasternal fossa	G4 and older had significantly higher TEWL than G1 ($p < 0.05$)
	G2: 21–25 years, $n = ''$		
	G3: 26–30 years, $n = ''$		
	G4: 31–35 years, $n = ''$		
	G5: 36–40 years, $n = ''$		
	G6: 41–45 years, $n = ''$		
	G7: 46–50 years, $n = ''$		
	G8: 51–55 years, $n = ''$		
	G9: 56–60 years, $n = ''$		
	G10: 61–66 years, $n = ''$		
	Chinese females		

[a]1 "Middle-aged" subject did not measure TEWL at this site
[b]1 "Elderly" subject did not measure TEWL at this site

45–55, and 65–80 years and observed no significant difference in TEWL between the groups [42]. Fluhr et al. compared TEWL in two age populations, comprising of 44 children 1–6 years and one of their adult parents 21–44 years, and found no significant differences between the groups [40]. Marrakchi and Maibach saw no significant difference in TEWL between ten individuals 24–34 years and ten individuals 66–83 years at nine anatomic sites [41]. Firooz et al. compared a more expansive group with ten people from each decade of life within the 10–60-year range and observed no significant differences in TEWL, as did Sato et al. comparing an elderly population with a middle-aged population in Tokyo at all anatomic sites measured [39, 43].

However, much of the literature reviewed found a decrease in TEWL in older individuals. Cua et al. investigated differences in TEWL between seven young adult females with a mean age of 25.9 years and eight elderly females with a mean age of 74.6 years and observed that the elderly population had a significantly lower basal TEWL. However, they measured TEWL on the forehead, upper arm, volar and dorsal forearm, postauricular area, palm, abdomen, upper back, thigh, and ankle and only saw a significant difference at the upper arm and abdomen. Nonetheless, mean TEWL was lower in the elderly at all sites, except the postauricular region [37]. Cua et al. conducted another study comparing 14 young adults with 15 elderly individuals at the same anatomic site as their first study and in this study also included the lower back. Again, the elderly population had significantly lower baseline TEWL at all the sites, except at the palm and the postauricular area the younger population had lower baseline TEWL [38]. This difference in relationship between age and TEWL based on anatomic site measured by the two Cua et al. studies may be attributed to the low sample size and potentially low power of their initial study. Also, their initial study only contained females, whereas the second study included women and men which may have impacted results [37, 38]. Wilhelm et al. found remarkably similar results in which they also measured at TEWL in 14 male and female young adults with a mean age of 26.7 years and another group of 15 male and female elderly individuals with a mean age of 70.5 years at the same anatomic sites as the second Cua et al. study. TEWL was significantly lower in the elderly population at all regions except the postauricular area and palm, consistent with Cua et al.'s second study [38, 45].

Conti et al. investigated a different age range by comparing subjects aged 12–60 and 61–92 years and found the older population had significantly lower TEWL values but only at certain sites measured including the epigastrium, buttocks, and calves [36]. Several other studies showed a similar decrease in TEWL with age [5, 35, 44]. Finally, Baumrin et al. took a slightly different approach and compared TEWL in infants of three different age groups (6 weeks to 3 months, 3–6 months, and 6–12 months) with female adults in the 18–35-year age range. Infants had higher TEWL than adults with a linear decrease in TEWL with age at all sites [34].

An outlier to the analysis above is Xie et al. in that the TEWL positively correlated with age. They measured TEWL in ten age groups (16–20, 21–25, 26–30, 31–35, 36–40, 41–45, 46–50, 51–55, 56–60, and 61–66 years) of Chinese females and individuals 31 years and older had significantly higher TEWL than the individuals in the youngest group and suggested this difference may be due to geographic and ethnic variations, since many of the other studies that concluded TEWL decreases with age were performed in America [46].

Anatomic Site

The effect of anatomic site on TEWL is also extensively studied (Table 15.3); many compared facial TEWL values with values on the extremities. Boireau-Adamezyk et al. investigated TEWL levels in 40 French women and elucidated the following relationship in TEWL: face > dorsal forearm = upper inner arm [35]. Mehta et al. measured TEWL in 500 Indians at the scalp, forehead, forearm, and leg. Scalp and forehead had significantly higher TEWL than the extremities, consistent with Boireau-Adamezyk et al.'s findings that the face has weaker barrier function than the extremities [5, 35].

Table 15.3 TEWL (transepidermal water loss): impact of anatomic site. Most studies found a significant relationship between site and TEWL. In general, the face has the highest TEWL, followed by the wrist, and then the abdomen and extremities. No conclusive relationship found regarding the abdomen and extremities. SD = standard deviation [5, 34, 35, 42, 47–51]

Study	Subjects (age range or mean ± SD, sample size, sex)	Site	Anatomic site and TEWL result
Rougier et al. [42]	20–30 years, 7–8 subjects per anatomic site, males	Forehead, postauricular, arm (upper outer), forearm (ventral elbow), forearm (ventral mid), forearm (ventral wrist), abdomen	Forearm (ventral elbow) < forearm (ventral mid) < arm (upper outer) ≤ abdomen < forearm (ventral wrist) < postauricular < forehead (no statistical significance noted)
Van Der Valk and Maibach [52]	22–64 years, $n = 10$, males and females	Volar forearm: cubital fossa, wrist fold, and three equidistant sites between	Significant variation in mean baseline TEWL from the wrist to elbow ($p < 0.05$); gradual decrease at the wrist to elbow and increase at the cubital fossa
Panisset et al. [51]	20–42 years, $n = 14$ Males and females	Ventral forearm: 3.5, 6.5, 9.5, 12.5, 15.5, 18.5, and 20.5 cm from fold of wrist at 1.5 cm on sides of a median line	Mean TEWL at the wrist significantly higher than all other sites ($p < 0.002$); no significant differences in TEWL between all other sites
Chilcott and Farrar [48]	18–28 years, $n = 17$ Males and females Caucasians	Volar forearms: five 2.5 cm diameter circular areas (1 cm apart and uppermost 4 cm from the antecubital fossa)	Most proximal site > midpoint ($p < 0.001$); most distal site > midpoint ($p < 0.01$)

Table 15.3 (continued)

Study	Subjects (age range or mean ± SD, sample size, sex)	Site	Anatomic site and TEWL result
Bock et al. [47]	25–54 years, $n = 25$ Males and Females	Volar forearm: "distal" site 5 cm from the wrist, "mid-volar" site, "proximal" site 5 cm from the cubital fossa	No significant difference in baseline TEWL between all sites
Machado et al. [49]	20–60 years, $n = 90$ Males and females Asian and Caucasian	Ventral wrist, ventral mid forearm close to ventral wrist (FA1), ventral mid forearm close to ventral elbow (FA2), ventral elbow, forehead[a], abdomen[b]	Forehead > wrist > FA1 = FA2 = elbow = abdomen ($p < 0.05$)
Mohammed et al. [50]	20–58 years, $n = 22$ Males and females Caucasian and Black	Cheek, abdomen, wrist, mid-ventral forearm	Cheek > wrist > abdomen = mid-ventral forearm ($p < 0.05$)
Boireau-Adamezyk et al. [35]	18–30 years, $n = 10$ 30–40 years, $n = "$ 40–55 years, $n = "$ 55–70 years, $n = "$ French females	Face, dorsal forearm, upper inner arm	Face > dorsal forearm = upper inner arm

(continued)

Table 15.3 (continued)

Study	Subjects (age range or mean ± SD, sample size, sex)	Site	Anatomic site and TEWL result
Baumrin et al. [34]	Infants (6 weeks to 12 months)	Dorsal forearm, ventral upper arm	Infants: ventral upper arm > dorsal forearm ($p = 0.008$)
	G1: 6 weeks to 3 months, $n = 12$		Adults: no significant difference
	G2: 3–6 months, $n = 11$		
	G3: 6–12 months, $n = 20$		
	Adults 18–35 years ($n = 60$)		
	All adult females		
Mehta et al. [5]	G1: 5–20 years, $n = 110$	Scalp, forehead, forearm, leg	Scalp and forehead > extremities ($p < 0.05$)
	G2: 21–35 years, $n = 169$		
	G3: 36–50 years, $n = 126$		
	G4: 51–70 years, $n = 95$		
	Indian males and females		

[a] $n = 84$
[b] $n = 59$

Many studies conducted an even more expanded comparison by examining at a variety of anatomic sites. Rougier et al. found the following relationship after measuring TEWL in various anatomic sites of 7–8 males: forearm (ventral elbow) < forearm (ventral mid) < arm (upper outer) ≤ abdomen < forearm (ventral wrist) < postauricular < forehead [42]. Machado et al. measured TEWL in six sites in a group of male and female Asians and Caucasians and determined the following relationship in TEWL: forehead > wrist > ventral mid forearm close to the ventral wrist = ventral mid forearm close to the ventral elbow = elbow = abdomen [49]. Mohammed et al. measured TEWL in 22 Caucasian and Black males and females and observed the following: cheek > wrist > abdomen = mid-ventral forearm [50]. Note that the face has the highest TEWL followed by the wrist, but the extremities and abdomen show conflicting results.

Several studies accomplished a more detailed approach and investigated whether TEWL differences exist between different areas within a general anatomic site. For example, many studies compared TEWL in different forearm areas. This is an area of significant interest since many investigations measure TEWL at the forearm. Panisset et al. compared TEWL in 14 males and females on the ventral forearm at 3.5, 6.5, 9.5, 12.5, 15.5, 18.5, and 20.5 cm up from fold of wrist. The wrist had a significantly higher TEWL than all the other sites with no significant differences between the other sites [51]. Van Der Valk and Maibach measured TEWL in four males and six females at a site next to the wrist fold, next to the cubital fossa, and three equidistant sites between and found the highest TEWL at the wrist and a gradual decrease towards the elbow. However, there was a slight increase at the site near the cubital fossa compared to the more distal site [52]. Conversely, Chilcott and Farrar determined TEWL in 17 male and female Caucasians at five 2.5 cm diameter circular areas 1 cm apart on the volar forearm; the most distal site and most proximal site had significantly higher TEWL than the midpoint [48]. Finally, Bock et al. measured TEWL in 25 males and females on the volar forearm at a distal, a mid-volar, and a proximal site—with no significant differences between any of the three sites [47]. With all studies yielding different results, a true correlation between TEWL and the placement on the forearm region cannot be derived.

Sex

Studies have found no significant impact of sex on TEWL at multiple sites (Table 15.4). These include Lammintausta et al. comparing seven white females and seven white males, Rougier et al. comparing groups of 7–8 males and females, Cua et al. comparing 14 Caucasian females and 15 Caucasian males, and Wilhelm et al. comparing 14 males and 15 females [38, 42, 45, 53].

However, others found a difference in TEWL based on sex. Conti et al. compared TEWL between 35 males and 58 females at 14 sites. Males had a greater TEWL than females at most sites; however, it was only significant at the cheek, upper back, and calf [36]. Chilcott and Farrar measured TEWL in eight Caucasian males and nine Caucasian females on the forearm, and males had a significantly higher TEWL than females, about 5% higher [48]. This contradicts Conti et al. who did not find a significant difference between males and females at the forearm. Firooz et al. measured TEWL in 25 males and 25 females, and overall males had significantly higher results than females when comparing the mean TEWL from multiple sites [39].

Two studies found age-related sex differences, but with conflicting results. Luebberding et al. studied six groups with the following age ranges: 20–29, 30–39, 40–49, 50–59, and 60–74 years. Each had 30 females and 30 males. Until the age of 50, men had significantly lower TEWL than women, regardless of site. However,

Table 15.4 TEWL (transepidermal water loss): impact of sex. Most found that males had higher baseline TEWL compared to females and only one study found the opposite. Studies that found no significant difference in TEWL based on sex were the oldest. SD = standard deviation [5, 36, 38, 39, 42, 45, 48, 53, 54]

Study	Subjects (age range or mean ± SD, sample size, sex)	Site	Sex and TEWL result
Lammintausta et al. [53]	19–65 years, $n = 7$, females	Right upper back above the scapula (3 areas)	No significant baseline differences
	16–64 years, $n = 7$, males		
	Caucasians		
Rougier et al. [42]	20–30 years, $n = 7$ or 8 per group, males and females	Upper-outer arm (eight males and seven females), forehead (seven males and eight females)	No significant differences
Cua et al. [38]	"Young" (24.9 ± 1.1 years), $n = 7$, females	Forehead, postauricular, upper arm, volar and dorsal forearm, palm, abdomen, thigh, ankle, upper back, lower back	No significant differences
	"Old" (75.3 ± 2.4 years), $n = 7$, females		
	"Young" (28.7 ± 0.5 years), $n = 7$, males		
	"Old" (73.8 ± 1.9 years), $n = 8$, males		
	Caucasians		
Wilhelm et al. [45]	"Young adult" (26.7 ± 2.8 years), $n = 7$, males	Forehead, dorsal aspect upper arm, dorsal and volar aspect forearm, postauricular region, palm, abdomen, upper and lower part of the back, extensor surface of the thigh, ankle	No significant differences
	"Young adult" (26.7 ± 2.8 years), $n = 7$, females		
	"Aged" (70.5 ± 13.8), $n = 8$, males		
	"Aged" (70.5 ± 13.8), $n = 7$, females		
Conti et al. [36]	2–92 years, $n = 93$	Forehead, cheek, extensor and flexor side of the forearm, antecubital fossa, abdomen, upper back, lumbar region, buttocks, pretibial area, calf, palm, dorsal hand, sole	Males > females
	35 males and 58 females		Significant at the cheek, upper back, and calf ($p < 0.05$)

Table 15.4 (continued)

Study	Subjects (age range or mean ± SD, sample size, sex)	Site	Sex and TEWL result
Chilcott and Farrar [48]	18–28 years, $n = 17$ Eight males and nine females Caucasians	Volar forearm (five 2.5 cm diameter circular areas 1 cm apart and uppermost area 4 cm from the antecubital fossa)	Males > females ($p < 0.05$)
Firooz et al. [39]	10–60 years, $n = 50$ 25 males and 25 females	Forehead, cheek, nasolabial fold, neck, forearm, dorsal side of the hand, palm, leg	Males > females ($p < 0.05$)
Luebberding et al. [54]	G1: 20–29 years, $n = 60$	Forehead, cheek, neck, volar forearm, dorsal hand	Independent of age: female > male ($p < 0.05$)
	G2: 30–39 years, $n = 60$		Age-dependent differences:
	G3: 40–49 years, $n = 60$		G1–G3: females > men of same age at the face, neck, and forearm ($p < 0.05$)
	G4: 50–59 years, $n = 60$ G5: 60–74 years, $n = 60$ 30 males and 30 females in each group		Older than 50 years: difference diminish with age at the face and neck but not the forearm
Mehta et al. [5]	G1: 5–20 years, $n = 61$, males	Scalp, forehead, forearm, leg	Median TEWL males > females at all ages except G4 ($p < 0.05$)
	G1: 5–20 years, $n = 49$, females		
	G2: 21–35 years, $n = 79$, males		
	G2: 21–35 years, $n = 90$, females		
	G3: 36–50 years, $n = 64$, males		
	G3: 36–50 years, $n = 62$, females		
	G4: 51–70 years, $n = 63$, males		
	G4: 51–70 years, $n = 32$, females		
	Indians		

this difference in TEWL diminished with age at most anatomic sites [54]. Mehta et al. studied four age groups (5–20, 21–35, 36–50, and 51–70 years) comprised of Indian females and males. Males had a significantly greater TEWL than females at all ages, except for the 51–70-year group where there was no significant difference [5].

Skin of Color

Much literature investigating the impact of skin of color on TEWL compared black skin and white skin. However, in another manuscript, we reviewed 26 articles and found conflicting results; several determined no significant difference in TEWL between black and white skin, some finding black skin to have a greater TEWL, and some finding white skin to have a greater TEWL [6].

Skin of color research has expanded beyond white and black skin and includes other groups, such as Hispanic and East Asian groups. However, we found a similar spread of results with varying significance and TEWL relationships between skin of color groups [6]. For example, Berardesca et al. determined baseline TEWL values in 15 Black volunteers with parents and grandparents that were described as Black, 12 white volunteers of Anglo-Saxon ancestry, and 12 Hispanic volunteers who were Mexican immigrants in Northern California and found no significant difference between baseline TEWL between the three groups [55]. On the other hand, Sugino et al. (abstract only) examined a wider expanse of various skin of color groups, with Black, Caucasian, Hispanic, and Asian participants and found TEWL values of the groups to be in the following order: Black > Caucasian ≥ Hispanic ≥ Asian [56].

Finally, we found that even within skin of color groups, for example, Asians, there were inconclusive results regarding whether TEWL differences exist between subgroups of these overarching skin of color categories, such as between Indonesians and Vietnamese individuals [6].

Circadian Rhythm

Spruit was the earliest to investigate whether time influences TEWL. He measured a subject's TEWL on their forearm at 8:00 and 16:00 every day from March 21 to April 13, 1970 (Table 15.5). TEWL was higher at 16:00 compared to 8:00 [60]. Reinberg et al. investigated this topic in detail measuring TEWL on the forearm for 48 h at 4:00, 9:00, 14:00, 19:00, and 23:00 in female Caucasians. There were troughs in TEWL at 14:00 and peaks during the night. This somewhat coincides with Spruit who found higher TEWL during the latter part of the day [59, 60]. Yosipovitch et al. took frequent measurements every 2 h in two sessions over a cumulative 24 h span in nine men and seven women, measuring TEWL at the forehead, upper back, forearm, and shins. TEWL had a significant time dependence at all sites, with a maximum TEWL around 20:00 and a minimum from 8:00 to 10:00 at most sites. However, shin had 2 peaks at 12:00 and 4:00. Yosipovitch et al. generated a curve of the circadian rhythm of TEWL on the forearm and forehead, which coincides with Spruit's findings that at 16:00 the TEWL is higher than at 8:00 [60, 61]. However, it did not have a trough at 14:00 that Reinberg et al. had found [59]. Ostermeier and Kerscher (abstract only) measured the cheek and forehead four times in a 12 h span in 24 individuals, and evening TEWL was higher than at all other time points [58].

Conversely, two studies observed a peak in TEWL in the morning, unlike the previously mentioned studies. Chilcott and Farrar measured TEWL every 2 h from

Table 15.5 TEWL (transepidermal water loss): impact of circadian rhythm. All studies found a relationship between time and baseline TEWL; however, findings were inconclusive due to the disparity in results. SD = standard deviation [48, 57–61]

Study	Subjects (age range or mean ± SD, sample size, sex)	Measurement times	Site	Circadian rhythm and TEWL result
Spruit [60]	$n = 1$[a]	8:00 and 16:00 from March 21 to April 13, 1970	Volar aspect of the forearm at three sites	Baseline water vapor loss: 16:00 > 8:00
Reinberg et al. [59]	27.9 ± 2.7 years, $n = 7$	48 h time span, Day 1 18:00 to Day 3 15:00 h	Flexor forearm	Troughs at 14:00 and peaks during night
	Females	Measurement times each day: 4:00, 9:00, 14:00, 19:00, 23:00		
	All Caucasian			
Yosipovitch et al. [61]	23–53 years, $n = 16$	Measured every 2 h in two sessions (daytime and nighttime) over a cumulative 24 h[b]	Forehead, upper back, forearm, shins	TEWL time dependent at all sites ($p \leq 0.05$)
	Males and females			Most subjects: max at the evening (~20:00); minimum in the morning (8:00–10:00) except the shins
				Shin: 2 peaks (12:00 and 4:00)
				All sites peak to trough difference significant ($p < 0.05$)
Chilcott and Farrar [48]	18–28 years, $n = 17$	Measured every 2 h from 9:00 to 17:00	Volar forearm (five 2.5 cm diameter circular areas 1 cm apart and uppermost 4 cm from the antecubital fossa)	Baseline TEWL: 9:00 > 17:00 ($p < 0.05$); 9% decrease
	Males and females			
	Caucasians			

(continued)

Table 15.5 (continued)

Study	Subjects (age range or mean ± SD, sample size, sex)	Measurement times	Site	Circadian rhythm and TEWL result
Le Fur et al. [57]	21–32 years, $n = 8$	Measured every 4 h for 48 h	Face, volar forearm	Circadian rhythm: circadian face ($p < 0.0005$), forearm ($p < 0.03$)
	Females			12 h rhythm for the face ($p < 0.05$) and forearm ($p < 0.0001$)
	Caucasians			8 h rhythm for the face ($p < 0.0005$) and forearm ($p < 0.0006$)
				Face: 2 peaks at 8:00 and 16:00; trough at 20:00–0:00
				Forearm: two peaks at 8:00 and 16:00; two troughs at 12:00 and 0:00
Ostermeier and Kerscher [58] [abstract]	21–39 years; $n = 24$	Measured four times in 12 h	Cheek, forehead	Evening higher than at all other times
	Sex not mentioned			

[a] Age and sex unknown
[b] 6 subjects not examined during daytime session

9:00 to 17:00 in eight male and nine female Caucasians on the forearms; TEWL at 9:00 was significantly higher than at 17:00 [48]. Le Fur et al. measured TEWL every 4 h for 48 h in eight female Caucasians on the face and volar forearm. There were 24 h, 12 h, and even 8 h significant rhythms on both sites. However, the face had two peaks at 8:00 and 16:00 and a trough at night from 20:00 to 0:00 and the forearm two peaks at 8:00 and 16:00 and two troughs at 12:00 and 0:00 [57].

Sleep

The impact of sleep on TEWL is a recently explored variable (Table 15.6). Altemus et al. investigated a 42 h sleep deprivation in 11 females compared to baseline, and there were no significant differences in TEWL on the forearm or face [8]. Choi et al. (abstract) investigated lack of sleep and alcohol on 20 Korean males, who frequently drink and did not get enough sleep. They compared TEWL after a good night of sleep to the morning after not having slept and drinking alcohol for 1 h the night before and found no significant TEWL differences [62].

Table 15.6 TEWL (transepidermal water loss): impact of sleep. Two of four studies found that sleep decreases baseline TEWL; however, the others found no significant differences in TEWL due to sleep. SD = standard deviation [8, 62–64]

Study	Subjects (age range or mean ± SD, sample size, sex)	Sleep	Site	Sleep and TEWL result
Altemus et al. [8]	18–29 years, $n = 11$ Females	42 h of sleep deprivation (compared to baseline)	Cheek, flexor forearm	No significant differences
Oyetakin-White et al. [64]	30–50 years, $n = 60$ Females	Poor sleepers ($n = 30$)	Upper inner arm	Baseline TEWL: poor sleepers > good sleepers ($p = 0.04$)
		PSQI > 5, sleep duration ≤ 5 h		
	Caucasians	Good sleepers ($n = 30$)		
		PSQI ≤ 5, sleep duration 7–9 h		
Choi et al. [62] [abstract]	30–36 years, $n = 20$	Measurement 1: Day 1— morning after good night sleep	Facial areas	No significant differences
	Males	Measurement 2: Day 2— drank 360 mL 17.5% alcohol for 1 h at night and measured the next morning after not sleeping		
	Koreans who often drink and lack sleep			
Jang et al. [63] [abstract]	"Old group" (mean age 47.9 ± 5.1 years): $n = 21$	Measurement 1: before sleep (after wash)	Not stated	Baseline TEWL: before sleeping > after sleeping
	Females	Measurement 2: after 7 h sleep in the morning		
	"Young group" (mean age 27.5 ± 2.8 years): $n = 11$	Measurement 3: after wash		
	Females			
	Koreans			

Conversely, Oyetakin-White et al. analyzed TEWL in poor and good Caucasian female sleepers. Poor sleepers were defined as having a Pittsburgh Sleep Quality Index (PSQI) greater than 5 and sleep duration of ≤ 5 h and good sleepers as having a PSQI of ≤ 5 and a sleep duration of 7–9 h. Poor sleepers had significantly higher baseline TEWL than good sleepers [64]. Jang et al. (abstract) found similar results in a group of 32 Korean women. They measured TEWL before sleeping and after washing to after 7 h of sleep the next morning. TEWL decreased post sleeping [63].

Food

Studies suggest that certain foods impact TEWL (Table 15.7). Hong et al. investigated TEWL impact of galacto-oligosaccharides (GOS) as found in infant formula as a supplement, milk products, certain beverages, and products [68]. Hong et al. compared TEWL levels in individuals receiving 1 g of GOS twice daily to those consuming 100% dextrin placebo and measured TEWL at the crow's feet area in 79

Table 15.7 TEWL (transepidermal water loss): impact of food. All studies found an impact of a specific food or food supplement on TEWL. SD = standard deviation [12, 65–67]

Study	Subjects (age range or mean ± SD, sample size, sex)	Food	Site	Food and TEWL result
Hong et al. [66]	32–68 years, $n = 79$	12 weeks	Crow's feet area	Week 4: GOS reduction from baseline > control reduction from baseline ($p < 0.05$)
	Males and females	Food: 1 g of galacto-oligosaccharides (GOS) 2×/day		Week 12: no significant difference between control W12 and control baseline
	Koreans with fine wrinkles at outer corner eyes	Control: 100% dextrin		GOS W12 < GOS baseline ($p < 0.05$)
Fukunaga et al. [65]	>20 years (mean age 43.6 ± 10.3 years): $n = 17$	Measurement 1: baseline	Forearm, cheek	Forearm: after ingestion GlcCer < before ingestion GlcCer ($p = 0.02$)
	Males and females	Measurement 2: 4 weeks after		Difference between before digestion and after digestion of control vs. GlcCer
		Food: 1.8 mg of glucosylceramide (GlcCer) 1× daily		GlcCer significantly lower than control ($p = 0.01$)
		Or		Cheek: no significant differences
		Placebo: same pill without GlcCer 1× daily		
		Measurement 3: after 4 weeks washout		
		Measurement 4: after 4 weeks GlcCer or placebo ingestion 1× daily (given the opposite treatment to what was given for Measurement 2)		

Table 15.7 (continued)

Study	Subjects (age range or mean ± SD, sample size, sex)	Food	Site	Food and TEWL result
Kuwano et al. [67]	25–52 years, $n = 36$	6 months	Face	GDL and placebo group: 6 months > baseline
	Males	Food: glucono-δ-lactone (GDL) 2000 mg/day		Rate of change TEWL compared to
	Japanese	Placebo: same pill without GDL		placebo > GDL ($p < 0.05$)
Vaughn et al. [12]	25–59 years, $n = 30$	4 weeks, 4 tablets 2× daily	Forehead, cheek	Placebo and turmeric: no significant differences
	Males and females	G1: Placebo		Herbal:
		G2: 500 mg/tablet turmeric		baseline > 4 weeks ($p = 0.003$)
		G3: 500 mg/tablet organic herbs		

Koreans with crow's feet, observing a significantly greater decrease in TEWL in those who consumed GOS compared to the placebo by Week 4. There was no significant TEWL difference in placebo group at Week 12 compared to baseline. There, however, was a significant difference in the GOS group compared to their baseline at Week 12 [66].

Fukunaga et al. compared TEWL in 17 individuals on the forearm and cheek after the subjects had consumed either a 1.8 mg of glucosylceramide (GlcCer) daily or a placebo. GlcCer occurs in foods like barley, rice, and corn. Individuals had significantly lower TEWL after consuming GlcCer compared to before consumption, and the difference in TEWL before consuming GlcCer to after consuming GlcCer was significantly lower than just taking the placebo. However, these differences were only at the forearm but not the cheek [65].

Kuwano et al. investigating the TEWL impact of glucono-δ-lactone (GDL), a food supplement and found naturally in wine and honey, had 36 Japanese males consume 2000 mg/day of GDL or placebo for 6 months. Both groups had higher TEWL levels compared to baseline. However, they attributed this to seasonal changes, as the weather changed to winter at the 6-month benchmark. The rate of TEWL change in the placebo group was significantly greater than the GDL group, suggesting GDL helped preserve barrier function in winter [67].

Vaughn et al. examined the TEWL effect of turmeric and herbal combination tablet consumption. Turmeric, a widely used spice in certain ethnic groups, and herbal supplements are often taken. Thirty participants were given either a placebo or a tablet containing 500 mg of turmeric or tablet containing 500 mg of an herbal combination—four tablets twice daily for 4 weeks. No significant differences were observed between the placebo and turmeric groups, but the herbal combination group had a significantly decreased TEWL after 4 weeks of consumption compared to baseline [12].

Body Mass Index (BMI)

Several studies investigated BMI and obesity's potential impact on TEWL (Table 15.8). Guida et al. compared forearm TEWL in an obese group defined by a BMI of ≥ 30 kg/m^2 to a control group with BMI ranging from 18.5 to 24.9 kg/m^2. Control had significantly greater BMI compared to the obese group, but there were no significant differences based on BMI level within the obese group. In addition, within the obese group, those with abdominal obesity had significantly lower TEWL compared to those without [69]. However, Nino et al. found contrasting results; they measured forearm TEWL in an overweight group with BMI between the 85th and 95th percentile and an obese group greater than the 95th percentile and compared it to the TEWL of a normal weight group. Those with abdominal obesity had

Table 15.8 TEWL (transepidermal water loss): impact of BMI. In three of four studies, either an increase in BMI or obesity led to an increase in TEWL. Opposing results were found regarding the impact of abdominal obesity on TEWL. SD = standard deviation [69–71, 79]

Study	Subjects (age range or mean ± SD, sample size, sex)	BMI/obesity	Site	BMI/obesity and TEWL result
Löffler et al. [70]	18–60 years, $n = 63$	G1: BMI < 25 kg/m^2 (underweight and normal)	Flexor forearm	G3 > G1 ($p < 0.05$); trend of increase from G1 to G3
	Males and females	G2: BMI 25–30 kg/m^2 (overweight)		Significant correlation between BMI and baseline TEWL ($p < 0.01$)
		G3: BMI > 30 kg/m^2 (obese)		
Guida et al. [69]	Obese (mean age 37.1 ± 13.1 years): $n = 60$	Obese: BMI $\geq$ 30 kg/m^2	Volar forearm	Control > obese ($p < 0.05$)
	Control (mean age 41.0 ± 12.3 years): $n = 20$	Control: BMI 18.5–24.9 kg/m^2		No significant TEWL differences based on BMI level in obese group
	Males and females			Obese group: without abdominal obesity > with abdominal obesity ($p < 0.05$)
Nino et al. [71]	Overweight and obese (age 8–15 years): $n = 65$	Overweight: BMI 85–95 percentile	Volar forearm	Obese > normal weight ($p < 0.05$)
	Normal weight (age 7–15 years): $n = 30$	Obese: BMI > 95 percentile		No significant differences according to BMI level
	Males and females	Normal weight		With abdominal obesity > without abdominal obesity ($p < 0.05$)
		Percentile based on age and sex		
Tavares et al. [79] [abstract]	20–46 years, $n = 51$ Females	All subjects obese or overweight	Face, breast, abdomen	Positive correlation between BMI and TEWL at all sites (between 0.282 and 0.601)

significantly higher TEWL than those without. Also, obese and overweight individuals had a significantly greater TEWL compared to normal weight individuals. They did not find significant correlation between TEWL and BMI value [71]. Löffler et al. found results similar to Nino et al.'s findings; they compared an underweight/normal group with a BMI under 25 kg/m^2, an overweight group of 25–30 kg/m^2, and an obese group with a BMI greater than 30 kg/m^2. The obese group had significantly greater TEWL than the normal/underweight group, but no significant difference between the overweight and normal/underweight group. They also, unlike the other two groups, found a significant positive correlation between BMI value and TEWL [70]. Finally, Tavares et al. (abstract only) investigated the correlation between BMI value and TEWL in obese and overweight subjects at the face, breast, and abdomen. There was a positive correlation between BMI and TEWL at all sites [79].

Smoking Status

The impact of smoking status on TEWL appears to be uncertain (Table 15.9). Muizzuddin et al. compared TEWL in active smokers, passive smokers, and nonsmokers. They defined active smoker as someone smoking one pack of cigarettes or

Table 15.9 TEWL (transepidermal water loss): impact of smoking status. The two studies have differing results, and therefore no conclusion can be made on whether smoking status impacts TEWL and if it does how. SD = standard deviation [9, 72]

Study	Subjects (age range or mean ± SD, sample size, sex)	Smoking status	Site	Smoking status and TEWL result
Muizzuddin et al. [9]	≥35 years, n = 100	Active smoker: ≥1 pack of cigarettes/day for >5 years	Cheek	Baseline TEWL: nonsmokers < active and passive (p < 0.001)
	People from New York, New Jersey, and Pennsylvania[a]	Passive smoker: never smoked and lived/worked with heavy smoker for 20 years		
		Nonsmokers: never smoked and not exposed to smoke except casually		
Xin et al. [72]	41–65 years, n = 99	Nonsmokers	Forearm	No significant TEWL differences between groups and no correlation between basal TEWL and years smoked
	Males	Light to moderate smokers: <20 cigarettes/day		
		Heavy smokers: ≥20 cigarettes/day		

[a] Sex not mentioned

more daily for more than 5 years. Passive smoker was defined as someone who never smoked but had lived or worked with a heavy smoker for 20 years. Nonsmoker was defined as those never smoking and was only exposed to smoke causally such as in public places.

Nonsmokers had significantly lower levels of TEWL compared to both active and passive smokers. No significant difference was observed between active and passive smokers [9]. Xin et al. found contradicting results where they analyzed TEWL in nonsmokers, light to moderate smokers who smoked less than 20 cigarettes a day, and heavy smokers who smoked 20 or more cigarettes per day. There was no significant difference in TEWL between the groups and no correlation between basal TEWL and years the individual had smoked [72].

Eccrine Sweating

Sweating can be the result of high temperature, physical activity, and emotion. Since temperature has been researched as a separate variable and subjects are usually not doing intensive physical activity during TEWL studies, we examined the impact of emotional sweating on TEWL. Being a part of an experiment and having one's TEWL measured can be potentially anxiety or emotion inducing; therefore, it is a relevant variable of interest. Pinnagoda et al. showed how emotional sweat impacted TEWL and used physical activity to induce sweating. However, prior to exercising, they measured baseline TEWL in the 44 men and women on the forearm with and without a topical agent used to inhibit sweating. In most cases, this difference pre-exercise in treated and untreated was not significantly different. Nonetheless, they found six "emotional sweaters," whose pre-exercise TEWL without a sweat inhibitor was significantly higher than the treated side [73].

Menstrual Cycle

The effect of the menstrual cycle and menopause on TEWL remains uncertain (Table 15.10). Harvell et al. measured TEWL in females on the day of maximal estrogen secretion, the day of maximal progesterone secretion, and the day of minimal estrogen/progesterone secretion. On the day of minimal estrogen/progesterone secretion, subjects had significantly higher TEWL than on the day of maximal estrogen secretion on the back and forearm. However, note that Harvell et al. determined these measurement days based on menstrual cycle start date and admitted there was inherent uncertainty when doing so. As a result, 67% of the data was obtained within a day of the expected event (i.e., day of maximal progesterone secretion), and 92% of the data was within 2 days [75]. Fujimura et al., on the other hand, investigated menopause effects by comparing TEWL in young and middle-aged females to postmenopausal females at multiple sites; there were no significant differences in TEWL based on menopause [74].

Table 15.10 TEWL (transepidermal water loss): impact of menstruation. Based on the findings of the two studies, menstrual cycle may impact TEWL, while menopause may not. SD = standard deviation [74, 75]

Study	Subjects (age range or mean ± SD, sample size, sex)	Menstrual cycle	Site	Menstrual cycle and TEWL result
Harvell et al. [75]	19–46 years, $n = 9$	Measurement days:	Volar forearm, interscapular area of the upper back	Baseline TEWL: day of minimal estrogen/progesterone secretion > day of maximal estrogen secretion at the forearm ($p = 0.021$) and back ($p = 0.037$)
	Females	Day of maximal estrogen secretion		Trend of higher TEWL from the day of maximal estrogen secretion to the day of minimal estrogen/progesterone secretion
		Day of maximal progesterone secretion		
		Day of minimal estrogen/progesterone secretion		
Fujimura et al. [74]	Younger group 21–39 years, $n = 31$	Premenopause: Younger and middle-aged group	Labia majora, groin, mons pubis, inner forearm, inner thigh	No significant differences between pre- and postmenopausal groups
	Middle-aged group 40–49 years, $n = 28$	Postmenopause: older group		
	Older postmenopausal group 47–60 years, $n = 40$			
	Females from Bangkok			

Discussion

Based on the summarized studies, several variables impact TEWL or may potentially impact TEWL measurements and therefore should be controlled for when conducting such experiments. Sample size and power should be a primary consideration where realistic, when conducting a TEWL experiment (and any experiment in general). Many TEWL experiments observed no significant correlation between their variable of interest and TEWL, but, without a power calculation, conclusions offered cannot be considered strong evidence or provide statistically acceptable significance due to the possibility of a type II error. Vaughn et al. was the only paper assessed here that explicitly stated that they conducted power calculation to determine the minimum necessary sample size [12]. Most sample sizes in other studies do not appear to include a significantly large sample size, and no statistical analysis or margins of error have been established by them. The absence of power calculation is an aspect that is lacking in much TEWL research. In addition, having a small sample size does not readily and accurately reveal real and important biological findings to the researchers.

Next, evaporimeter standardization and technician training have a clear impact on the measurements and are important variables that should be controlled for. Room temperature has a positive correlation with TEWL. Pinnagoda et al. recommended a room temperature of 20–22 °C to avoid potential fluctuations in measurements and avoid sweating [17]. Rogiers et al. suggested a room temperature below 22 °C; however, at 18 °C, it may be impossible to test due to persons complaining of cold and not wanting to continue the study [76]. Many TEWL studies follow this temperature guideline and conduct TEWL measurement in temperature-controlled environments or with sweat inhibitors to eliminate potential adverse impact of a high temperature environment [57, 66, 73].

Climatic factors are critical in the measurement of TEWL. As discussed previously, evidence exists that temperature has an impact on TEWL. Relative humidity has also been described as being a complex but important variable in determining TEWL and advised to be kept close to but lower than 50% [76]. Therefore, we decided to determine how many of the inspected papers controlled for climatic conditions during TEWL measurement and, if so, were the conditions described. Abstracts were not included as it could not be determined from the limited information provided whether climatic factors were controlled. Words such as "standardized," "maintained," and "use of air conditioning" were considered to indicate a controlled environment. Of the 57 papers inspected, 33 controlled for and identified the temperature and relative humidity of the test environment and one paper controlled for and identified only temperature; two papers stated that they controlled for climatic conditions but did not describe them; 16 papers did not control for climatic conditions but measured and reported temperature and relative humidity in the test area; and five papers did not control for or report climatic conditions. Overall, around 60% of the papers reviewed controlled for these variables. Such conditions are critical variables that must be controlled for in all studies. Furthermore, the methods of control varied from air conditioning to climatic chambers to undescribed methods [8, 47, 48]. Standardization of how climatic factors are controlled is also important in validating results as some methods may be more effective than others. Finally, it is important to note that even within the controlled studies variation existed in how much "control" was placed on the climatic conditions. For example, Mehta et al. stated that they maintained the temperature and relative humidity, but the reported limits were 20–27 °C and 10–60%, respectively [5]. On the other hand, Xie et al. also controlled for these conditions but maintained the testing conditions at 20 ± 1 °C and 55 ± 3% relative humidity [46]. While most of the papers with identified controls had tighter limits like Xie et al., it is important to standardize the acceptable amount of variation in temperature and relative humidity when controlling for climatic conditions.

The environment that the subjects experience impacts TEWL, but no consistent relationship has been determined. Studies compared TEWL during winter and summer; most determined that during winter humans have higher TEWL values. Wei et al. suggested this reduction in skin barrier function may be the result of changes in levels and ratios of stratum corneum lipids and keratin levels that occur during the winter [30].

Some had conflicting results with skin having higher TEWL in summer compared to winter. Song et al. suggested this may be due to an increase in skin hydration that helps persevere the skin barrier because of the often increase in humidity during summer [29]. Additionally, when evaluating TEWL over all seasons, it appears that in general summer and winter cause significantly higher TEWL than autumn and spring. This further validates the notion that season impacts TEWL and should be controlled for. Next, only one study was conducted on altitude impact with no significant effect [33]. However, power analysis was not conducted, and more studies investigating the relationship between altitude and TEWL are needed.

Physiological factors considered age; most concluded that TEWL decreases with age, especially as one reaches their 60s–70s. This has been illustrated in a review by Rogiers et al. that suggested that significant differences in TEWL may occur during certain periods of life; however, they found no significant difference overall [76]. Several studies observed no significant difference with age, but such studies were far less in number. Some like those by Rougier et al. and Marrakchi and Maibach had small sample sizes [41, 42]. Fluhr et al. had eldest participants at 44 years, while many studies found significant differences in TEWL at much older ages [40]. Baumrin et al. did find a significant difference in adults of a younger age, but they compared adults to infants, while Fluhr et al. compared adults to children [34, 40]. One possible explanation for this is that elderly stratum corneum has more skin barrier function as well as decreased permeability. In contrast, premature infant skin has increased permeability due to a lack of fully developed skin barrier function, affecting TEWL. Furthermore, the amount of photodamage increases with age, which can affect skin barrier function as well [77].

Xie et al. was the only contrasting result, that older subjects have higher TEWL values. They suggest this discrepancy may be due to geographic or ethnic differences since most studies, other than theirs, that concluded that the elderly had lower TEWL were conducted in America. This was also the only study where the anatomic site studied was the neck [46]. Several studies saw site-specific differences in age effects on TEWL, so it is possible that the effect of age on TEWL changes based on anatomic site. Boireau-Adamezyk et al. suggested that this change in TEWL with increasing age may be partly due to a thickening of the stratum corneum with age, as observed in their study [35].

A definite relationship between TEWL and anatomic site exists; however, the exact relationship between every anatomic site's TEWL value remains unclear since the data varies. In general, the face had highest TEWL values followed by the wrist and then abdomen and extremities. Data regarding the extremities and torso is inconclusive. This conclusion, however, differs from the order identified in previous older literature such as in the Rogiers et al. review of literature from 1977 to 1988, supplementing the need for an update [76]. Furthermore, some even suggest significant differences in TEWL in different regions on a singular anatomic site, such as the forearm. Although data regarding the TEWL on different sites of the forearm is inconclusive and often contradicts each other, it is important to explore and substantiate any potential relationship. Forearm is a widely used site for TEWL measurement, and therefore such variation in site on the forearm in TEWL could lead to discrepancy in the data. Rogiers et al. even suggested to avoid some sites like the palm and the wrist due to high interindividual variability at such locations [76].

Most studies analyzing the relationship between sex and TEWL determined that males had higher TEWL values than females. A possible explanation by Firooz et al. is that males tend to engage in more outdoor activities and have more damaged skin [39]. Only one study had opposing results. However, note that this study collected data for females in autumn of 2009 and males in autumn of 2011 [54]. Potential climate differences, timing differences, or instrument differences could have impacted their results. Several found no significant relationship between sex and TEWL. Interestingly, these were the oldest studies conducted on sex and TEWL reviewed and all had small sample sizes [38, 42, 45, 53].

Based on the data regarding race or ethnicity and TEWL, no clear conclusion can be drawn, as there is much variation in the data with no majority findings. Controlling for other related variables, such as the ones listed here, could help reveal a more defined relationship between race/ethnicity and TEWL.

All studies investigating the impact of time and circadian rhythm on TEWL determined differences in TEWL based on time. However, there is disparity in the data regarding the actual rhythm itself, with some studies seeing forearm TEWL peaks at the night and others finding peaks in the morning. Yosipovitch et al., for example, proposed that peaks at night could be a result of some unknown circadian cellular or metabolic activity in the epidermis during night [61]. In addition, some studies suggest that different TEWL circadian rhythm curves exist based on anatomic site measured [57, 61]. Differing levels of cortisol offer a possible explanation for the peaks in TEWL in the morning. A previous study examined the effect of psychological stress and how it deteriorates skin barrier function. Psychological stress was associated with increased levels of salivary cortisol 30 min after awakening, which is generally considered the time cortisol peaks. In addition, this psychological stress was connected to increases in basal TEWL and stratum corneum hydration, while stratum corneum integrity was decreased [78].

Based on studies analyzed, it appears that more sleep does result in lower TEWL values. However, data is limited, and two of the four studies investigated found no significant TEWL sleep impact. Therefore, more data is needed for a definite conclusion.

The literature suggests that certain foods may impact TEWL. However, each study analyzed one specific food product, and there was no commonality of food products across the studies, making it difficult to make well-defined conclusions regarding the impact of individual foods on TEWL. Further research is needed on specific foods to provide clearer guidelines for TEWL studies.

There was limited variation in data regarding the impact of BMI and obesity on TEWL. In three of four studies, an increase in BMI or obesity led to a TEWL increase. Löffler et al. suggested this could be due to increased sweat gland activity in obese individuals at rest [70]. Conversely, Nino et al., who found increased TEWL in those with abdominal obesity compared to those without, suggested the roles of adipokines causing replacement of the stratum corneum and leptin promoting fibroblast proliferation and collagen synthesis could explain the increased TEWL in obese patients [71]. Interestingly, Guida et al. had the opposite results to Nino et al., but referenced the exact same mechanisms of adipokines and leptin activity as a potential cause for lower TEWL values in obese individuals [69, 71]. Further data regarding the impact of obesity and abdominal obesity on TEWL is warranted.

Smoking impact on TEWL is also not conclusive given the scarcity of data and discrepancy in results, with one study suggesting that not only smoking but even being exposed to excessive smoking increases TEWL and another finding no TEWL impact of smoking [9, 72]. Thus, this is another area for further data.

Emotional eccrine sweating impacts TEWL results and significantly increases measured values. Adequate rest time for the patient, multiple "dummy" measurements, and application of a sweat inhibitor are all potential methods to control this variable.

Finally, menstrual cycle may impact on TEWL, while menopause has no effect. However, once again, there is insufficient evidence for a well-defined conclusion. It is therefore imperative that additional research should be conducted on the impact of menstruation and menopause on TEWL.

Conclusion

TEWL research is a widely studied field that despite more than 60 years of evidence continues to show variation in results and, in some instances, conflicting results. We outline variables impacting or may potentially impacting, TEWL and stress matching and controlling for these, should reduce the conflicting results, as noted here. Doing so will determine real and biologically important relationships regarding stratum corneum barrier function and variables, such as sex and age.

Acknowledgements None.

Declarations
Funding: Basic Science, Clinical, and Translational Research Summer Funding provided by the University of Rochester School of Medicine and Dentistry.

Conflicts of Interest/Competing Interests (Include Appropriate Disclosures)   Not applicable.

Consent to Participate   Not applicable.

Consent for Publication   Not applicable.

Availability of Data and Material (Data Transparency)   All literature is open and available to the public.

Code Availability (Software Application or Custom Code)   Not applicable.

Author's Contributions   Equal participation by Dr. Howard Maibach and Reva Peer: Anuk Burli contributed to discussion as well as editing.

References

1. Elias PM. Skin barrier function. Curr Allergy Asthma Rep. 2008;8:299–305. https://doi.org/10.1007/s11882-008-0048-0.
2. Fluhr JW, Feingold KR, Elias PM. Transepidermal water loss reflects permeability barrier status: validation in human and rodent in vivo and ex vivo models. Exp Dermatol. 2006;15:483–92. https://doi.org/10.1111/j.1600-0625.2006.00437.x.
3. Fujimura T, Miyauchi Y, Shima K, Hotta M, Tsujimura H, Kitahara T, Takema Y, Palungwachira P, Laohathai D, Chanthothai J, Nararatwanchai T. Ethnic differences in stratum corneum functions between Chinese and Thai infants residing in Bangkok, Thailand. Pediatr Dermatol. 2018;35:87–91. https://doi.org/10.1111/pde.13335.
4. Grice K, Bettley FR. The effect of skin temperature and vascular change on the rate of transepidermal water loss. Br J Dermatol. 1967;79:582–8. https://doi.org/10.1111/j.1365-2133.1967.tb11421.x.
5. Mehta HH, Nikam VV, Jaiswal CR, Mehta HB. A cross-sectional study of variations in the biophysical parameters of skin among healthy volunteers. Indian J Dermatol Venereol Leprol. 2018;84:521. https://doi.org/10.4103/ijdvl.IJDVL_1151_15.
6. Peer RP, Maibach HI. Did human evolution in skin of color enhance TEWL barrier? Arch Dermatol Res. 2022;314(2):121.
7. Kottner J, Lichterfeld A, Blume-Peytavi U. Transepidermal water loss in young and aged healthy humans: a systematic review and meta-analysis. Arch Dermatol Res. 2013;305:315–23. https://doi.org/10.1007/s00403-012-1313-6.
8. Altemus M, Rao B, Dhabhar FS, Ding W, Granstein RD. Stress-induced changes in skin barrier function in healthy women. J Invest Dermatol. 2001;117:309–17. https://doi.org/10.1046/j.1523-1747.2001.01373.x.
9. Muizzuddin N, Marenus K, Vallon P, Maes D. Effect of cigarette smoke on skin. J Soc Cosmet Chem. 1997;48:235–42.
10. Holder DJ, Marino MJ. Logical experimental design and execution in the biomedical sciences. Curr Protoc Pharmacol. 2017;76:A3G1–A3G26. https://doi.org/10.1002/cpph.20.
11. Hillebrand GG, Wickett R. Epidemiology of skin barrier function: host and environmental factors. In: Walters KA, Roberts MS, editors. Dermatologic, cosmeceutic, and cosmetic development therapeutic and novel approaches. Boca Raton, FL: CRC Press; 2007. p. 129–56.
12. Vaughn AR, Clark AK, Notay M, Sivamani RK. Randomized controlled pilot study of dietary supplementation with turmeric or herbal combination tablets on skin barrier function in healthy subjects. J Med Food. 2018;21:1260–5. https://doi.org/10.1089/jmf.2018.0015.
13. Young MM, Franken A, du Plessis JL. Transepidermal water loss, stratum corneum hydration, and skin surface pH of female African and Caucasian nursing students. Skin Res Technol. 2019;25:88–95. https://doi.org/10.1111/srt.12614.
14. Wilson D, Berardesca E, Maibach HI. In vitro transepidermal water loss: differences between black and white human skin. Br J Dermatol. 1988;119:647–52. https://doi.org/10.1111/j.1365-2133.1988.tb03478.x.

15. Wilson DR, Maibach HI. TEWL and the newborn. In: Peter E, Berardesca E, Maibach HI, editors. Bioengineering of the skin: water and the stratum corneum, vol. 1. Boca Raton, FL: CRC Press Inc.; 1994. p. 115–27.

16. Pinnagoda J, Tupker RA, Coenraads PJ, Nater JP. Comparability and reproducibility of the results of water loss measurements: a study of 4 evaporimeters. Contact Dermatitis. 1989;20:241–6. https://doi.org/10.1111/j.1600-0536.1989.tb03139.x.

17. Pinnagoda J, Tupker RA, Agner T, Serup J. Guidelines for transepidermal water loss (TEWL) measurement. A report from the Standardization Group of the European Society of Contact Dermatitis. Contact Derm. 1990;22:164–78. https://doi.org/10.1111/j.1600-0536.1990. tb01553.x.

18. De Paepe K, Houben E, Adam R, Wiesemann F, Rogiers V. Validation of the VapoMeter, a closed unventilated chamber system to assess transepidermal water loss vs. the open chamber Tewameter. Skin Res Technol. 2005;11:61–9. https://doi.org/10.1111/j.1600-0846.2005. 00101.x.

19. ServoMed Evaporimeters. Operation handbook. Stockholm: ServoMed; 1981.

20. Nilsson GE. Measurement of water exchange through skin. Med Biol Eng Comput. 1977;15:209–18. https://doi.org/10.1007/BF02441040.

21. Cravello B, Ferri A. Relationships between skin properties and environmental parameters. Skin Res Technol. 2008;14:180–6. https://doi.org/10.1111/j.1600-0846.2007.00275.x.

22. Lamke LO, Wedin B. Water evaporation from normal skin under different environmental conditions. Acta Derm Venereol. 1971;51:111–9.

23. Chen C-P, Hwang R-L, Chang S-Y, Lu Y-T. Effects of temperature steps on human skin physiology and thermal sensation response. Build Environ. 2011;46:2387–97. https://doi. org/10.1016/j.buildenv.2011.05.021.

24. Black D, Del Pozo A, Lagarde JM, Gall Y. Seasonal variability in the biophysical properties of stratum corneum from different anatomical sites. Skin Res Technol. 2000;6:70–6. https://doi. org/10.1034/j.1600-0846.2000.006002070.x.

25. De Paepe K, Houben E, Adam R, Hachem JP, Roseeuw D, Rogiers V. Seasonal effects on the nasolabial skin condition. Skin Pharmacol Physiol. 2009;22:8–14. https://doi. org/10.1159/000159772.

26. Kikuchi K, Kobayashi H, Le Fur I, Tschachler E, Tagami H. The winter season affects more severely the facial skin than the forearm skin: comparative biophysical studies conducted in the same Japanese females in later summer and winter. Exog Dermatol. 2002;1:32–8. https:// doi.org/10.1159/000047989.

27. Li X, Galzote C, Yan X, Li L, Wang X. Characterization of Chinese body skin through in vivo instrument assessments, visual evaluations, and questionnaire: influences of body area, intergeneration, season, sex, and skin care habits. Skin Res Technol. 2014;20:14–22. https://doi. org/10.1111/srt.12076.

28. Muizzuddin N, Ingrassia M, Marenus KD, Maes DH, Mammone T. Effect of seasonal and geographical differences on skin and effect of treatment with an osmoprotectant: Sorbitol. J Cosmet Sci. 2013;64:165–74.

29. Song EJ, Lee JA, Park JJ, Kim HJ, Kim NS, Byun KS, Choi GS, Moon TK. A study on seasonal variation of skin parameters in Korean males. Int J Cosmet Sci. 2015;37:92–7. https:// doi.org/10.1111/ics.12174.

30. Wei KS, Stella C, Wehmeyer KR, Christman J, Altemeier A, Spruell R, Wimalasena RL, Fadayel GM, Reilman RA, Motlagh S, Stoffolano PJ, Benzing K, Wickett RR. Effects of season stratum corneum barrier function and skin biomarkers. J Cosmet Sci. 2016;67:185–203.

31. Yang J, Tu Y, Man MQ, Zhang Y, Cha Y, Fan X, Wang Z, Zeng Z, He L. Seasonal variations of epidermal biophysical properties in Kunming, China: a self-controlled cohort study. Skin Res Technol. 2020;26:702. https://doi.org/10.1111/srt.12857.

32. Ye C, Chen J, Yang S, Yi J, Chen H, Li M, Yin S, Lai W, Zheng Y. Skin sensitivity evaluation: what could impact the assessment results? J Cosmet Dermatol. 2020;19:1231–8. https://doi. org/10.1111/jocd.13128.

33. Lee M, Jung Y, Kim E, Lee HK. Comparison of skin properties in individuals living in cities at two different altitudes: an investigation of the environmental effect on skin. J Cosmet Dermatol. 2017;16:26–34. https://doi.org/10.1111/jocd.12270.

34. Baumrin E, Mukansi MM, Sibisi C, Mosam A, Stamatas GN, Dlova NC. Epidermal barrier function in healthy black South African infants compared with adults. Pediatr Dermatol. 2018;35:e425–6. https://doi.org/10.1111/pde.13675.

35. Boireau-Adamezyk E, Baillet-Guffroy A, Stamatas GN. Age-dependent changes in stratum corneum barrier function. Skin Res Technol. 2014;20:409–15. https://doi.org/10.1111/srt.12132.

36. Conti A, Schiavi ME, Seidenari S. Capacitance, transepidermal water loss and causal level of sebum in healthy subjects in relation to site, sex and age. Int J Cosmet Sci. 1995;17:77–85. https://doi.org/10.1111/j.1467-2494.1995.tb00111.x.

37. Cua AB, Wilhelm KP, Maibach HI. Cutaneous sodium lauryl sulphate irritation potential: age and regional variability. Br J Dermatol. 1990;123:607–13. https://doi.org/10.1111/j.1365-2133.1990.tb01477.x.

38. Cua AB, Wilhelm KP, Maibach HI. Frictional properties of human skin: relation to age, sex and anatomical region, stratum corneum hydration and transepidermal water loss. Br J Dermatol. 1990;123:473–9. https://doi.org/10.1111/j.1365-2133.1990.tb01452.x.

39. Firooz A, Sadr B, Babakoohi S, Sarraf-Yazdy M, Fanian F, Kazerouni-Timsar A, Nassiri-Kashani M, Naghizadeh MM, Dowlati Y. Variation of biophysical parameters of the skin with age, gender, and body region. Sci World J. 2012;2012:386936. https://doi.org/10.1100/2012/386936.

40. Fluhr JW, Pfisterer S, Gloor M. Direct comparison of skin physiology in children and adults with bioengineering methods. Pediatr Dermatol. 2000;17:436–9. https://doi.org/10.1046/j.1525-1470.2000.01815.x.

41. Marrakchi S, Maibach HI. Biophysical parameters of skin: map of human face, regional, and age-related differences. Contact Dermatitis. 2007;57:28–34. https://doi.org/10.1111/j.1600-0536.2007.01138.x.

42. Rougier A, Lotte C, Corcuff P, Maibach H. Relationship between skin permeability and corneocyte size according to anatomic site, age, and sex in man. J Soc Cosmet Chem. 1988;39:15–26.

43. Sato N, Kitahara T, Fujimura T. Age-related changes of stratum corneum functions of skin on the trunk and the limbs. Skin Pharmacol Physiol. 2014;27:181. https://doi.org/10.1159/000353912.

44. Wen X, Jiang X. Study on the relationship between neck skin and age, season. J Clin Dermatol. 2011;40:601–5.

45. Wilhelm KP, Cua AB, Maibach HI. Skin aging. Effect on transepidermal water loss, stratum corneum hydration, skin surface pH, and casual sebum content. Arch Dermatol. 1991;127:1806–9. https://doi.org/10.1001/archderm.127.12.1806.

46. Xie X, Wang Y, Zeng Q, Lv Y, Hu R, Zhu K, Liu C, Lai W, Guan L. Characteristic features of neck skin aging in Chinese women. J Cosmet Dermatol. 2018;17:935–44. https://doi.org/10.1111/jocd.12762.

47. Bock M, Wulfhorst B, John SM. Site variations in susceptibility to SLS. Contact Dermatitis. 2007;57:94–6. https://doi.org/10.1111/j.1600-0536.2007.01159.x.

48. Chilcott RP, Farrar R. Biophysical measurements of human forearm skin in vivo: effects of site, gender, chirality and time. Skin Res Technol. 2000;6:64–9. https://doi.org/10.1034/j.1600-0846.2000.006002064.x.

49. Machado M, Salgado TM, Hadgraft J, Lane ME. The relationship between transepidermal water loss and skin permeability. Int J Pharm. 2010;384:73–7. https://doi.org/10.1016/j.ijpharm.2009.09.044.

50. Mohammed D, Matts PJ, Hadgraft J, Lane ME. Variation of stratum corneum biophysical and molecular properties with anatomic site. AAPS J. 2012;14:806–12. https://doi.org/10.1208/s12248-012-9400-3.

51. Panisset F, Treffel P, Faivre B, Lecomte PB, Agache P. Transepidermal water loss related to volar forearm sites in humans. Acta Derm Venereol. 1992;72:4–5.

52. Van der Valk PG, Maibach HI. Potential for irritation increases from the wrist to the cubital fossa. Br J Dermatol. 1989;121:709–12. https://doi.org/10.1111/j.1365-2133.1989.tb08212.x.
53. Lammintausta K, Maibach HI, Wilson D. Irritant reactivity in males and females. Contact Dermatitis. 1987;17:276–80. https://doi.org/10.1111/j.1600-0536.1987.tb01477.x.
54. Luebberding S, Krueger N, Kerscher M. Skin physiology in men and women: in vivo evaluation of 300 people including TEWL, SC hydration, sebum content and skin surface pH. Int J Cosmet Sci. 2013;35:477–83. https://doi.org/10.1111/ics.12068.
55. Berardesca E, de Rigal J, Leveque JL, Maibach HI. In vivo biophysical characterization of skin physiological differences in races. Dermatologica. 1991;182:89–93. https://doi.org/10.1159/000247752.
56. Sugino K, Imokawa G, Maibach HI. Ethnic difference of stratum corneum lipid in relation to stratum corneum function. J Invest Dermatol. 1993;100:587.
57. Le Fur I, Reinberg A, Lopez S, Morizot F, Mechkouri M, Tschachler E. Analysis of circadian and ultradian rhythms of skin surface properties of face and forearm of healthy women. J Invest Dermatol. 2001;117:718–24. https://doi.org/10.1046/j.0022-202x.2001.01433.x.
58. Ostermeier M, Kerscher M. Diurnal rhythm of our skin: myth or reality? evaluation by using biophysical measurements. Akt Dermatol. 2018;44:539.
59. Reinberg AE, Touitou Y, Soudant E, Bernard D, Bazin R, Mechkouri M. Oral contraceptives alter circadian rhythm parameters of cortisol, melatonin, blood pressure, heart rate, skin blood flow, transepidermal water loss, and skin amino acids of healthy young women. Chronobiol Int. 1996;13:199–211. https://doi.org/10.3109/07420529609012653.
60. Spruit D. The diurnal variation of water vapour loss from the skin in relation to temperature. Br J Dermatol. 1971;84:66–70. https://doi.org/10.1111/j.1365-2133.1971.tb14198.x.
61. Yosipovitch G, Xiong GL, Haus E, Sackett-Lundeen L, Ashkenazi I, Maibach HI. Time-dependent variations of the skin barrier function in humans: transepidermal water loss, stratum corneum hydration, skin surface pH, and skin temperature. J Invest Dermatol. 1998;110:20–3. https://doi.org/10.1046/j.1523-1747.1998.00069.x.
62. Choi J, Kim S, Han J, Kim E. 1275 The effect of drinking and sleep deprivation on the men skin. J Investig Dermatol. 2018;138:S217. https://doi.org/10.1016/j.jid.2018.03.1291.
63. Jang S, Han J, Jeon H, Kim A, Kim E. 295 A study of skin characteristic after sleeping according to age. J Investig Dermatol. 2019;139:S51. https://doi.org/10.1016/j.jid.2019.03.371.
64. Oyetakin-White P, Suggs A, Koo B, Matsui MS, Yarosh D, Cooper KD, Baron ED. Does poor sleep quality affect skin ageing? Clin Exp Dermatol. 2015;40:17–22. https://doi.org/10.1111/ced.12455.
65. Fukunaga S, Wada S, Sato T, Hamaguchi M, Aoi W, Higashi A. Effect of torula yeast (Candida utilis)-derived glucosylceramide on skin dryness and other skin conditions in winter. J Nutr Sci Vitaminol (Tokyo). 2018;64:265–70. https://doi.org/10.3177/jnsv.64.265.
66. Hong YH, Chang UJ, Kim YS, Jung EY, Suh HJ. Dietary galacto-oligosaccharides improve skin health: a randomized double blind clinical trial. Asia Pac J Clin Nutr. 2017;26:613–8. https://doi.org/10.6133/apjcn.052016.05.
67. Kuwano T, Kawano S, Kagawa D, Yasuda Y, Inoue Y, Murase T. Dietary intake of glucono-delta-lactone attenuates skin inflammation and contributes to maintaining skin condition. Food Funct. 2018;9:1524–31. https://doi.org/10.1039/c7fo01548h.
68. Torres DPM, Gonçalves MPF, Teixeira JA, Rodrigues LR. Galacto-oligosaccharides: production, properties, applications, and significance as prebiotics. Compr Rev Food Sci Food Saf. 2010;9:438–54. https://doi.org/10.1111/j.1541-4337.2010.00119.x.
69. Guida B, Nino M, Perrino NR, Laccetti R, Trio R, Labella S, Balato N. The impact of obesity on skin disease and epidermal permeability barrier status. J Eur Acad Dermatol Venereol. 2010;24:191–5. https://doi.org/10.1111/j.1468-3083.2009.03503.x.
70. Löffler H, Aramaki JU, Effendy I. The influence of body mass index on skin susceptibility to sodium lauryl sulphate. Skin Res Technol. 2002;8:19–22. https://doi.org/10.1046/j.0909-752x.
71. Nino M, Franzese A, Ruggiero Perrino N, Balato N. The effect of obesity on skin disease and epidermal permeability barrier status in children. Pediatr Dermatol. 2012;29:567–70. https://doi.org/10.1111/j.1525-1470.2012.01738.x.

72. Xin S, Ye L, Man G, Lv C, Elias PM, Man MQ. Heavy cigarette smokers in a chinese popula-tion display a compromised permeability barrier. Biomed Res Int. 2016;2016:9704598. https://doi.org/10.1155/2016/9704598.

73. Pinnagoda J, Tupker RA, Coenraads PJ, Nater JP. Transepidermal water loss with and without sweat gland inactivation. Contact Dermatitis. 1989;21:16–22. https://doi.org/10.1111/j.1600-0536.1989.tb04679.x.

74. Fujimura T, Sato N, Ophaswongse S, Takagi Y, Hotta M, Kitahara T, Takema Y, Palungwachira P. Characterization of vulvar skin of healthy Thai women: influence of sites, age and meno-pause. Acta Derm Venereol. 2013;93:242–5. https://doi.org/10.2340/00015555-1534.

75. Harvell J, Hussona-Saeed I, Maibach HI. Changes in transepidermal water loss and cutane-ous blood flow during the menstrual cycle. Contact Dermatitis. 1992;27:294–301. https://doi.org/10.1111/j.1600-0536.1992.tb03283.x.

76. Rogiers V, Group E. EEMCO guidance for the assessment of transepidermal water loss in cosmetic sciences. Skin Pharmacol Appl Ski Physiol. 2001;14:117–28. https://doi.org/10.1159/000056341.

77. Grice JE, Moghimi HR, Ryan E, Zhang Q, Haridass I, Mohammed Y, Roberts MS. Non-formulation parameters that affect penetrant-skin-vehicle interactions and percuta-neous absorption. In: Dragicevic N, Maibach HI, editors. Percutaneous penetration enhancers drug penetration into/through the skin. Berlin: Springer; 2017. https://doi.org/10.1007/978-3-662-53270-6_4.

78. Choe SJ, Kim D, Kim EJ, Ahn JS, Choi EJ, Son ED, Lee TR, Choi EH. Psychological stress deteriorates skin barrier function by activating 11beta-hydroxysteroid dehydrogenase 1 and the HPA axis. Sci Rep. 2018;8:6334. https://doi.org/10.1038/s41598-018-24653-z.

79. Tavares L, Palma L, Santos O, Almeida MA, Bujan MJ, Rodrigues LM. Body mass index and association with in vivo skin physiology. Paper presented at the World Congress of the International Society for Biophysics and Imaging of the skin (ISBS), Copenhagen, Denmark; 2012.

Chapter 16
Relationships Between Skin of Color and the TEWL Barrier

Reva P. Peer, Anuk Burli, and Howard I. Maibach

Introduction

A major role skin has in human survival is its function as a barrier against excessive water loss. Transepidermal water loss (TEWL), a widely accepted objective measure of this function, documents the amount of water lost from the body by non-eccrine sweat diffusing across the stratum corneum [1]. The stratum corneum provides barrier properties and other protection functions, including, but not limited to, controlling transcutaneous water loss [2]. Therefore, a higher TEWL would indicate increased water diffusion from the skin and consequently a decrease in stratum corneum water barrier function.

Since the 1960s, we and others compared TEWL between racial, ethnic, and skin pigmentation groups [3–5]. Stratum corneum differences have been observed between skin of color groups and Caucasian skin, e.g., Weigand et al. determined that the stratum corneum in Black skin is more compact and cohesive than white skin [6]. Therefore, the idea of differences in TEWL between skin of color and Caucasian groups appears plausible. After our migration from our origin in Africa, *Homo sapiens* skin color has evolved and diversified. Here, we attempt to answer the question, in *Homo sapiens* evolution, post migration from Africa, has skin of color and Caucasian skin in relationship to TEWL provided an advantage to any group?

The last major peer review evaluation of studies investigating relationships between TEWL and skin of color was conducted 10 years ago and may benefit from an update. While TEWL is a widely studied objective measurement, studies that

R. P. Peer (✉) · A. Burli
School of Medicine and Dentistry, University of Rochester, Rochester, NY, USA
e-mail: Reva_Peer@urmc.rochester.edu

H. I. Maibach
Department of Dermatology, University of California San Francisco,
San Francisco, CA, USA
e-mail: Howard.Maibach@ucsf.edu

© The Author(s), under exclusive license to Springer Nature
Switzerland AG 2022
A. M. Feschuk et al. (eds.), *Dermal Absorption and Decontamination*,
https://doi.org/10.1007/978-3-031-09222-0_16

investigate TEWL in skin of color often contain conflicting information, and literature is sparse in certain skin of color groups compared to others. For example, many
studies were conducted on primarily Caucasian and Black skin, as they are easily
visually distinguishable, while studies measuring TEWL in other peoples of color
do exist, they are limited, and few have undergone peer review [7].

Evaluating these objective studies is essential in forming plausible conclusions
based on limited and sometimes conflicting data and to understand the current state
of knowledge in the research community regarding properties of skin of color.
Analyzing this data and elucidating the gaps in our knowledge regarding skin of
color are also important because it will provide direction for the research community on topics that will require more investigation. Here, we highlight these gaps in
knowledge and provide an updated appraisal of studies analyzing skin of color and
TEWL to determine if any advantage regarding TEWL has emerged throughout
evolution.

Materials and Methods

We searched Embase; PubMed; Google; Google Scholar; the Miner Library Online
Database of the University of Rochester in Rochester, NY, USA; standard dermatology textbooks; and the dermatology library at the University of California, San
Francisco, CA, USA. Keywords in searches included words pertaining to skin of
color (i.e., skin of color, race, ethnicity, Caucasian, Black, African American,
Hispanic, Asian) and stratum corneum barrier function (i.e., stratum corneum,
TEWL, skin, skin barrier function, water loss). These references were reviewed, and
relevant publications were procured. Only data regarding basal TEWL from each
study was reviewed and presented. Although we recognize race and ethnicity can be
considered controversial terms, many studies use racial and ethnic categories to
describe the individuals studied. Therefore, we use the same categorical terms when
referencing these studies in order to describe them.

Results

From the 1980s to the present, there have been 26 studies examining skin of color
differences and stratum corneum function—TEWL with conflicting results
(Table 16.1).

Table 16.1 Skin of color differences in stratum corneum capacity—transepidermal water loss (TEWL). No clear conclusion on the potential impact of skin of color on TEWL [3, 5, 8–31]

Study	Technique	Subjects	Site	Results
De Luca et al. [12]— abstract only	In vivo	Somalian 29	Not documented in abstract	No significant differences
		White European not stated		
		Age not stated		
Goh and Chia [16]	In vivo	Chinese 15	Right scapular region	No significant differences
		(10 males, mean age = 30.8 years, range 18–38 years; five females, mean age = 25.6 years, range 20–34 years)		
		Malaysian 12		
		(7 males, mean age = 25.7 years, range 19–37 years; five females, mean age 27.8 years, range 18–39 years)		
		Indian 11		
		(6 males, mean age = 26.5 years, range 18–35 years; five females, mean age = 30.2 years, range 24–34 years)		
Berardesca and Maibach [10]	In vivo	Hispanic male 7 (age 27.8 ± 4.5 years)	Upper back	No significant differences
		White male 9 (age 30.6 ± 8.8 years)		
Berardesca and Maibach [3]	In vivo	Black male 10	Back	No significant differences
		(age 29.9 ± 7.2 years)		
		White male 9		
		(age 30.6 ± 8.8 years)		
Wilson et al. [5]	In vitro	10 Blacks (mean age 38.6 years)	Inner thigh	TEWL for Blacks greater than Caucasians ($p < 0.01$)
		12 Caucasians (mean age 41.1 years)		
		(age range 5–72 years for both)		

(continued)

Table 16.1 (continued)

Study	Technique	Subjects	Site	Results
Berardesca et al. [9]	In vivo	Black 15	Volar and dorsal forearm	No significant TEWL difference between Black, White, and Hispanics at either site
		(mean age 46.7 ± 2.4 years)		
		White 12		
		(mean age 49.8 ± 2 years)		
		Hispanics 12 (mean age 48.8 ± 2 years)		
Kompaore et al. [18]	In vivo	Black African 7 (all male)	Volar forearm	Baseline TEWL:
		French Caucasian eight (six males and two females)		Black and Asian > Caucasian ($p < 0.01$); no significant difference between Black and Asian
		Asian 6 (all male)		
		(age 23–32 years for all)		
Sugino et al. [25]— abstract only	In vivo	Black, Caucasian, Hispanic, and Asian (number and age of subjects not specified)	Not documented	Baseline TEWL:
				Black > Caucasian ≥ Hispanic ≥ Asian
Reed et al. [23]	In vivo	Skin type V/VI:	Volar forearm	No significant differences between Asian and White; skin type V/VI displayed higher basal TEWL than type II/III without statistical significance
		African American 4		
		Filipino 2		
		Hispanic 1		
		Skin type II/III:		
		Asian 6		
		Caucasian 8		
		(age 22–38 years for all)		
Warrier et al. [26]	In vivo	Black female 30	Left and right medical cheeks, mid-volar forearms, lateral mid-lower legs	Baseline TEWL:
		White female 30		Black < White on the cheeks and legs ($p < 0.05$); same relationship on the forearm without statistical significance
		(age 18–45 years, all)		
Berardesca et al. [11]	In vivo	Black African American women 8	Mid-volar forearm	No difference in baseline TEWL
		White European women 10		
		(mean age 42.3 ± 5 years for all)		

Table 16.1 (continued)

Study	Technique	Subjects	Site	Results
Singh et al. [24]	In vivo	Black 10	Volar forearm	Baseline TEWL:
		Caucasian 10		Caucasian > Asian > Hispanic > Black ($p < 0.01$)
		Hispanic 10		
		Asian 10		
		(age 18–80 years for all)		
Aramaki et al. [8]	In vivo	Japanese female 22	Forearm	Baseline TEWL: Japanese < German ($p < 0.05$)
		(mean age 25.8 years)		
		German female 22		
		(mean age 26.9 years)		
Yosipovitch et al. [30]	In vivo	Chinese 13	Volar forearm	No significant differences
		Malays 7		
		Indians 10		
		Caucasians 9		
		(mean age 34 ± 8 years for all)		
Grimes et al. [17]	In vivo	African American women 18	Inner forearm	No significant differences
		White women 19		
		(age 35–65 years for both)[a]		
Fotoh et al. [13]	In vivo	Sub-Saharan African Black or Caribbean Black women 25 (mean age 24.04 years), African or Caribbean mixed races from intermarriage between Black African or Black Caribbean and White European Caucasian 25 (mean age 24.7 years), and European Caucasian women 25 (mean age 23.12 years)	Forehead and volar forearm	No significant differences
		(age 20–30 years for Black Africans or Caribbeans and European Caucasians and 20–32 years for African or Caribbean mixed race)		

(continued)

Table 16.1 (continued)

Study	Technique	Subjects	Site	Results
Muizzuddin et al. [21]	In vivo	African American female 73 (mean age 35.1 ± 7.5 years)	Right and left facial cheek	Baseline TEWL:
		Caucasian female 119 (mean age 36.0 ± 6.0 years)		East Asians and Caucasians > African Americans ($p < 0.001$); Caucasians > East Asian ($p < 0.001$)
		East Asian female (first-generation immigrants to New York from China, Japan, and Korea) 149 (mean age 30.2 ± 5.8 years)		
Yamashita et al. [29]	In vivo	Japanese Asian 92 (mean age 41.1 ± 12.8 years)	Cheek, dorsal aspect of the hand, inner upper arm	Baseline TEWL:
		French Caucasian 104 (mean age 40.4 ± 14.4 years)		French > Japanese at the dorsal hand and upper arm ($p < 0.01$); no significant difference in cheek, but same relationship found
Lee et al. [19]	In vivo	Indonesian female 200 (100 from Jakarta and 100 from Bandung) (mean age 27.4 ± 4.6 years)	Forehead and cheek front (left)	Singapore > Indonesian for the cheek ($p < 0.05$); Vietnam > Indonesia for the forehead ($p < 0.001$); Vietnam > Singapore for the forehead ($p < 0.01$); no other significant relationships
		Vietnamese female 100 (mean age 26.5 ± 4.8 years)		
		Singaporean female (Chinese origin) 97 (mean age 27.0 ± 4.1 years)		
Pappas et al. [22]	In vivo	African American	Facial skin	Baseline TEWL:
		Caucasian		Caucasian > African American ($p < 0.05$); with trend of Caucasian > Northern Asian > African American
		Northern Asian		
		($n = 17$–21 for all) (age 20–45 years)		

Table 16.1 (continued)

Study	Technique	Subjects	Site	Results
Galzote et al. [15]	In vivo	Females from Harbin, China, 106	Mid portions of both cheek and forehead	Subjects from Harbin, China, have the greatest mean value for TEWL (no significance stated)
		Females from Shanghai, China, 100		
		Females from New Delhi, India, 100		
		Females from Seoul, South Korea, 116		
		Females from Sendai, Japan, 108		
		(all born and currently residing in respective country) (age 14–75 years)		
Voegeli et al. [27]	In vivo	Black African female 4	30 areas on the left side of the face (forehead, check, jaw, and eye areas)	Overall general trend in TEWL: Indian > Chinese > Black African > Caucasian; however, significance only in Indian > Caucasian ($p < 0.001$), Chinese > Caucasian ($p < 0.001$), Black Africans > Caucasian ($p < 0.01$)
		Indian female 4		
		Chinese female 4		
		Caucasian female 4		
		(all mean age: 21.8 ± 1.1 years)		
Voegeli et al. [28]	In vivo	$N = 60$	Right facial cheek and postauricular area	Basal TEWL: Albino African females > Black African and Caucasian females ($p < 0.0001$) for both sites; Black Africans and Caucasians no significant difference
		Three age-matched groups:		
		Albino African female (mean age 40.3 ± 2.9 years)		
		Black African female (mean age 38.2 ± 2.3 years)		
		Caucasian female (mean age 44.6 ± 3.1 years)		

(continued)

Table 16.1 (continued)

Study	Technique	Subjects	Site	Results
Mack et al. [20]	In vivo	Beijing, China (ethnic Chinese), 120 children, 40 adult females	Dorsal forearm and upper inner arm	Baseline TEWL: children from Beijing > children in Mumbai and Skillman in both sites with no p value provided; no significant difference in adults and between white and American groups
		Skillman, New Jersey:		
		White 84 children, 18 adult females		
		African American 88 children, 19 female adults		
		Mumbai, India (ethnic South Asian)		
		105 children, 40 adult females (children age 3–49 months; adult women mean age 31 years)		
Fujimura et al. [14]	In vivo	Thai 30	Inner thigh, buttock, inner upper arm	Baseline TEWL:
		Chinese 30		Chinese > Thai at all sites ($p < 0.001$)
		(age 6–24 months)		
Young et al. [31]	In vivo	African American female 19	Palmar and dorsal hands and volar forearms	No significant difference
		Caucasian female 31		
		(age 18–40 years)		

[a] All with moderate photodamage on the face

No TEWL Differences

Much skin of color literature began with and remains dominated by a comparison between Black skin and white skin. However, even within this major subset of literature, results are conflicting. Several studies determined no significant difference in TEWL between Black and white skin. De Luca et al. (abstract only) measured TEWL in 29 young and healthy Somalian people and white Europeans and did not find significant difference in this parameter between the groups [12]. Berardesca and Maibach, with ten Black male and nine white male volunteer subjects, and in a later study by Berardesca et al., with eight Black African American women volunteers with skin type VI and ten white Caucasian women volunteers with skin types I and II, saw no differences in baseline TEWL [3, 11]. Larger sample sizes such as Grimes et al. that measured TEWL in 18 African American women and 19 white women both with moderate photodamage on the face and Young et al. that ascertained TEWL in 19 African American and 31 Caucasian first year female nursing students also found no significant differences in TEWL between the groups [17, 31].

Reed et al., taking a different approach from previous studies, examined differences in skin properties of individuals with various degrees of skin pigmentation, as well as individuals in different racial groups. They compared seven individuals with skin types V and VI (four African Americans, two Filipinos, and one Hispanic) and 14 individuals with skin types II/III (six Asians and eight Caucasians) and noted no differences in baseline TEWL between the two groups. They also measured basal TEWL in six Asian and eight Caucasians both with skin types II/III and discovered no significant difference between these two subgroups as well [23].

Voegeli et al. utilized a similar approach to Reed et al. by investigating differences in skin properties based on facial skin pigmentation. In three age-matched groups with 60 females, Albino African females, Black African females, and Caucasian females, they measured TEWL in two anatomic sites, one sun exposed (facial cheek) and one not sun exposed (postauricular area). The two ethnic groups had different Fitzpatrick skin phototypes (II/III and V/VI). They compared intra-ethnic skin properties between the Albino African and Black African subjects and discovered that Albino Africans had a significantly higher basal TEWL relative to the other two groups; however, there was no difference in basal TEWL between the Black African female subjects and the Caucasian subjects at both sites. Therefore, they found no significant difference in basal TEWL based on ethnicity but observed an intra-ethnic difference in basal TEWL with different skin pigmentation. They suggested this difference could be due to stratum corneum UV damage, but that this was not likely since this difference in TEWL was seen in the non-photo-exposed site as well [28].

Fotoh et al. examined TEWL differences between ethnic groups and is the only study that includes a mixed-race group. They assessed TEWL in 25 sub-Saharan African Black or Caribbean Black women, 25 African or Caribbean mixed-race women, and 25 European Caucasian women. The mixed-race women were from intermarriages between white European Caucasians and Black Africans or Black Caribbean individuals. This study therefore not only examined differences in skin of color but also ethnic differences as African Black or Caribbean and mixed-race individuals are both defined as having Fitzpatrick skin type VI, whereas European Caucasian have type III, IV, or V. They assumed that Black and mixed-race individuals do not respond to UV light similarly and further subdivided the VI category into VIa for mixed-race individuals and VIb for Black individuals. All subjects had been living in the same region for at least 6 months. Furthermore, they investigated differences in TEWL in these ethnic populations at a photo-exposed site (the forehead) and a non-photo-exposed site (the volar forearm) and found no significant difference in baseline TEWL between any of the three ethnic groups at both sites [13].

TEWL Differences

Several studies observed a significant difference between Black and white skin. Wilson et al. found that the baseline mean TEWL of Black skin subjects was greater than the TEWL of white Caucasian skin. This study differs from the others discussed since it is the only observation conducted in vitro on skin samples taken from refrigerated cadavers of 12 Caucasians and ten Black Americans of Afro-Caribbean ethnic origin that were age and gender matched. A potential benefit of conducting an in vitro study is that it is not affected by environmental factors or individual factors such as emotional eccrine sweating [5].

Conversely, an in vivo study by Warrier et al. observed conflicting opposite results in their study when they assessed TEWL in 30 Black females and 30 white females at three different anatomic sites. The baseline TEWL was significantly greater in white females than Black females on the cheeks and the legs, opposite to what Wilson et al. found. TEWL was also greater in the white females on the forearm but did not reach significance [26].

While much skin of color research and TEWL research began by studying differences between white and Black skin, studies have expanded beyond these two categories and have examined such differences in other groups like Asian and Hispanic populations. Berardesca and Maibach compared baseline TEWL values in seven Hispanic males and nine white males [10]. Berardesca et al. determined baseline TEWL values in 15 Black volunteers with parents and grandparents that were self-described as Black race, 12 white volunteers of Anglo-Saxon ancestry, and 12 Hispanic volunteers who were Mexican immigrants in Northern California. It was not noted how long the Hispanic volunteers had lived in Northern California [9]. In both studies, they noticed no difference between baseline TEWL between any of the three groups [9, 10].

Kompaore et al. measured TEWL in seven African Black who lived in France for at least 6 years, eight French Caucasians, and six Asian subjects who had been living in France for at least 6 years and found that Black and Asian subjects had a significantly higher TEWL than Caucasian participants [18]. Sugino et al. (abstract only) described a wider expanse of skin of color groups, with Black, Caucasian, Hispanic, and Asian participants, and found TEWL values of the groups to be in the following order: Black > Caucasian ≥ Hispanic ≥ Asian [25]. Both studies determined TEWL levels to be higher in Black skin compared to white Caucasian skin, which was similar to the findings by Wilson et al.; however, Kompaore et al.'s conclusion differed from Wilson et al.'s findings related to the Asian participants [5, 18, 25].

Singh et al. elucidated TEWL values in ten Black, ten Caucasian, ten Hispanic, and ten Asian individuals and discovered baseline TEWL levels to be significantly different with the following order: Caucasian > Asian > Hispanic > Black. Although there are significant differences, when examining this study in relation to previous studies, we note even more variation in the relative magnitudes of Asian and Hispanic TEWL values compared to other racial and ethnic groups [24]. Furthermore, this study's conclusions were opposite regarding the relative TEWL values between Caucasian and Black individuals to what was listed in the studies by Wilson et al., Kompaore et al., and Sugino et al. [5, 18, 24, 25].

Aramaki et al. assessed TEWL in 22 Japanese women living in Germany for 1–5 years and 22 German women and observed a significantly lower basal TEWL in Japanese women versus German women [8]. Muizzuddin et al. analyzed TEWL values in 73 African American females from the New York tristate area, 119 Caucasian females, most of whom were local from the tristate area, and a subset living in the United Kingdom, and 149 East Asian females who were first-generation immigrants to New York from China, Japan, and Korea. They determined that the East Asian and Caucasian groups had a significantly higher TEWL than African Americans and also noted Caucasian subjects to have a higher TEWL than East Asian participants [21].

Yamashita et al. examined characteristics of skin between 92 Japanese individuals living in Japan and 104 French Caucasians living in France in multiple anatomic sites, both sun exposed and non-exposed. Baseline TEWL was significantly greater in French individuals than Japanese at the dorsal hand and upper arm but showed no difference on the cheek [29]. This generally coincides with Aramaki et al.'s and Muizzuddin et al.'s findings that European Caucasians have a higher TEWL than East Asians [8, 21]. However, note that these individuals live in two different geographical environments and measures were conducted in two different countries. Furthermore, TEWL was measured using instruments made by different companies in France and Japan. However, Yamashita et al. stated that they used the results of a validation study to convert the measured TEWL values of one instrument to what its equivalent would be in the other [29].

Pappas et al. described a pilot study that measured baseline TEWL values in African Americans, Caucasians, and Northern Asians. Each group had a sample size of 17–21 individuals. Caucasians had significantly greater baseline TEWL than African American subjects. They concluded a trend of TEWL with the following order Caucasian > Northern Asian > African American. However, no statistical difference was reported between Northern Asians and the other groups [22].

Voegeli et al. utilized a novel approach to measuring TEWL in ethnic groups: they measured TEWL in 30 different areas on the left side of the face including the forehead, cheek, jaw, and eye areas and then took these values to generate continuous color maps that they superimposed on digital images of the subjects' faces. Different colors were used to represent the physiological value of the TEWL at that location. The study included four Chinese, four Indian, four Caucasian, and four Black African female subjects. They assessed the overall TEWL among the four ethnic groups, TEWL for each region they measured (i.e., jaw, forehead, etc.), and TEWL for each of the 30 sites they measured. When describing overall TEWL, they noticed the following trend: Indians > Chinese > Black Africans > Caucasians. However, significance was only determined between Caucasians and each of the other three groups. When looking at differences in TEWL between the four ethnic groups at various areas of the face and at different individual sites on the face, it became more complex, as there was large variation in the data depending on which site was measured. For example, there was a significant difference in TEWL between Indian and Black Africans in the cheek region, but no difference in any other region. Another example is that there was a significant difference in TEWL between African Blacks and Caucasians at the oblique jaw but not at the lateral jaw. This study highlighted how anatomic site may play an important role in the relationship between ethnicity and skin of color and TEWL [27].

Although categories such as Asian and Hispanic have often been used in skin of color studies discussed above, there are different subgroups within these broad, overarching categories that have varying ancestries and skin colors. Several studies investigated these subpopulation categories specifically within the Asian population to determine if differences in skin properties exist between these groups. Goh and Chia analyzed skin properties in 15 Chinese, 12 Malaysian, and 11 Indian volunteers from a STD clinic in Singapore. Although they focused on skin irritation, they documented baseline TEWL between the three groups in unirritated skin and observed no significant difference between these groups [16]. Yosipovitch et al. also investigated skin properties in Asian groups and Caucasians living in Singapore included 13 Chinese, seven Malaysian, ten Indian, and nine Caucasian participants with similar ages and found no significant difference in TEWL between the groups [30].

Lee et al. measured skin biophysical properties in 200 Indonesian females living in Jakarta (100 people) and Bandung (100 people), 100 Vietnamese women living in Ho Chi Minh, and 97 Singaporean women of Chinese origin on the cheek and forehead. They, unlike Goh and Chia and Yosipovitch et al., determined significant differences between Asian ethnic groups. Singaporean Chinese women had significantly higher TEWL than Indonesian women on the cheek only. In addition, Vietnamese women had significantly higher TEWL than the Indonesian and Singaporean Chinese subjects on the forehead only. Note that all measurements were taken in different geographical environments. However, the same devices were used to measure TEWL in all groups, and the study was conducted within the same season [19].

Galzote et al. characterized facial skin in Asian populations during two different seasons, as well as compared the mean TEWL value between the populations for both seasons. They had 106 female participants from China living in Harbin and 100 from Shanghai, 100 females from India living in New Delhi, 116 females from South Korea living in Seoul, and 108 females from Japan living in Sendai. The only difference noted between the TEWL measurements within these Asian population groups was that subjects from Harbin, China, had the greatest mean TEWL relative to the other groups. No significance was stated. Although the study was conducted in different countries, the same instruments were used at all testing sites, operators followed protocols to ensure consistency between sites, and all testing sites were temperature- and humidity-controlled environments [15].

Mack et al. not only examined skin properties in various Asian populations but differences within and among children and adults. Their study consisted of 120 children and 40 adult females that were ethnically Chinese living in Beijing, 84 children and 18 adult females that were ethnically white living in New Jersey, 88 children and 19 adult females that were African Americans living in New Jersey, and 105 children and 40 adult females that were ethnically South Asian living in Mumbai, India, and observed no difference in TEWL between any of the adult groups [20].

On the other hand, children from Beijing had a higher TEWL than those in Mumbai and New Jersey. This coincides with their other findings that the stratum corneum barrier is different in children versus adults and the properties of the stratum corneum change with age. Children tended to have higher TEWL than adult. Therefore, it is possible that there is a difference in TEWL between different ethnic groups during childhood that does not exist in adulthood [20].

Finally, Fujimura et al. investigated differences in stratum corneum functions in younger individuals as well. The study consisted of 30 Thai infants and 30 Chinese infants whose ages ranged from 6 to 24 months old. Both Thai and Chinese infants resided in Bangkok, Thailand. They measured TEWL at the thigh, buttock, and upper arm and found TEWL to be significantly greater in Chinese infants compared to Thai infants at all sites [14].

Discussion

The United States will soon be a nation of color; the US Census Bureau predicts that minority populations will surpass persons identifying as non-Hispanic white by the year 2044 [32]. Since these demographics are anticipated to change over time, so will the need for addressing the medical and health needs of this diversifying skin of color patient population. However, the foundation of much of our knowledge is based on consumer research conducted on a predominately Caucasian male study population [33]. Furthermore, the physician demographic in the United States itself lacks significant Black and Hispanic representation, both major minority groups [34]. It is thus important to understand and elucidate the physiologic, morphologic, and biochemical differences in skin properties between the skins of color and white skin that occurred throughout evolution. Understanding any potential variation would allow us to help explain differences in skin functionality and determine how to best manage and treat skin-related disorders in skin of color populations.

The term skin of color encompasses so-called racial and ethnic groups who have skin color different from what is considered "white" or "Caucasian skin." These skin of color groups may share similar skin properties and disease presentations. Race and ethnicity have often been considered as biological risk factors for certain health conditions and often viewed as controversial and problematic terms. Racial categories such as "Asian" often encompass groups of people that are genetically, phenotypically, and culturally different [35]. Furthermore, defining an individual's race can be a potentially complex process since individuals can have multiple different racial backgrounds.

Ethnicity, on the other hand, most commonly defines groups with a shared culture background. Therefore, ethnicity can be more representative of the environmental and societal factors that influence a group of people. Although these terms are not ideal and we believe skin of color to be a more useful term to describe these biological changes that have occurred through evolution, much of the literature on skin of color uses terms such as race and ethnicity. Classifications were needed to stratify differences between skin of color populations, and such terminology was commonplace in the studies we reviewed and in the literature in general. As a result, we also referred to the terms race and ethnicity based on what was used in the literature itself, recognizing its inherent issues.

Based on this extensive data reviewed, we cannot ascertain how evolution has affected stratum corneum function in skin of color. There is considerable variation in the results with multiple studies contradicting one another for all peoples of color discussed. This coincides with other literature reviews that failed to generate a clear conclusion regarding the relationship between TEWL and skin of color [36, 37]. On the other hand, Rawlings made the conclusion that Asians in general have the lowest TEWL and Black individuals in general have higher TEWL values. However, this overview does not include much of the current literature [38]. Machado et al. stated that the literature suggests there is no significant difference in TEWL for different ethnic groups. This study does not include more recent studies. In addition, they stated one potential issue that needed consideration was that most studies had small sample sizes [39].

The literature further suggests there may even be variation in TEWL within the overarching racial categories that many studies employ. For example, the category of Asian was often used in studies as a singular ethnic or racial group. However, the Asian populations consist of many culturally and ethnically diverse groups. Several studies suggested there may be variation between Asian subpopulations such as Chinese, Malay, Indian, and Thai groups, potentially due to biological differences and in some studies geographical differences [14, 15, 19, 20]. However, the data regarding these differences was limited, so no definite conclusion could be made. Nonetheless, if such differences exist, this may potentially impact the findings of studies that employ broad categorical groups such as Asian or Hispanic.

Taken together, no conclusion can be made regarding skin of color and stratum TEWL function. This is concerning given the importance of stratum corneum function in preserving life. If differences do exist between skin of color, it is critical to identify and understand them to provide adequate and necessary care for peoples of color.

Our analysis of the studies suggests that the variations in results and even entirely conflicting results may be a result of uncontrolled experimental variables that should potentially be controlled for when measuring TEWL. One such factor listed is the relative anatomic site measured. Rougier et al. described TEWL in several sites and observed the following order of differences: forearm (ventral elbow) < forearm (ventral mid) < arm (upper outer) ≤ abdomen < forearm (ventral wrist) < postauricular < forehead [40]. Pinnagoda et al. suggested that these site differences in TEWL were due to regional differences in skin structure such as the epidermis and distribution of eccrine sweat glands [41]. In addition, there is a difference in skin thickness and stratum corneum layers in different anatomic regions [42]. Many studies described here measured TEWL in a variety of locations. It is possible that stratum corneum differences in skin of color may exist in certain anatomic sites but not others. It is also possible that certain skin of color groups may have higher TEWL values compared to others at one site and lower TEWL values at another site. This was highlighted by Voegeli et al., who found significant differences in TEWL in certain areas of the face and not others between different ethnic groups. In addition, they developed continuous color maps based on the magnitude of TEWL values they measured at each facial site and then superimposed these maps on faces for each of the ethnic groups. They observed clear differences in TEWL color map patterns for each of the four different groups [27]. Therefore, anatomic site may be an important variable in TEWL measurement and could help explain the variation in the data.

Another factor we listed was sample size. The wide range of the sample size within the studies, ranging from single digits to triple digits, could impact the power of each study and therefore should be considered when assessing the significance of the various studies. Machado et al. pointed out this potential issue in their review as well [39].

Individual factors such as emotional eccrine sweating can also have an impact on TEWL as this can increase the amount of water vapor passing through the stratum corneum. The testing conditions under which TEWL is measured could potentially be anxiety provoking or stressful for a patient and cause emotional eccrine sweating. Pinnagoda et al. observed that emotional sweaters can have $1-1.8$ g/m^2 higher TEWL levels ($p < 0.001$) during rest compared to TEWL levels at rest using a topical sweat inactivator [43]. Therefore, it is possible that individuals who experience such sweating may cause fluctuation in the data and affect the results of the study.

Furthermore, differing ages between subjects in each study can contribute to different TEWL measurements. Skin age can affect TEWL as elderly stratum corneum has both more skin barrier function and decreased permeability. In contrast, premature infant skin has increased permeability due to a lack of fully developed skin barrier function, affecting TEWL [44]. In addition, skin diseases such as psoriasis and atopic dermatitis influence TEWL as well, yet different skin diseases are more common in different age groups [42]. Further research must be conducted to assess how to best understand TEWL with regard to differing ages as well as how skin pathology affects this measurement.

UV radiation (UVR) may also impact skin of color differences in TEWL during the aging process. Exposure to UVR damages the skin barrier, as seen in sunburns, and therefore potentially leads to a greater TEWL [45]. Darker skin contains more melanin which provides greater protection against UVR and is one of the major factors determining skin pigmentation [46]. Consequently, higher levels of melanin and thus darker skin have been selected for in populations near the equator that are exposed to higher UVR [47, 48]. However, modern migrations have allowed people of fairer skin to live in geographic areas with high UVR that they are not fully adapted too. During the aging process, both constitutive pigmentation and photoaging are impacted and can increase an individual's susceptibility to UVR damage. Constitutive pigmentation takes a major role in reducing DNA damage and skin cancer from UVR, but it decreases with aging [49–51]. This is because the number of active melanocytes decreases in individuals above 30 years by 10–20% per decade [52, 53]. As a result, individuals with white skin who already have lesser amount of melanin at baseline are more likely to be susceptible to UVR as they age. They may therefore have higher TEWL compared to their same age darker skin counterparts in sun-exposed areas. Furthermore, photoaging has been found in clinical studies to be delayed by 10–20 years in the skin of color population, and therefore people with fairer skin are more likely to experience premature skin ageing and skin damage [54]. For these reasons, UVR exposure during aging may be impacting white skin more than darker skin in sun-exposed areas and leading to higher TEWL levels in white skin compared to their same age darker skin counterpart.

Environmental factors such as room temperature and season can also impact TEWL. Changes and fluctuations in the temperature of the room where measurements are being taken can lead to changes in TEWL [55]. Muizzuddin et al. studied TEWL of the cheek during the summer and winter on 40 Caucasian females and noted significant changes in TEWL: TEWL during winter was greater than summer [56].

In addition, technical factors could impact TEWL. For example, variation in TEWL measurements exists not only between instruments made by different companies but also between individual instruments made by the same company. This variation in instruments made by the same company is often due to age. Therefore, while an individual instrument will have reproducible results, it may have different results from an older or newer instrument of the same type and made by the same company. Newer machines appear to respond faster with less stabilization, whereas older machines take longer and appear to measure lower TEWL readings [57].

Conclusion

Taken together, no clear distinction in TEWL in skin of color or Caucasian skin is possible to make today. It is important we gain more clarity on this topic, as it may give more insight into other evolutionary changes in skin of color and Caucasian skin. In addition, such differences in skin of color and Caucasian skin may be clinically relevant and necessitate distinct methods of care or treatments for individuals of color and Caucasians. A separate manuscript follows detailing confounding variables that, if controlled in future studies, should help provide a clear answer [58].

Acknowledgements None.

Declarations
Funding: Basic Science, Clinical, and Translational Research Summer Funding provided by the University of Rochester School of Medicine and Dentistry.

Conflicts of Interest/Competing Interests (Include Appropriate Disclosures)   Not applicable.

Consent to Participate   Not applicable.

Consent for Publication   Not applicable.

Availability of Data and Material (Data Transparency)   All literature is open and available to the public.

Code Availability (Software Application or Custom Code)   Not applicable.

Author's Contributions   Equal participation by Reva Peer and Dr. Howard Maibach: Anuk Burli helped with discussion and editing.

References

1. Fluhr JW, Feingold KR, Elias PM. Transepidermal water loss reflects permeability barrier status: validation in human and rodent in vivo and ex vivo models. Exp Dermatol. 2006;15:483–92. https://doi.org/10.1111/j.1600-0625.2006.00437.x.
2. Elias PM. Skin barrier function. Curr Allergy Asthma Rep. 2008;8:299–305. https://doi.org/10.1007/s11882-008-0048-0.
3. Berardesca E, Maibach HI. Racial differences in sodium lauryl sulphate induced cutaneous irritation: black and white. Contact Dermatitis. 1988;18:65–70. https://doi.org/10.1111/j.1600-0536.1988.tb02741.x.
4. Grice K, Bettley FR. The effect of skin temperature and vascular change on the rate of transepidermal water loss. Br J Dermatol. 1967;79:582–8. https://doi.org/10.1111/j.1365-2133.1967.tb11421.x.
5. Wilson D, Berardesca E, Maibach HI. In vitro transepidermal water loss: differences between black and white human skin. Br J Dermatol. 1988;119:647–52. https://doi.org/10.1111/j.1365-2133.1988.tb03478.x.
6. Weigand DA, Haygood C, Gaylor JR. Cell layers and density of Negro and Caucasian stratum corneum. J Invest Dermatol. 1974;62:563–8. https://doi.org/10.1111/1523-1747.ep12679412.
7. Wesley NO, Maibach HI. Racial (ethnic) differences in skin properties: the objective data. Am J Clin Dermatol. 2003;4:843–60. https://doi.org/10.2165/00128071-200304120-00004.
8. Aramaki J, Kawana S, Effendy I, Happle R, Loffler H. Differences of skin irritation between Japanese and European women. Br J Dermatol. 2002;146:1052–6. https://doi.org/10.1046/j.1365-2133.2002.04509.x.
9. Berardesca E, de Rigal J, Leveque JL, Maibach HI. In vivo biophysical characterization of skin physiological differences in races. Dermatologica. 1991;182:89–93. https://doi.org/10.1159/000247752.
10. Berardesca E, Maibach HI. Sodium-lauryl-sulphate-induced cutaneous irritation. Comparison of white and Hispanic subjects. Contact Dermatitis. 1988;19:136–40. https://doi.org/10.1111/j.1600-0536.1988.tb05512.x.
11. Berardesca E, Pirot F, Singh M, Maibach H. Differences in stratum corneum pH gradient when comparing white Caucasian and black African-American skin. Br J Dermatol. 1998;139:855–7. https://doi.org/10.1046/j.1365-2133.1998.02513.x.
12. De Luca R, Balestrieri A, Dinle Y. [Measurement of cutaneous evaporation. 6. Cutaneous water loss in the people of Somalia]. Boll Soc Ital Biol Sper. 1983;59:1499–1501.
13. Fotoh C, Elkhyat A, Mac S, Sainthillier JM, Humbert P. Cutaneous differences between Black, African or Caribbean Mixed-race and Caucasian women: biometrological approach of the hydrolipidic film. Skin Res Technol. 2008;14:327–35. https://doi.org/10.1111/j.1600-0846.2008.00299.x.
14. Fujimura T, Miyauchi Y, Shima K, Hotta M, Tsujimura H, Kitahara T, Takema Y, Palungwachira P, Laohathai D, Chanthothai J, Nararatwanchai T. Ethnic differences in stratum corneum func-

tions between Chinese and Thai infants residing in Bangkok, Thailand. Pediatr Dermatol. 2018;35:87–91. https://doi.org/10.1111/pde.13335.

15. Galzote C, Estanislao R, Suero MO, Khaiat A, Mangubat MI, Moideen R, Tagami H, Wang X. Characterization of facial skin of various Asian populations through visual and non-invasive instrumental evaluations: influence of seasons. Skin Res Technol. 2014;20:453–62. https://doi.org/10.1111/srt.12140.

16. Goh CL, Chia SE. Skin irritability to sodium lauryl sulphate--as measured by skin water vapour loss-by sex and race. Clin Exp Dermatol. 1988;13:16–9. https://doi.org/10.1111/j.1365-2230.1988.tb00641.x.

17. Grimes P, Edison BL, Green BA, Wildnauer RH. Evaluation of inherent differences between African American and white skin surface properties using subjective and objective measures. Cutis. 2004;73:392–6.

18. Kompaore F, Marty JP, Dupont C. In vivo evaluation of the stratum corneum barrier function in blacks, Caucasians and Asians with two noninvasive methods. Skin Pharmacol. 1993;6:200–7. https://doi.org/10.1159/000211136.

19. Lee MR, Nam GW, Jung YC, Park SY, Han JY, Cho JC, Suh KD, Hwang JK. Comparison of the skin biophysical parameters of Southeast Asia females: forehead-cheek and ethnic groups. J Eur Acad Dermatol Venereol. 2013;27:1521–6. https://doi.org/10.1111/jdv.12042.

20. Mack MC, Chu MR, Tierney NK, Ruvolo E Jr, Stamatas GN, Kollias N, Bhagat K, Ma L, Martin KM. Water-holding and transport properties of skin stratum corneum of infants and toddlers are different from those of adults: studies in three geographical regions and four ethnic groups. Pediatr Dermatol. 2016;33:275–82. https://doi.org/10.1111/pde.12798.

21. Muizzuddin N, Hellemans L, Van Overloop L, Corstjens H, Declercq L, Maes D. Structural and functional differences in barrier properties of African American, Caucasian and East Asian skin. J Dermatol Sci. 2010;59:123–8. https://doi.org/10.1016/j.jdermsci.2010.06.003.

22. Pappas A, Fantasia J, Chen T. Age and ethnic variations in sebaceous lipids. Dermato-Endocrinology. 2013;5:319–24. https://doi.org/10.4161/derm.25366.

23. Reed JT, Ghadially R, Elias PM. Skin type, but neither race nor gender, influence epidermal permeability barrier function. Arch Dermatol. 1995;131:1134–8.

24. Singh J, Gross M, Sage B, Davis HT, Maibach HI. Effect of saline iontophoresis on skin barrier function and cutaneous irritation in four ethnic groups. Food Chem Toxicol. 2000;38:717–26. https://doi.org/10.1016/s0278-6915(00)00058-2.

25. Sugino K, Imokawa G, Maibach HI. Ethnic difference of stratum corneum lipid in relation to stratum corneum function. J Invest Dermatol. 1993;100:587.

26. Warrier AG, Kligman AM, Harper RA, Bowman J, Wickett RR. A comparison of black and white skin using noninvasive methods. J Soc Cosmet Chem. 1996;47:229–40.

27. Voegeli R, Rawlings AV, Seroul P, Summers B. A novel continuous colour mapping approach for visualization of facial skin hydration and transepidermal water loss for four ethnic groups. Int J Cosmet Sci. 2015;37:595–605. https://doi.org/10.1111/ics.12265.

28. Voegeli R, Rawlings AV, Summers B. Facial skin pigmentation is not related to stratum corneum cohesion, basal transepidermal water loss, barrier integrity and barrier repair. Int J Cosmet Sci. 2015;37:241–52. https://doi.org/10.1111/ics.12189.

29. Yamashita Y, Okano Y, Ngo T, Buche P, Sirvent A, Girard F, Masaki H. Differences in susceptibility to oxidative stress in the skin of Japanese and French subjects and physiological characteristics of their skin. Skin Pharmacol Physiol. 2012;25:78–85. https://doi.org/10.1159/000335259.

30. Yosipovitch G, Goon ATJ, Chan YH, Goh CL. Are there any differences in skin barrier function, integrity and skin blood flow between different subpopulations of Asians and Caucasians. Exog Dermatol. 2002;1:302–6.

31. Young MM, Franken A, du Plessis JL. Transepidermal water loss, stratum corneum hydration, and skin surface pH of female African and Caucasian nursing students. Skin Res Technol. 2019;25:88–95. https://doi.org/10.1111/srt.12614.

32. Colby SL, Ortman JM. Projections of the size and composition of the U.S. population: 2014 to 2060. Washington, DC: US Census Bureau; 2014.
33. Oh SS, Galanter J, Thakur N, Pino-Yanes M, Barcelo NE, White MJ, de Bruin DM, Greenblatt RM, Bibbins-Domingo K, Wu AH, Borrell LN, Gunter C, Powe NR, Burchard EG. Diversity in clinical and biomedical research: a promise yet to be fulfilled. PLoS Med. 2015;12:e1001918. https://doi.org/10.1371/journal.pmed.1001918.
34. Castillo-Page L. Diversity in the physician workforce facts & figures 2010. Washington, DC: Association of American Medical Colleges; 2010.
35. Shoo BA, Kashani-Sabet M. Melanoma arising in African-, Asian-, Latino- and Native-American populations. Semin Cutan Med Surg. 2009;28:96–102. https://doi.org/10.1016/j.sder.2009.04.005.
36. Darlenski R, Fluhr JW. Influence of skin type, race, sex, and anatomic location on epidermal barrier function. Clin Dermatol. 2012;30:269–73. https://doi.org/10.1016/j.clindermatol.2011.08.013.
37. Richards GM, Oresajo CO, Halder RM. Structure and function of ethnic skin and hair. Dermatol Clin. 2003;21:595–600. https://doi.org/10.1016/s0733-8635(03)00081-0.
38. Rawlings AV. Ethnic skin types: are there differences in skin structure and function? Int J Cosmet Sci. 2006;28:79–93. https://doi.org/10.1111/j.1467-2494.2006.00302.x.
39. Machado M, Hadgraft J, Lane ME. Assessment of the variation of skin barrier function with anatomic site, age, gender and ethnicity. Int J Cosmet Sci. 2010;32:397–409. https://doi.org/10.1111/j.1468-2494.2010.00587.x.
40. Rougier A, Lotte C, Corcuff P, Maibach H. Relationship between skin permeability and corneocyte size according to anatomic site, age, and sex in man. J Soc Cosmet Chem. 1988;39:15–26.
41. Pinnagoda J, Tupker RA, Agner T, Serup J. Guidelines for transepidermal water loss (TEWL) measurement. A report from the Standardization Group of the European Society of Contact Dermatitis. Contact Derm. 1990;22:164–78. https://doi.org/10.1111/j.1600-0536.1990.tb01553.x.
42. Feldmann RJ, Maibach HI. Regional variation in percutaneous penetration of 14C cortisol in man. J Invest Dermatol. 1967;48:181–3. https://doi.org/10.1038/jid.1967.29.
43. Pinnagoda J, Tupker RA, Coenraads PJ, Nater JP. Transepidermal water loss with and without sweat gland inactivation. Contact Dermatitis. 1989;21:16–22. https://doi.org/10.1111/j.1600-0536.1989.tb04679.x.
44. Grice JE, Moghimi HR, Ryan E, Zhang Q, Haridass I, Mohammed Y, Roberts MS. Non-formulation parameters that affect penetrant-skin-vehicle interactions and percutaneous absorption. In: Dragicevic N, Maibach HI, editors. Percutaneous penetration enhancers drug penetration into/through the skin. Berlin: Springer; 2017. https://doi.org/10.1007/978-3-662-53270-6_4.
45. Rees JL. The genetics of sun sensitivity in humans. Am J Hum Genet. 2004;75:739–51. https://doi.org/10.1086/425285.
46. Visscher MO. Skin color and pigmentation in ethnic skin. Facial Plast Surg Clin North Am. 2017;25:119–25. https://doi.org/10.1016/j.fsc.2016.08.011.
47. Jablonski NG. The evolution of human skin colouration and its relevance to health in the modern world. J R Coll Physic Edinb. 2012;42:58–63. https://doi.org/10.4997/JRCPE.2012.114.
48. Jablonski NG, Chaplin G. The evolution of human skin coloration. J Hum Evol. 2000;39:57–106. https://doi.org/10.1006/jhev.2000.0403.
49. Gilchrest BA, Eller MS, Geller AC, Yaar M. The pathogenesis of melanoma induced by ultraviolet radiation. N Engl J Med. 1999;340:1341–8. https://doi.org/10.1056/NEJM199904293401707.
50. Tadokoro T, Kobayashi N, Zmudzka BZ, Ito S, Wakamatsu K, Yamaguchi Y, Korossy KS, Miller SA, Beer JZ, Hearing VJ. UV-induced DNA damage and melanin content in human skin differing in racial/ethnic origin. FASEB J. 2003;17:1177–9. https://doi.org/10.1096/fj.02-0865fje.
51. Yamaguchi Y, Coelho SG, Zmudzka BZ, Takahashi K, Beer JZ, Hearing VJ, Miller SA. Cyclobutane pyrimidine dimer formation and p53 production in human skin after repeated

UV irradiation. Exp Dermatol. 2008;17:916–24. https://doi.org/10.1111/j.1600-0625.2008. 00722.x.

52. Gilchrest BA, Blog FB, Szabo G. Effects of aging and chronic sun exposure on melanocytes in human skin. J Invest Dermatol. 1979;73:141–3. https://doi.org/10.1111/1523-1747. ep12581580.

53. Quevedo WC, Szabo G, Virks J. Influence of age and UV on the populations of dopa-positive melanocytes in human skin. J Invest Dermatol. 1969;52:287–90.

54. Del Bino S, Duval C, Bernerd F. Clinical and biological characterization of skin pigmentation diversity and its consequences on UV impact. Int J Mol Sci. 2018;19:2668. https://doi. org/10.3390/ijms19092668.

55. Potts RO. Stratum corneum hydration: experimental techniques and interpretations of results. J Soc Cosmet Chem. 1986;37:9–33.

56. Muizzuddin N, Ingrassia M, Marenus KD, Maes DH, Mammone T. Effect of seasonal and geographical differences on skin and effect of treatment with an osmoprotectant: sorbitol. J Cosmet Sci. 2013;64:165–74.

57. Pinnagoda J, Tupker RA, Coenraads PJ, Nater JP. Comparability and reproducibility of the results of water loss measurements: a study of 4 evaporimeters. Contact Dermatitis. 1989;20:241–6. https://doi.org/10.1111/j.1600-0536.1989.tb03139.x.

58. Peer RP, Maibach HI. Unbearable transepidermal water loss (TEWL) experimental variability: why? Arch Dermatol Res. 2022;314(2):99.

Chapter 17
Zinc Oxide Nanoparticles In Vitro Human Skin Decontamination

Yachao Cao, Xiaoying Hui, Akram Elmahdy, Hanjiang Zhu,
and Howard I. Maibach

Introduction

Recent interest in the use of solid sorbent decontaminants, such as nano-crystalline metal oxides, is based on their large surface area (relative to their small particle sizes) available to adsorb chemicals and the numerous highly reactive sites on the surface to catalyze chemicals [1–3]. Common nano metal oxides including CaO [3], MgO [4–6], Al_2O_3 [7], and ZnO NP ([8–12]) have been explored for their adsorbent and catalyst capacities for defense applications, such as nuclear, biological, and chemical warfare agents (CWA) [13–20].

ZnO NP is a nano metal oxide adsorbent widely used in environmental catalysis. ZnO NPs possess numerous Lewis and Bronsted acid sites that create a high adsorption capacity for a wide range of hazardous components and used for discovering decontamination and detoxification of many chemical warfare agents and/or their simulants ([8, 10, 11, 12]). There is limited research available to understand detailed mechanisms of this process.

We examine ZnO NP functions as a reducing (catalytic) agent for decontamination and detoxification of POX, a model chemical of organophosphate pesticide and

Y. Cao
Department of Dermatology, School of Medicine, University of California San Francisco, San Francisco, CA, USA

School of Mechanical Engineering, Hebei University of Science and Technology, Shijiazhuang, China

X. Hui (✉) · A. Elmahdy · H. Zhu
Department of Dermatology, School of Medicine, University of California San Francisco, San Francisco, CA, USA

H. I. Maibach
Department of Dermatology, University of California San Francisco, San Francisco, CA, USA
e-mail: howard.maibach@ucsf.edu

A. M. Feschuk et al. (eds.), *Dermal Absorption and Decontamination*,
https://doi.org/10.1007/978-3-031-09222-0_17

315

a CWA simulant with various ZnO nanoparticle sizes and shapes, and different carrier mediums in an in vitro human skin permeation system and/or in vitro human stratum corneum binding device. Radioactivity of [^{14}C]-POX was used to trace the degree of skin binding and permeation, and acetyl cholinesterase activity was counted to detect the degree of enzyme inhibition and/or reactivation with and without ZnO NPs being present. We expect this design to gain mechanistic insights and knowledge in developing clinically useful ZnO NP based human skin surface decontamination and detoxification technology.

Material and Method

Test Chemicals and Reagents

Model Toxic Chemical and Topical Formulation

[^{14}C]-Paraoxon (POX) (purities > 97%, 50 mCi/mmol), non-radiolabeled POX, and [7-^{14}C]-benzoic acid (55 mCi/mmol) were obtained from American Radiolabeled Chemicals, Inc. (St. Louis, MO, USA). Non-labeled POX and trace amounts of [^{14}C]-POX were mixed in ethanol to a final topical solution, 2% (w/v) concentration and 0.5 µCi/10 µL radioactivity.

Reactive Regents

Three forms of zinc oxide nanoparticles (ZnO, MW 81.39) were used. The solid nanopowder (particle size < 100 nm) and water dispersion (≤40 nm, 20% wt in H_2O) were purchased from Sigma-Aldrich (St Louis, MO). Porous nanopowder (<100 nm) was gifted by Dr. Jin Zhang, Department of Chemistry, UCSC. The nanotubes (length in the range of 100–200 nm and diameter approximately 50–75 nm) were provided by Prof. Oomman K. Varghese, Department of Physics, University of Houston.

All other nanopowders, bismuth(III) oxide (Bi_2O_3) (MW 465.96 and Particle size 90–210 nm), silver(I) oxide (Ag_2O) (231.74 and <100), iron(II, III) oxide (Fe_3O_4) (231.53 and 50–100), copper(II) oxide (CuO) (79.55 and <50), and titanium(IV) oxide (TiO_2) (79.87 and 21) were from Sigma-Aldrich (St Louis, MO).

Polymer materials polyvinyl acetate (PVAc) (MW 86.09), polyvinylprrrolidone (PVP) (40,000), and pluronic F127 (Poloxamer 407) (~12,600) were gifted by BASF (Budd Lake, NJ).

Benzoic acid and acetylcholinesterase (AChE) from Electrophorus electricus (Type VI-S, lyophilized powder, 200–1000 units/mg protein) and AChE Activity Assay Kit were from Sigma-Aldrich (St Louis, MO), and phosphate buffered saline (PBS) tablet, reagent-grade ethanol, HPLC-grade water, polyethylene glycol were from Fisher Scientific (Pittsburg, PA).

Soluene-350® tissue solubilizer and ULTIMA GOLD™ scintillation cocktails were obtained from PerkinElmer Life and Analytical Sciences (Boston, MA, USA).

Receptor fluid (RF) was prepared by mixing PBS aqueous solution (0.01 M, pH 7.4) and PEG in ratio of 94:6 (v/v) to a final 6% PEF in PBS solution.

Human Skin Preparations

Human skin samples for in vitro skin research, approved by the UCSF Human Research Committee were dermatomed from five human adult cadavers (ages 67–82 years) within 24 h after death at the UCSF Anatomy Laboratory. Thigh skin is recommended for in vitro skin exposure assessment and modeling studies since it provides realistic dermal absorption values [21]. Dermatomed skin sample, in approximate 500-µm thickness contains SC, "viable" epidermis, and partial dermis layers. Collected skin samples were stored at 0–4 °C and used within 4 weeks of storage.

To minimize variance, each skin sample's physical condition, thickness, and transepidermal water loss (TEWL) rate were examined with a 5–30× binocular stereo microscope (American Optical Corp., Buffalo, NY), digital caliper (Fisher Scientific), and an evaporimeter (Delfin Technologies Ltd., Kuopio, Finland), respectively, to ensure skin integrity prior to study. TEWL values higher than 15 g/h m^2 for a skin sample were not utilized [22].

Acetylcholinesterase Activity Assay Protocol

Principle: Modified Ellman method [23] in which thiocholine, produced by AChE, reacts with 5,5′-dithiobis(2-nitrobenzoic acid) to form an colorimetric (412 nm) product, proportional to the AChE activity present. One unit of AChE is the amount of enzyme that catalyzes the production of 1.0 µmol of thiocholine per minute at room temperature at pH 7.5.

Detailed AChE assay procedure was published online by Sigma-Aldrich. Briefly described as follows.

1. Preparation: (a) Working Reagent: 200 mL of Assay Buffer mixed with 2 mg of Reaction. (b) Samples: Working Reagent mixed with receptor fluid in 1:4 (v/v) ratio.
2. Measurement: (a) Set a 96 well plate to SpectraMax Microplate Reader (Molecular Device, San Jose, CA) and set up absorbance at 412 ± 5 nm. (b) Incubate all samples at room temperature for 2 min, and then take the initial absorbance reading at 412 nm as A412initial. (c) Continue to incubate the plate at room temperature for 10 min, and then take the final measurement as A412final.
3. AChE activity calculation:

   Activity of receptor fluid in units of AChE inhibited by 1 L of receptor fluid (units AChE/L) determined by following formulation:

AChE Activity(units/L)

$$= (A412\text{final} - A412\text{initial}) / (A412\text{calibrator} - A412\text{blank}) \times n \times 200$$

*200 = equivalent activity (units/L) of the Calibrator when assayed is read at 2 and 10 min. n = dilution factor. A412calibrator = Absorbance of the calibrator at 10 min. A412blank = Absorbance of the blank at 10 min.

Inhibition and Reactivation of Acetylcholinesterase Activity

AChE working solution incubated with [^{14}C]-POX testing solution or plus additional reactive reagents—nanoparticles or polymers at the same time or later in designed ratios. The mixed incubation solutions were placed in a shaking water bath (Fisher Scientific Isotemp Shaking Water Bath) at 37 °C for defined times. Aliquots of the incubation solution were collected at designed times during the process to measure radioactivity and AChE activity.

1. Inhibition Kinetics of AChE Activity

    Stock solution of paraoxon (2%) was diluted by AChE suspended in phosphate buffer to a final 0.5% concentration, and incubated 37 °C. At designed time intervals, aliquots of the incubation solution were collected to measure AChE activity level until the activity was reduced up to 95% of its initial level. The decline curve of AChE activity was predicted by calculation of the average values measured from each time point via a four parameter logistic curve fitting model (MyCurve Fit—Online Curve Fitting, https://mycurvefit.com). The Eq. (17.1) used to calculate best curve fitting is

$$y = d + \frac{a - d}{1 + \left(\dfrac{x}{c}\right)^{b}} \tag{17.1}$$

*x = the independent variable and y = the dependent variable just as in the linear model above. The four estimated parameters are: a = the minimum value that can be obtained (i.e., what happens at 0 dose); d = the maximum value that can be obtained (i.e., what happens at infinite dose); c = the point of inflection (i.e., the point on the S shaped curve halfway between a and d); b = Hill's slope of the curve (i.e., this is related to the steepness of the curve at point c).

2. Reactivation Kinetics of Inhibited AChE Activity

    The above AChE inhibited incubation solution was then mixed with solid nanopowders or polymers in designed concentration range. Aliquots of 50 μL of reactivation cocktail were withdrawn at specified time intervals (30–120 min) to measure AChE activities.

3. AChE reactivation calculation:

   (a) Preparation of two standard curves: <u>negative control</u>—different concentrations of AChE (no POX); <u>positive control</u>—one concentration of AChE, different concentrations of POX.
   (b) Using above standard corves to measure POX-reactivation reagent binding radio (% AChE inhibited).
   (c) Reactivation kinetic calculation: a simple linear regression (17.2) is used to determine the degree of AChE activity recovery.

$$y = ax + b \qquad (17.2)$$

   *x = the independent variable (i.e., what you control, such as, dose, concentration, etc.); y = the dependent variable (i.e., what you measure as the signal); a = the slope of the fitted line; and b = the intercept of the dependent axis.

ZnO NPs Binding Affinity

The experiment measures binding affinity of ZnO solid or porous nanoparticles to paraoxon is briefly introduced as follows. Saturated POX containing trace amount of [^{14}C]-POX in PBS solution (3.64 mg/mL of water at 20 °C, pH = 7. https://pubchem.ncbi.nlm.nih.gov/compound/Paraoxon) was placed in a beaker. Different quantities of binding materials ZnO nanoparticles, solid or porous from 1, 2, 4, 6, 8, and 10 g earth mixed in the same PBS solution in a dialysis tube. The dialysis device has a dialysis tube placed in the beaker with model chemical solution and incubates in a water bath at 37 °C for up to 24 h to reach equilibrium (Fig. 17.1). Binding rate

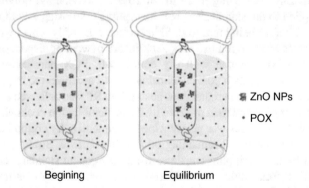

Begining   Equilibrium

Fig. 17.1 Illustration of ZnO NPs—POX binding process. Model chemical—[^{14}C]-Paraoxon (2%) in PBS solution placed in a glass beach and then a dialysis tubing containing PBS solution and ZnO or other nanoparticles in the same beach. Then, the beach containing these samples incubated in a water bath at 37 °C for 24 h to reach equilibrium. All samples were counted individually for radioactivity to determine binding rates. A small glass beach containing

was calculated as chemical concentration in the dialysis tubing (µg chemical/g nanoparticles). In another experiment, binding affinities of solid, nanotube, and porous ZnO NPs to [^{14}C]-benzoic acid were tested.

In Vitro Skin Absorption and Decontamination of [^{14}C]-POX

Human dermatomed skin sample was mounted on a continuous flow-through glass diffusion cell (PermeGear, Inc., Hellertown, PA). The donor chamber of the cell (above the skin, 1 cm^2 surface area) remained open to air and received dosing formulation. The receiving chamber (below the skin, 3 mL in volume) was filled to capacity with receptor fluid, 6% PEG in PBS (0.01 M, pH 7.4). The buffer saline was pumped through the diffusion cell at a rate of 4 mL/h via a Pump Pro MPL (Watson-Marlow, Inc., Wilmington, MA). The cell was maintained at approximately 32 °C using a LAUDA heating circulator (LAUDA, Lauda-Königshofen, Germany).

1. In vitro skin absorption and penetration
    A ten micro-liter (10 µL) solution of [^{14}C]-POX was dosed on this 1 cm^2 skin area and allowed to air-dry. The applied dose partitioned into SC, diffused to epidermis and dermis, and finally into the receiving chamber, where the receptor fluid was fully filled and stirred magnetically at ~600 RPM. All skin layer samples and receptor fluid samples were collected at designed times to determine permeation kinetics.
2. In vitro skin surface decontamination
    Skin surface dose application was the same as the above. After designated time post dose, the skin was decontaminated as follows: ZnO NP solid powder (5 mg, dry particles), ZnO NP dispersion (25 µL in water), ZnO NP solid powder (5 mg in 25 µL of water, or ethanol, or 10% carboxymethyl polymer solution), or porous ZnO NP (5 mg in 25 µL of 10% carboxymethyl polymer solution) were applied to the skin surface half hour post POX dosing and remained there for 30 min before being removed. Skin surface was softly wiped with a dry cotton ball three times to remove residual ZnO NP powder or dispersion. Skin sample controls were wiped with dry cotton ball. POX permeation assay was continued for up to 24 h post chemical dosing to ascertain the impact of decontamination process on percutaneous absorption. RF was collected at 30 min, 1 h, and then every 2 h and then mixed with liquid scintillation cocktail. The surface of control skin samples was gently wiped twice with a dry cotton ball to recover the fraction of chemical remaining on the skin surface. Stratum corneum was removed by tape stripping ten times using D-Squame standard sampling disc (Cuderm). Dermis and viable epidermis were separated by heat treatment [24] and placed individually into vials with 2 mL of Soluene 350 Tissue Solubilizer (PekinElmer Life and Analytical Sciences, Boston, MA, USA) for total tissue digestion. The test chemical was extracted overnight at room temperature with shaking.

3. Combination of ZnO NPs wipe and DDGel decontamination in vitro DDGel (dermal decontamination gel) preparation was described in WO 2017/053594 Al, 2017; Cao et al. [25, 26]. Briefly, DDGel was prepared freshly as follows: weighing Kollidon SR (3 g), lutrol (1 g), carboxymethyl cellulose (0.3 g), Fuller's earth (2.5 g), and bentonite (0.5 g); dissolved with 2 mL of water and 10 mL of ethanol, mixed well into a light gray color gel.

A 1 cm² cotton pad pre-wetted with 20 µL of distilled water followed by spreading of solid ZnO NPs (5 mg) on the surface. 30 min after the initiation of the experiment (received topical application of POX), the ZnO NPs wipe was applied on the dosed skin surface with gentle massages for 30 s, followed by patch removal. Then DDGel (~0.15 g) was immediately applied to the same skin surface and removed approximately 15 min after the gel completely dried on the surface.

Radioactivity Measurements

Test samples were measured for radioactivity with a PerkinElmer Tri-Carb 2900TR liquid scintillation spectrometer (PerkinElmer Life and Analytical Sciences, Inc., Waltham, MA, USA) calibrated with background control scintillation cocktail standards.

All in vitro experiment samples were collected and mixed with scintillation cocktail for radioactivity quantification.

Accuracy and reliability of liquid scintillation spectrometry were ensured weekly by calibration via running manufacturer provided internal quench and calibration standards. Liquid scintillation spectrometer was automatically-calibrated before samples were counted on the instrument counting deck at all times.

Data Analysis and Regression

Mass balance calculations were performed to ascertain recovery degree [27]. Total chemical amount in a given tissue was calculated based on the total sample volume or weight and chemical concentration in that sample. To enhance and ensure data comparability across treatments (control, powder, and dispersion), the assayed decontamination and absorption data were normalized by total recovery for each diffusion cell and then statistically analyzed and compared.

Chemical amounts (labeled and non-labeled paraoxon) were expressed as percent of dose (% dose) recovered from receptor fluid, skin surface, stratum corneum, viable epidermis, and dermis. All data are shown as mean ± SD ($n = 5$ replicates). A normality test (Kolmogorov–Smirnov) was conducted on all data: the data were found not normally distributed (non-Gaussian); a Student's t-test ($p < 0.05$) was applied to check if decontaminant of powder or dispersion system significantly reduced the chemical amounts in various compartments of the skin and the RF (mimics the blood in systemic circulation) when compared to the control.

Decontamination efficacy was determined as a percentage difference in the total amount of an agent that permeated after 24-h exposure between controls (equivalent to 100%) and decontaminated skin.

Results

In Vitro AChE Activity, Inhibition and Reactivation

Time response curve of AChE inhibition by presenting POX is illustrated in Fig. 17.2. The enzyme activity quickly declined from initial time (as 100% activity at 0 min, prior to adding paraoxon) to 6% 5 min post POX mixed with the incubation of 0.5% (w/v) POX solution. The curve then slightly decreased, and later plateaued at 2–3% of the initial activity until the end of the experiment (15 min post).

The inhibition kinetic of AChE activity was analyzed with a four parameter logistic curve fitting model (MyCurve Fit—Online Curve Fitting, https://mycurve-fit.com) to illustrate the decline curve:

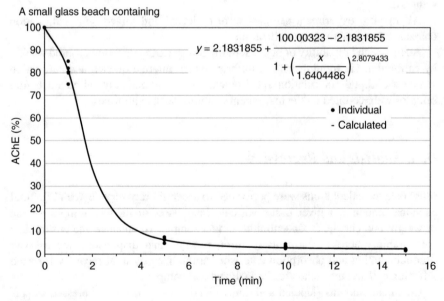

Fig. 17.2 Time-dependent AChE inhibited by paraoxon (μmol/mL). The enzyme activity quickly reduced from initial time (as 100% before adding paraoxon) to 6% after 5 min incubation of 0.5% (w/v) POX solution. By 10–15 min post, AChE only remains approximate 2% of activity. Each symbol (solid circle) represents an individual value of five samples. The AChE activity declining kinetics calculated via four parameter logistic curve fitting model (MyCurve Fit—Online Curve Fitting, https://mycurvefit.com)

$$y = 2.18 + \frac{100.00 - 2.18}{1 + (x/1.64)^{2.81}}$$

Figure 17.3 evaluated detoxification capacity of individual solid nanopowders (Bi_2O_3, Ag_2O, Fe_3O_4, ZnO, CuO, or TiO_2), or polymers (PVAc, PVP, or F127) against POX inhibition of AChE activity in a 2 h in vitro incubation period. The capacity was estimated by comparison of AChE activity per unit of testing reagent applied (gm) and a linear AChE activity curve in a positive control (containing a set of POX concentrations). Therefore, the final capacity was expressed as units of "paraoxon detoxified (µg inactivated)" per gram of decon reagents. Among these testing reagents, ZnO NPs have the highest detoxification capacity followed by PVAc. These two are statistically higher than any other reagents tested in the experiment ($p < 0.05$) but there is no statistical difference between these top two ($p > 0.05$).

Figure 17.4a–d gave decontamination/detoxification capacities of selected reagent from previous experiment (Fig. 17.3) such as solid nanopowders ZnO (Fig. 17.4a) and TiO_2 (Fig. 17.4b), polymers PVAc (Fig. 17.4c) and PVP (Fig. 17.4d) in reactivation of POX inhibited AChE. These agents added to previously inhibited AChE solution (the same procedure as introduced in Fig. 17.2, 15 min inhibition incubation). The enzyme was gradually reactive after mixing with these

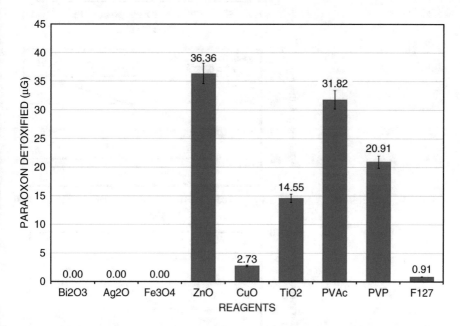

Fig. 17.3 shows maximum detoxification capacities of selected reagents (nanopowders and polymers) to [^{14}C]-paraoxon calculated via reactivation of AChE measurement after in vitro incubation for 2 h. The capacity was expressed as "paraoxon detoxified (µg inactivated) per gram of decon reagents applied". Among the reagents, ZnO NPs had highest detoxification capacity than others ($p < 0.05$) except that of PVAc polymer ($p > 0.05$). Each bar represents the mean ± S.D. of five replicates

Fig. 17.4 Time course of
AChE reactivation by
adding 5 g of ZnO NPs (**a**),
TiO$_2$ NPs (**b**), PVAc (**c**), or
PVP (**d**) in previously
AChE activity inhibited
solution (see Fig. 17.2) at
20 min post-initial. From
60 to 120 min, AChE
activity was linearly
reactivated. The orders of
reactivation are ZnO
(highest) followed by
PVAc, PVP, and TiO$_2$.
Each symbol and line
represents the mean of five
experiments

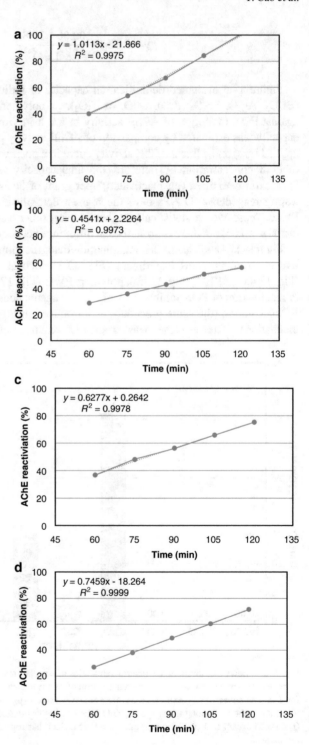

nanopowders or polymers. A linear increase of AChE activity was then observed during 60–120 min incubations after the inhibition initiated. The linear data demonstrated that ZnO NPs having the highest rate of AChE reactivation.

Binding Affinity of ZnO Nanoparticles

Two physical structural differences of ZnO nanoparticles in solid and porous formats were compared in their binding capacities to [14C]-POX. Saturated POX solution was mixed with a set of quantities of ZnO NPs of 1, 2, 4, 6, 8, and 10 g in a dialysis device and incubated for 24 h. Figure 17.5a, b showed the best linear fitting curves of dose–response relationship occurred when the quantities of ZnO NPs (in both physical structures) were used from 2 to 8 g ranges. Average binding rate of POX in the porous ZnO NP group was slightly higher than that of solid ones but not statistically significant ($p > 0.05$).

In Vitro Skin Penetration and Decontamination

In vitro skin penetrating rates of [14C]-POX and surface decontamination efficiencies of ZnO NPs are presented in Tables 17.1 and 17.2. Vehicle effect on solid ZnO NPs prepared in different topical formulations—dry powder, water dispersion (commercial product), and in ethanol or water (freshly prepared prior to the experiment) on decontamination of [14C]-POX is evaluated in Table 17.1. Quantification of POX retained in epidermis and dermis (as amount absorbed in skin 24 h post dose) and penetrated into the receptor fluid (as amount diffusing through skin layer) gives important skin toxicological indexes for the capacity of test chemical that eventually permeates into the human body and the degree of systemic poisoning. Mass balances of applied [14C]-POX recovery for all testing groups are 90% or higher, except the control at 82%.

Table 17.2 compared skin decontamination efficacies of two structurally different ZnO NPs, porous, and solid in vitro. These two ZnO NPs were freshly mixed with CMC polymer solution (10%, w/v) to be surface decontamination formulations. Two controls were no surface decontamination and a CMC polymer solution alone. Each formulation was then wiped on the [14C]-POX dosed skin surface at 30 min post-topical application. Results show that the recovered [14C]-POX (as % dose) from removed surface residue and skin absorbed samples in CMC polymer, porous, and solid ZnO NPs groups were significantly different than those in the control ($p < 0.05$). However, in skin penetration samples, which represent amount of the toxic chemicals penetrating into the deep tissue or systemic circulation, the CMC polymer groups were similar to the control ($p > 0.05$), whereas the porous and solid ZnO NPs groups showed significant effects when compared to the control ($p < 0.05$). CMC polymer has been reported to have surface cleaning and decontamination functions, from Fig. 17.6.

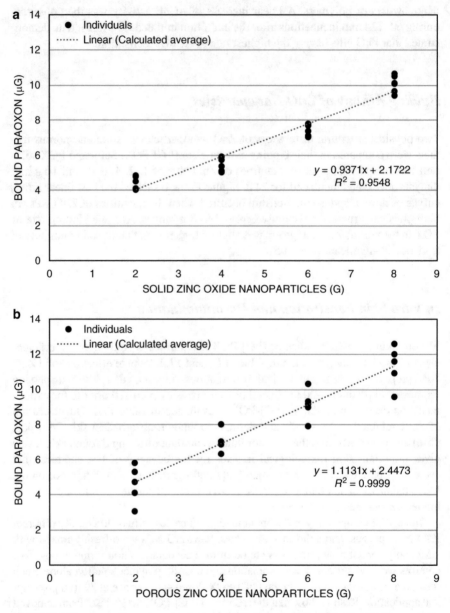

Fig. 17.5 (**a, b**) show a linear dose–response curve. Solid and porous ZnO NPs' binding capabilities are proportional to their concentrations. Overall cumulated bound POX in porous group is statistically higher than that of solid group ($p < 0.05$). Each symbol represents the mean ± S.D. of five replicates

Table 17.1 Vehicle effect on ZnO NP skin decontamination of paraoxon in vitro

	Radioactivity of [^{14}C]-paraoxon as percent dose recovered				
	Control[a] (no decon)	Dry powder[b]	Water dispersion[c]	Powder + ethanol[d]	Powder + water[e]
Skin surface					
Decontamination	–	79 ± 11	57 ± 4.0	72 ± 2.0	63 ± 1.5
Two tape strips	45 ± 5.7	4.2 ± 0.9	4.6 ± 1.7	1.9 ± 0.5	2.7 ± 1.7
In skin					
Stratum corneum	4.5 ± 0.8	0.3 ± 0.2	7.2 ± 0.6	3.2 ± 0.2	4.2 ± 0.5
Epidermis	6.3 ± 0.2	2.0 ± 0.5	5.3 ± 0.7	0.7 ± 0.2	1.0 ± 0.2
Dermis	9.1 ± 1.5	5.1 ± 0.3	8.6 ± 2.6	0.8 ± 0.1	0.4 ± 0.1
Through skin					
Receptor fluid	7.8 ± 1.0	2.9 ± 0.6	6.4 ± 1.0	0.4 ± 0.1	1.3 ± 0.6
Summery					
Surface removed[f]	45 ± 5.7	83 ± 12[a]	62 ± 5.8[a]	74 ± 1.3[a]	66 ± 0.6[a]
Skin absorbed	16 ± 1.2	7.1 ± 0.6[a, c, d, e]	13.9 ± 2.6[b, d, e]	1.5 ± 0.8[a, b, c]	1.4 ± 0.4[a, b, c]
Skin penetrated	7.8 ± 1.0	2.9 ± 0.6[a, c, d, e]	6.4 ± 1.0[b, d, e]	0.4 ± 0.1[a, b, c, e]	1.3 ± 0.6[a, b, c, d]
Mass balance	82 ± 3.7	97 ± 13	104 ± 11[a]	92 ± 0.9	91 ± 0.7

Vehicle effect on solid ZnO NPs prepared in different topical formulations—dry powder, water dispersion (commercial product), and in ethanol or water (freshly prepared prior to the experiment) on decontamination of [^{14}C]-POX. ZnO NPs in freshly prepared ethanol or water mediums or even in dry status gave statistically significance ($p < 0.05$) in reduce amount of POX skin absorbed and penetrated (to the systemic). Whereas using ZnO NPs in water dispersion did not decrease POX skin absorption and penetration when compared to the control ($p > 0.05$). Each number represents the mean ± SD of five replicates

[a]Statistical significant ($p < 0.05$)of recovered ^{14}C radioactivity between the control and one of other treated groups

[b]Statistical significant ($p < 0.05$) of recovered ^{14}C radioactivity between the dry powder group and one of others

[c]Statistical significant ($p < 0.05$) of recovered ^{14}C radioactivity between the water dispersion group and one of others

[d]Statistical significant ($p < 0.05$)of recovered ^{14}C radioactivity between the ethanol group and one of others

[e]Statistical significant ($p < 0.05$) of recovered ^{14}C radioactivity between the (fresh) water group and one of others

Table 17.2 Comparison of skin decontamination efficacies of two structurally different ZnO NPs, porous and solid in vitro when polymer used as medium

	Radioactivity of [^{14}C]-paraoxon as percent dose recovered			
	Control (no decon)[a]	Carboxymethyl polymer only[b]	Porous ZnO NPs in polymer[c]	Solid ZnO NPs in polymer[d]
Skin surface				
Decontamination	–	61 ± 6.7	57 ± 2.2	70 ± 7.5
Two tape strips	30 ± 5.2	4.9 ± 1.4	7.5 ± 3.8	6.1 ± 1.7
In skin				
Stratum corneum	23 ± 4.5	12 ± 0.3	14 ± 0.3	13 ± 1.4
Epidermis	12 ± 4.0	4.6 ± 2.1	5.6 ± 0.1	6.5 ± 0.5
Dermis	20 ± 3.2	11 ± 0.7	12 ± 0.3	12 ± 1.7
Through skin				
Receptor fluid	10 ± 1.5	6.9 ± 1.2	5.6 ± 1.5	4.4 ± 0.8
Summery				
Surface removed	30 ± 5.2	66 ± 4.2[a]	64 ± 2.7[a]	77 ± 4.2[a]
Skin absorbed	32 ± 3.6	16 ± 1.4[a]	18 ± 0.2[a]	18 ± 1.2[a]
Skin penetrated	10 ± 1.5	7.2 ± 1.2	5.6 ± 1.5[a]	4.8 ± 0.4[a]
Mass balance	95 ± 4.3	90 ± 4.8	98 ± 6.4	97 ± 1.1

Two structurally different ZnO NPs—solid and porous freshly prepared with CMC polymer solution (10%, w/v) to decontaminate skin surface POX. CMC polymer solution alone and no surface decontamination also performed as controls. Each number represents the mean ± SD of five replicates

ZnO solid and porous in CMC polymer solution showed statistically high in removing surface POX residues, reducing skin absorbed, and decreasing skin penetrated when compared those in the control ($p < 0.05$) but no differences when compared to the polymer alone group ($p > 0.05$). The data suggest that CMC polymer possibly blocked the surface area of the nanoparticle to reduce effective catalytic sites

Table 17.3 evaluates the combination efficacy of pre-wipe with or without ZnO NPs powder following DDGel application on decontamination of POX on skin in vitro. The amount of [^{14}C]-POX removed from skin surface by the ZnO NPs wipe and DDGel group was statistically higher than that of wipe alone plus DDGel group ($p < 0.05$). With such high decontamination efficiency, amounts of [^{14}C]-POX recovered in and through the skin samples in ZnO NPs wipe and DDGel group were statistically lower than those in wipe alone plus DDGel group and the control ($p < 0.05$).

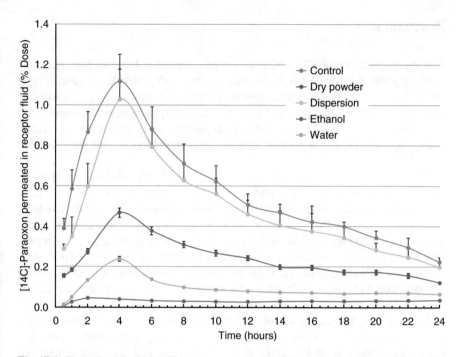

Fig. 17.6 Illustration of vehicle effect on paraoxon in vitro skin permeation process. Whether the control or ZnO NPs decontamination with different carriers, skin permeation peaks are occurred at four post-dose application. The graph shows that skin surface decontamination

Table 17.3 Comparison of the wipe effect with or without additional ZnO NP in skin decontamination in vitro

Decon/cleaning steps	Radioactivity of paraoxon as percent dose recovery (%D)		
	ZnO NPs Wipe + DDGel[a]	Wipe + DDGel[b]	Control[c]
Decon efficiency[d]			
Wipe	51 ± 9[b]	28 ± 4	–
DDGel	35 ± 8	36 ±3	–
Penetrated			
Absorbed in skin	13 ± 2[b, c]	22 ± 3[c]	47 ± 2
Permeated through skin	0.04 ± 0.00[b, c]	0.06 ± 0.02[c]	0.3 ± 0.0
Total recovery	100 ± 4	94 ± 9	98 ± 2
AchE activity (μmol/min/L)	7.2 ± 0.8[c]	7.6 ± 1.1[c]	3.3 ± 0.4

Wiping up prior DDGel application with ZnO NPs increases removal of skin surface contaminants and decreases the chemicals retained in the skin are significantly ($p < 0.05$). Each number represents the mean ± SD of three replicates
[b]Statistical significant ($p < 0.05$) between the ZnO NP wipe + DDGel and the wipe + DDGel groups
[c]Statistical significant ($p < 0.05$) observed from either Wipe + ZnO NP/DDGel or wipe + DDGel group to the control ($p < 0.05$)
[d]Total recovery of [14C]-POX from surface decontamination (wipe and DDGel) and the first two SC tape strips (as removable surface residues)

Discussion

Zinc oxide nanoparticle (ZnO NP), an inorganic metal oxide with high chemical stability, photostability, and high electrochemical coupling coefficient, can be used for applications such as catalysts, optical materials, UV absorbers, gas sensors, or other areas. ZnO NP as a potential adsorbent is widely used in environmental and toxic chemical catalysis [33]. Its use in such capacities depends on its microstructural properties including specific surface area, morphology, and particles size [28, 29].

For example, the particle has different shapes (rod-like and isometric) and is commonly used in the manufacture and application of materials with sizes of up to 100 nm. The particle has two structural forms, solid and porous. The solids have large surface area relative to their small diameter size, therefore a large surface to size ratio, so solid NPs have high catalytic activity. ZnO NPs with a porous structure, however, have advantages over the solid ones because of their high specific surface area. As a result, ZnO NPs in both solid and porous structures can safely be used in a lower concentration with a higher efficiency [30], and provide more opportunity for the diffusion and adsorption of target molecules and hydroxyl radicals during reactions [31].

This study explored the effect of ZnO NP in decontamination and detoxification of $[^{14}C]$-paraoxon ($[^{14}C]$-POX) and observed its efficiency when compared to other nanoparticles such as Bi_2O_3, Ag_2O, Fe_3O_4, CuO TiO_2, and polymers (PVAc and PVP), etc. (Figs. 17.3 and 17.4). The major objective was to investigate how ZnO NPs' physical properties (solid and porous) and their carrier vehicles (water, organic solvent, and/or polymers) altered in vitro skin decontamination and detoxification capacities of ZnO NPs when $[^{14}C]$-POX was employed as a model chemical.

Solid and porous ZnO NPs bound to $[^{14}C]$-POX in aqueous medium in linear proportion, and the total cumulative amount bound in the porous group was statistically higher than that of the solid group ($p < 0.05$) (Fig. 17.5a, b). Similar observations were made in a pilot experiment that measured in vitro $[^{14}C]$-benzoic acid binding rates to human stratum corneum (SC) with presentation of ZnO NPs in three different morphologies and sizes as solid (<100 nm), nanotube (100–200 nm), and porous (<100 nm) in aqueous medium for a 24 h incubation. Amounts of solid, nanotube, and porous ZnO NPs bound with $[^{14}C]$-benzoic acid with binding rates of 4.6 ± 1.7, 10 ± 2.6, and $13 \pm 4.4\%$, respectively, which supported the importance of morphology, surface area, and particle size of ZnO NPs in determination of their decontamination capacities.

During the study we observed differences of decontamination efficacy when the ZnO NP carrier medium switched from freshly prepared water or ethanol to timed water dispersion (commercial product) or polymers (Table 17.1 and Fig. 17.6). A 24-h permeation curve of $[^{14}C]$-POX from skin surface to the receptor fluid (represented as amount in the deep tissue or systemic circulation) illustrated that an absorption peak occurred 4 h post-topical application (or 210 min after skin surface decontamination) in the dry powder, water dispersion, or freshwater groups but not in the fresh ethanol group (Fig. 17.6). Note that ZnO NP in water dispersion almost lost its binding capacity. As a result, its permeation curve and the peak were as high as those of the control group. Its peak was about four times higher than that of the fresh-water group. The latter had the second lowest 24-h permeation curve and peak. These data suggest that freshly prepared ethanol as ZnO NP carrier is an efficient medium for skin surface decontamination followed by fresh water. Table 17.1 provided more evidence for the determination of the highest decontamination capacity of ZnO NP formulation prepared freshly in ethanol followed by water. In the case of a long time in aqueous medium, such as water dispersion or other liquid mediums, ZnO NP could become unstable or its surface catalyst sites could interfere with these liquids and then loose its binding and/or adsorbent capacities to the skin surface chemicals.

Table 17.2 showed in an in vitro experiment, carboxymethyl polymer used as ZnO NP (solid or porous) carrier medium to decontaminate skin surface [^{14}C]-POX resi-due (Table 17.2). The amounts of POX absorbed in and through the skin in these two groups had no statistical differences when compared with that of the polymer control ($p > 0.05$). This phenomenon resembles our previous report that polymers (Kollidon SR, lutrol, and/or carboxymethyl cellulose) could decrease the decontaminant capac-ity of MOF (metal organic framework) significantly [32], as polymers block MOF surface activity areas and therefore reduce the number of binding sites (Fig. 17.7).

To maximize ZnO NPs' decontamination/detoxification capacities, an attempted combination of ZnO NP, wetted wiping patch, and DDGel (dermal decontamination

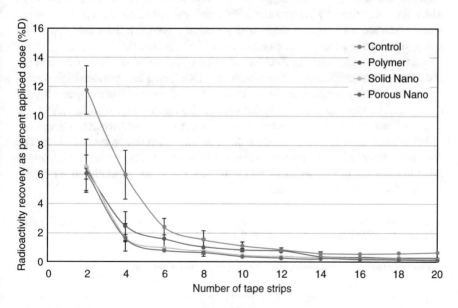

Fig. 17.7 Comparison of skin decontamination efficacies of two structurally different ZnO NPs, porous and solid in vitro stratum corneum tape strips. These two ZnO groups and CMC polymer alone groups had similar surface decontamination capacities ($p > 0.05$) but statistically higher than that of the control in first 1–5 trips ($p < 0.05$). The data further suggest, as discussed in Table 17.2, that CMC polymer possibly blocked the surface area of the nanoparticle to reduce effective cata-lytic sites

gel) methods was studied. This new skin decontamination package combines multiple technologies: a small volume of water surface wetting, ZnO NP dry adsorbent wiping patch, and DDGel, a quick drying strippable film [32], to produce a powerful and effective method of cleaning surface chemicals, reducing local and systemic absorption, and decreasing or blocking chemical toxicity. The cotton fiber-based absorbent has no interfering interaction with NPs, yet still provides additional benefits such as porosity reactivity that allow liquidized chemicals for fast transportation and/or absorption as well as particulate filtration. Thus, the ZnO NP absorbent wiping patch works cooperatively to adsorb/absorb, bind, and hydrolyze the surface chemical contaminant. DDGel further extracts the chemical residue in the stratum corneum reservoir to prevent deep penetration. As shown in Table 17.3, wiping with freshly water wetted ZnO NP cotton wipe prior to DDGel application resulted in statistically significant decontamination of [^{14}C]-POX in terms of the amount removed from the skin surface, reduced amount absorbed in skin, and decreased amount permeated into the receptor fluid (as in systemic circulation) compared to the wipe + DDGel method, as well as the control ($p < 0.05$).

In conclusion, this study shows ZnO NPs effectively removing toxic chemicals from SC, reducing further penetration into epidermal and dermal layers, and thus reducing absorption into systemic circulation. ZnO NP efficiency in the conduction of chemical decontamination and detoxification processes is related to its high chemical stability, photostability, and high electrochemical coupling coefficient, which are determined by the nanoparticles' intact microstructural properties such as specific surface area, morphology, and particles sizes [33]. This study provides appropriate carrier mediums to enhance ZnO NPs' capacities.

This result suggests that the ZnO NPs coupled with an appropriate carrier medium, and other decontamination methods such as DDGel, etc., can provide high decontamination efficacy versus chemical toxicants and offer a significant opportunity for further development as a new skin decontamination technology against CWAs and other toxicants that pose a dermal exposure risk in military and civilian settings.

We do not wish to overgeneralize these results. Skin decontamination studies have been internationally evaluated since World War I. Comparative evaluations using in vitro and in vivo methods will hopefully clarify the most effective chemistry systems for each toxic chemical.

Funding This research was supported by Defense Threat Reduction Agency (DTRA) Grant: HDTRA1-14-0005 UCSF (BRBAA11-PerC-9-2-0054-Base).

Conflict of Interest The authors did not report any conflict of interest.

References

1. Saxena A, Srivastava AK, Singh B, Goyal A. Removal of sulphur mustard, sarin and simulants on impregnated silica nanoparticles. J Hazard Mater. 2012;211–212:226–32.
2. Sharma N, Kakkar R. Recent advancements on warfare agents/metal oxides surface chemistry and their simulation study. Adv Mater Lett. 2013;4:508–21.

3. Wagner GW, Bartram PW, Koper O, Klabunde KJ. Reactions of VX, GD and HD. J Phys Chem B. 1999;103:3325–8.
4. Maddah B, Chalabi H. Synthesis of MgO nanoparticales and identification of their destructive reaction product by 2-chloroethyl ethyl sulfide. J Nanosci Nanotechnol. 2012;8:157–64.
5. Sellik A, Pollet T, Ouvry L, Briançon S, Fessi H, Hartmann DJ, Renaud FN. Degradation of paraoxon (VX chemical agent simulant) and bacteria by magnesium oxide depends on the crystalline structure of magnesium oxide. Chem Biol Interact. 2017;267:67–73. https://doi.org/10.1016/j.cbi.2016.11.023.
6. Vu AT, Jiang S, Ho K, Lee JB, Lee CH. Mesoporous magnesium oxide and its composites: preparation, characterization, and removal of 2-chlorothyl ethyl sulfide. Chem Eng J. 2015;269:82–93.
7. Bisio C, Carniato F, Palumbo C, Safronyuk SL, Starodub MF, Katsev AM, Marchese L, Guidotti M. Nanosized inorganic metal oxides as heterogeneous catalysts for the degradation of chemical warfare agents. Catal Today. 2016;277:192–9. https://doi.org/10.1016/j;cattod.2015.12.023.
8. Giannakoudakis DA, Florent M, Wallace R, Secor J, Karwacki C, Bandosz TJ. Zinc peroxide nanoparticles: surface, chemical and optical properties and the effect of thermal treatment on the detoxification of mustard gas. Appl Catal B Environ. 2018;226:429–40.
9. Mahato TH, Prasad GK, Singh B, Acharya J, Srivastava AR, Vijayaraghavan R. Nanocrystalline zinc oxide for the decontamination of sarin. J Hazard Mater. 2009;165:928–32.
10. Prasad GK, Mahato TH, Singh B, Ganesan K, Pandey P, Sekhar K. Detoxification reactions of sulphur mustard on the surface of zinc oxide nanosized rods. J Hazard Mater. 2007;149:460–4.
11. Houšková V, VáclavŠtengl SB, Murafa N, Kalendová A, Opluštil F. Nanostructure materials for destruction of warfare agents and eco-toxins prepared by homogeneous hydrolysis with thioacetamide: Part 1—zinc oxide. J Phys Chem Solids. 2007;68:716–20. https://doi.org/10.1016/j.jpcs.2006.12.012.
12. Armin Kiani, Kamran Dastafkan. Zinc oxide nanocubes as a destructive nanoadsorbent for the neutralization chemistry of 2-chloroethyl phenyl sulfide: A sulfur mustard simulant. Journal of Colloid and Interface Science. 2016;271–9.
13. Hosono H. Recent progress in transparent oxide semiconductors: materials and device application. Thin Solid Films. 2007;515:6000–14.
14. Klingshirn C. ZnO NP: material, physics and applications. Chem Phys Chem. 2007;8:782–803.
15. Prasad GK. Silver ion exchanged titania nanotubes for decontamination of 2-chloroethyl phenyl sulphide and dimethyl methyl phosphonate. J Sci Ind Res. 2009;68:379–84.
16. Prasad GK. Decontamination of 2-chloro ethyl phenyl sulphide using mixed metal oxide nanocrystals. J Sci Ind Res. 2010;69:835–40.
17. Sadeghi M, Hosseini MH. Nucleophilic chemistry of the synthesized magnesium oxide (magnesia) nanoparticles via microwave@sol-gel process for removal of sulfurous pollutant. Int J Bio-Inorg Hybrid Nanomater. 2012;1:175–82.
18. Sadeghi M, Hosseini H. A novel method for the synthesis of CaO nanoparticle for the decomposition of sulfurous pollutant. J Appl Chem Res. 2013;7:39–49.
19. Sadeghi M, Hosseini MH, Tafi H. Synthesis and characterization of $ZnCaO_2$ nanocomposite catalyst and the evaluation of its adsorption/destruction reactions with 2-CEES and DMMP. Int J Bio-Inorg Hybrid Nanomater. 2013;2:281–93.
20. Vidyasagar CC, Arthoba NY, Venkatesh TG, Viswanatha R. Solid-state synthesis and effect of temperature on optical properties of Cu–ZnO NP, Cu–CdO and CuO nanoparticles. Powder Technol. 2011;214:337–43.
21. EFSA (European Food Safety Authority). Guidance on dermal absorption. EFSA J. 2012;10(4):2665. http://onlinelibrary.wiley.com/doi/10.2903/j.efsa.2012.2665/epdf. Accessed 10 May 2022
22. De Paepe K, Houben E, Adam R, Wiesemann F, Rogiers V. Validation of the VapoMeter, a closed unventilated chamber system to assess transepidermal water loss vs. the open chamber Tewameter. Skin Res Technol. 2005;11(1):61–9.
23. Holas O, Musilek K, Pohanka M, Kuca K. Reviews: the progress in the cholinesterase quantification methods. Expert Opin Drug Discovery. 2012;7:1207–23.

24. Zou Y, Maibach HI. Dermal-epidermal Separation methods: research implications. Arch Dermatol Res. 2017;310:1–9.
25. Cao Y, Elmahdy A, Zhu H, Hui X, Maibach H. Binding affinity and decontamination of dermal decontamination gel to model chemical warfare agent simulants. J Appl Toxicol. 2018a;38(5):724–33.
26. Cao Y, Hui X, Elmahdy A, Maibach H. In vitro human skin permeation and decontamination of diisopropyl methylphosphonate (DIMP) using Dermal Decontamination Gel (DDGel) and Reactive Skin Decontamination Lotion (RSDL) at different time points. Toxicol Lett. 2018b;299:118–23.
27. Bucks AWD. Predictive approaches II mass-balance procedure. In: Shah V, Maibach HI, Jenner J, editors. Topical drug bioavailability, bioequivalence, and penetration. Boston, MA: Springer; 2013. p. 197–207. https://doi.org/10.1007/978-1-4899-1262-6.
28. Khan I, Saeed K, Khan I. Review: nanoparticles: properties, applications and toxicities. 2019. Arab J Chem. 2019;12:908–31.
29. Sadeghi M, Yekta S, Ghaedi H. Decontamination of chemical warfare sulfur mustard agent simulant by ZnO nanoparticles. Int Nano Lett. 2016;6:161–71.
30. Siddiqi KS, Rahman A, Tajuddin HA. Properties of zinc oxide nanoparticles and their activity against microbes. Nanoscale Res Lett. 2018;13:141.
31. Tu and Tuan. A facile and fast solution chemistry synthesis of porous ZnO nanoparticles for high efficiency photodegradation of tartrazine. Vietnam J Chem. 2018;56(2):214–9.
32. Cao Y, Hui X, Maibach H. Effect of superabsorbent polymers (SAP) and metal organic frameworks (MOF) wiping sandwich patch on human skin decontamination and detoxification in vitro. Toxicol Lett. 2021;337:7–17.
33. Kolodziejczak-Radzimska A, Jesionowski T. Zinc oxide—from synthesis to application: a review. Materials. 2014;7(4):2833–81.
34. Kiani A, Dastafkan K. Zinc oxide nanocubes as a destructive nanoadsorbent for the neutralization chemistry of 2-chloroethyl phenyl sulfide: a sulfur mustard simulant. J Colloid Interface Sci. 2016;478:271–9.
35. X Hui, Zhu HJ, Maibach HI. Compositions and methods of using the same for decontamination of skin. WO 2017/053594 Al. 2017. https://patentimages.storage.googleapis.com/93/d6/9a/7ea54588cc95c8/WO2017053594A1.pdf. Accessed 10 May 2022

Index

Printed in the United States
by Baker & Taylor Publisher Services